THE
Ms. GUIDE
TO A
WOMAN'S
HEALTH

THE
Ms. GUIDE
TO A
WOMAN'S
HEALTH

The Most Up-to-date Guide to
a Woman's Health and Well-being

CYNTHIA W. COOKE, M.D.
SUSAN DWORKIN

Illustrations by Judith Glick

Doubleday & Company, Inc.
Garden City, New York
1979

The following people have contributed their time and expertise in reading and commenting on various sections of the manuscript. Great thanks is given to them. The final opinions in the book are those of the authors.

Janet Abrahm, M.D.
Ellen Berman, M.D.
Jean Brown, M.S., C.N.M.
C. Gene Cayten, M.D.
Maryann Coombe
William Crombleholme, M.D.
Peter Cullen, M.D.
Sandra Doughty, M.S.N.
Linda Echols, M.S.N.
Kenneth Frank, M.D.
Robert Guintoli, M.D.

George Huggins, M.D.
Beatrice Kauffman
Suzanne Braun Levine
Michael Mennuti, M.D.
William Pearlman, Ph.D.
Joel Polin, M.D.
Rose Schneiderman, M.S.W.
Marie Smith, A.B.
Pamela Wilson, M.D.
Chung Wu, M.D.

The authors give special thanks to Nina Finklestein of *Ms.* magazine and Betty Prashker of Doubleday for their great help and encouragement during the preparation of the manuscript.

This book is being published simultaneously in hard and paper covers.

Library of Congress Cataloging in Publication Data

Cooke, Cynthia W.
The Ms. guide to a woman's health.

Bibliography: p. 411
Includes index.
1. Women—Health and hygiene. 2. Gynecology—
Popular works. 3. Obstetrics—Popular works.
I. Dworkin, Susan, joint author. II. Ms. III. Title.
[DNLM: 1. Gynecology—Popular works. WP120 C772m]
RG121.C763 1979   613'.04'244
ISBN: 0-385-03961-1
Library of Congress Catalog Card Number 76–52003

CONTENTS

side effects. Diaphragm. Cervical caps. Foams, creams,
and jellies. Condoms. Withdrawal. Rhythm, by calen-
dar, by temperature, by testing the cervical mucus.
Sterilization. Abstinence.

CHAPTER FOUR   93

INFERTILITY

Infertility in women and its possible causes. Abnor-
malities of the ovaries, Fallopian tubes, uterus, cervical
mucus. Habitual abortion. Infertility in men and its
possible causes. Testicular abnormalities and other
causes of decreased sperm count. Abnormal sperm
transport. Abnormal sexual function. Infertility in cou-
ples. Immunologic problems. Fertility work-up. Tests
in women, in men, for couples. Psychological aspects
of infertility. Treatments for infertility. Drugs, surgery.
Artificial insemination. Test-tube babies. Cloning.
Adoption.

CHAPTER FIVE   115

HAVING CHILDREN

Conception and the development of pregnancy. Tests
for pregnancy. Prenatal care. Diet and exercise. Minor
discomforts of pregnancy. Normal labor and delivery.
Anesthesia, induction of labor, forceps, midwives,
emergency delivery. Normal postpartum course.
Breast-feeding. Abnormal pregnancy and childbirth.
Abnormal presentations. Multiple births. Miscarriage.
Ectopic pregnancy. Prematurity. Caesarean section.
Anemia. Toxemia. Rh disease. Medically high-risk
pregnancies. Alcohol, smoking, drugs, and pregnancy.
Infectious diseases. Tests to monitor high-risk preg-
nancies.

*Dysmenorrhea. Premenstrual syndrome. Pelvic conges-
tion syndrome. Major surgical procedures: D & C, hysterectomy, indications. Fibroids. Ovarian cysts, polycystic ovaries. Polyps, Bartholin's abscess. Endometriosis. Breast cancer, causes and therapy. Fibrocystic
disease of breast. Cervical cancer. Pap tests. Endometrial cancer. DES and its problems. Anemia. Arthritis. Varicose veins.*

CHAPTER TWELVE   385

SEXUAL HEALTH

*Varieties of normal sexual activities. The normal sex-
ual response. Sexual dysfunction, male and female.
Treatment of sexual problems. How to choose a good
sex therapist. Physical illness and sexual dysfunction.
Rape. How to get proper postassault treatment. Medical and legal aspects.*

CHAPTER THIRTEEN   403

ROUTINE HEALTH CARE FOR WELL WOMEN

*The political and social aspects of determining your
own process for health care. Routine examinations and
screening tests for well women.*

THE
Ms. GUIDE
TO A
WOMAN'S
HEALTH

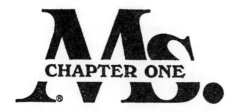

CHAPTER ONE

WELL-WOMAN CARE

This book is written by a woman doctor and a woman patient, and it has two underlying purposes:

—to help women think their way through to a sweeping revision in standards for their own health;

—to give them a *plan* for staying healthy and coping with illness, so they can survive the crisis that currently seethes in the American health care system.

Ever since one can remember, good health has been synonymous with "normality." Wellness entitles you to equality. Anyone who isn't well has to *prove* that she is equal.

That's why handicapped people have never enjoyed equal rights in this country.

That's why the aged and infirm have such trouble being taken seriously.

In the same way, the idea that women are less healthy than men for so many years of their lives is a springboard for grave social, political, and psychological inequalities. The idea of simple femaleness as a compromised state of health must now be stricken from medical mythology—and the first people who have to learn that lesson are the women for whom this book is written.

It is time for women to do serious battle with the notion that they are sick when they are menstruating, sick when they are pregnant, sick when they are going through menopause. *These are not sicknesses.* They are normal, healthy stages of life, completely consistent with wellness. If a woman feels rotten because of them, she should be able to say "I feel rotten" without classifying herself as an invalid who is too "sick" to play ball or too "sick" to be President.

If a woman accepts the idea that the natural cycles of a healthy body make her "sicker" than men, there will be no end to the men ready to accept the idea and victimize her with it.

Our book, then, is concerned with the wellness of women, with their good health—for we are healthy most of the time—and secondarily, with their ill health.

Just as so much of pediatrics has become a matter of "well-baby care," gynecology should by all rights be a matter of "well-woman care." In fact, it is already, with its routine Pap smears, urinalysis, and pelvic exams. But the gynecologists and their patients have not faced up to this fact, for reasons often thoroughly neurotic. For example, doctors doing maintenance work on healthy women do not enjoy as much power as doctors prescribing cures to people who think they are sick. And nobody likes to give up power. On the other side of the desk, patients may feel keenly the loss of the comfortable old dependency on doctors, companion to all the other outworn and outdated dependencies of women—for which the strongest of us may harbor a nostalgia that is far beneath us.

The attitude of the insurance companies toward well-woman care is a rather pointed example of the lack of equity toward women in the health care system.

Insurance companies sometimes refuse to cover medical procedures such as childbirth and abortion for unmarried women; many refuse to cover abortion for married women as well. Thus, the companies are telling us that these are not legitimate medical conditions, the responsibility for which must be shared by the fathering half of the population.

On the other hand, insurance companies maintain that the higher rate of visitation to doctors and other health care providers by women under forty makes them "sicker" than men—therefore, they must pay much higher rates for disability insurance. The fact is that the majority of these visits are made for well-woman care: they center around pregnancy, contraception, and childbirth. Why should a woman pay higher insurance rates than a man just because she pays more routine attention to keeping herself well than a man does?

Most chapters in this book are devoted to stages of life in which particular modes of care are pertinent—and for most women, most health care is *non-medical*. Hygiene. Diet. Menstrual protection. Birth control.

The chapters dealing with disorders of women try to elucidate a *process* by which a woman can deal with her illness.

Doctors and hospitals always have a process. They know what to do, step by step, in case of mastectomy, breech birth, venereal disease. It helps the frightened patient immeasurably to know the routine hospital/doctor process, and in addition, to have a process of her own. How to choose the best doctor for her particular illness. How many opinions to get; from where. What the cost of the illness will be. Whether her insurance will cover it. How much pain is to be expected; how much bleeding is to be expected. How long a recuperation to plan for. Which emotional after effects can be predicted and where to seek counseling to assuage them.

In short, we have tried to instruct the woman on *how to be sick*—so that even in the gravest emergency, she is still mistress of her own body and her own fate.

SURVIVING THE HEALTH CARE CRISIS

Doctors have occupied godlike heights above their patients for so long that the current assault on their collective power has created much psychological chaos in doctor-patient relationships. Because of the consciousness-raising of the women's movement, gynecologists have been singled out for particular scrutiny.

The long-dormant hostility against doctors by patients who feel that they are paying too much for unguaranteed service has been brought to the surface by several different factors. First, there is the matter of cost. More and more people feel that good health is a matter of right; more and more people resent the fact that, in this country today, the rich are still cured of illnesses from which the poor routinely die. Second, the growing population of elderly people, living on fixed incomes and requiring constant medical care they cannot afford, is a virtual hotbed of resentment against private medicine and its soaring cost. Third, there has been an explosion of medical information for non-medical people. In all the media, we constantly receive information for laymen. This book is an example. Patients know more than they have ever known before; the mystery that once surrounded doctoring is broken; yet we still do not know enough to doctor ourselves, and we never will.

Each of these developments contributes in its own way to a fourth: the proliferation of patient self-help groups.

People with Parkinson's disease have organized; people with cancer; families of people with cancer; people with diabetes, arthritis, genetic disorders; the dying have organized, so effectively that they have finally won the priceless right to refuse treatment (e.g., the family of Karen Ann Quinlan). The handicapped have finally organized, so that they are winning for themselves some of the rights they should have enjoyed long ago.

In this way, fellow sufferers bring themselves a comfort few doctors can provide.

They have also begun to lobby for government allocations of research and development funds to help their cause, finally beginning to change the closed manner in which those decisions were traditionally made.

Perhaps all this ferment and discontent will bring changes for the better.

Perhaps a decent health insurance system can be devised so that citizens will receive the care they need without facing bankruptcy. Perhaps hospital care can somehow be standardized at a high level, so that those with money to get to hospitals of good repute will not enjoy so great an advantage over those who must go to what is close and hope for the best.

All these wonderful things may happen—but they certainly won't happen quickly.

Therefore, we have tried to guide our readers in the best choice of methods to bring them safely through the chaos—now.

We want women to stop buying bedside manner alone from their doctors. Personality was something nobody was graded on in medical school.

We want women to insist on courtesy and warmth in labor rooms; to know how much lab work is necessary and how much simply pads a bill; to exercise a healthy suspicion of surgery and physicians who prescribe it without adequate attention to less risky alternatives.

We believe that women must take advantage of the information explosion and hold themselves equally responsible with their doctors for knowledge of their own bodies and maintenance of their own good health. No longer can the patient cower behind her own ignorance, praising her doctor for all good, blaming her doctor for all evil. The doctor too must voluntarily abandon his godlike posture, lest he be dethroned by an enraged public.

A more egalitarian division of power between patient and doctor requires that the language barrier between them be broken. On the one hand, a woman has to learn the medical terms; on the other hand, her doctor has to learn to speak in plain English as much as possible.

Throughout this book, we have written out the medical terms phonetically. And we ask our readers to say them out loud a couple of times, wherever they appear. Only in this way can the language of medicine be desanctified, so that words like osteoporosis and diethylstilbesterol become merely words again instead of insurmountable barriers between people who should be talking to each other more, not less.

This book is about medical facts, not about politics and economics— but there are some political and economic conditions that must be mentioned if a woman is to find her own process for continuing health care.

The growth of the notion of malpractice is an additional imbalance in a society in which care is already rendered unequally according to wealth.

Let no patient imagine that malpractice insurance was invented to protect her against the mistakes of doctors. It was invented to protect doctors and hospitals against the wrath of injured patients, and enriches no one except the insurance companies. If you fall into the hands of an incompetent physician, whatever you or your family can collect in a suit will be small comfort indeed. Besides, *you* are paying for your doctor's malpractice insurance to begin with. Medical practitioners and hospitals pass the cost of their insurance back to the public as surely as auto companies pass back the cost of the air pollution equipment that the public demanded they install.

Like reparations after a war, malpractice payments may help to build the future. They do not heal the maimed or raise the dead, and of course, they do nothing to stop the war. Certainly, it's clear that patients who bring frivolous suits against hospitals and doctors are unlikely to win, and the exercise of the right to sue, therefore, does little more than raise costs all around. Most practitioners have this insurance. Whether or not it has lowered the *mistake* rate is a matter of conjecture. If you ever do decide to sue, be sure that you are equipped not just with a passion for vengeance but for nothing less than *justice*—and get yourself a great lawyer. You can be sure that those you are suing will have the very best.

SOCIAL FACTORS THAT ARE CHANGING HEALTH CARE

Those who fought for non-discriminatory practices for medical schools have won a little. In the next two decades or so, 20–40 per cent of graduating physicians may be female. In addition, women should keep in mind that less than 50 per cent of the physicians in this country now belong to the traditionally conservative American Medical Association—and that at recent conventions, young doctors with a changed social conscience have voiced their opposition to that organization's policies.

Group practice is another growing innovation in medical sociology. In a group practice, you have your regular doctor—but should she or he be unavailable, another member of the group will be covering. This means that the doctor can take a vacation, read a book, junk the beeper, enjoy some of the amenities that keep the rest of us human despite the trials of our work. For patients, a side effect of group practice is that it lessens the dependency on the "one and only" doctor. You learn that if your doctor is off, another doctor will probably do just as well, at least for interim treatment.

We recommend that patients have alternative doctors. It's part of the process that is independence; it helps a doctor to function more as a human being and less as a god-substitute.

In an era of concern about the environment, women must realize that medicine, particularly research into new drugs and treatments, is conditioned by environmental factors far out of any one physician's control.

Therefore, women should never believe any medical fact—not even those put forth in this book—for all time. The environment has been made so unstable by pollution and the emissions of industry, and just as much by changing social and sexual mores, by evolving concepts of liberty and the legislation that follows upon them, that medical practice cannot help but be fluid. That's why the Food and Drug Administration is constantly re-evaluating long-accepted medicines. After all, who knows how an old drug will mix with a new idea?

The process we suggest here is to stay open-minded, to read constantly and constantly re-evaluate what you thought was true. Newspapers tend to be sensational in their treatment of "new" medical discoveries; medical trade journals tend to be overly conservative in their welcome to new ideas. The women's magazines, the monthlies, and some well-considered consumer-education spots on television and radio are the best guide, because they are filtered through the sensibilities of the patients who produce them.

CHOOSING A DOCTOR

The process for selecting a doctor and a mode of treatment differs for every eventuality. And *each* process for *each* eventuality is suggested in detail throughout this book.

Suffice it to say here that a woman should never decide on a doctor or a mode of treatment of a serious illness without at least one or two other opinions. The opinion of another doctor is fine. When choosing a physician, the opinions of other women who have sought health care or experienced the same ailment are excellent. The patient self-help groups are invaluable selection aids. Keep in mind that doctors are often reluctant to criticize each other. Don't wait for doctors to become the willing judges of their peers; you could wait a lifetime. Use the best tool available now—the experience of other women who have gone through the same thing.

Remember, finally, that doctors are not today what they were yesterday. They are changing—because of the same pressures that change patients. *In fact, many of our feminist recriminations against physicians*

*become outdated by the time we have done enough con-
sciousness-raising to articulate them.* Medicine may be shot through
with social evils, but when you're suffering, you have no time to do battle with social evils. That's for when you're well.

Battle the social evils, therefore, *before* the fact of illness. Keep in
mind that millions of women, all over this country, and millions of
men, elderly people, handicapped people, younger physicians and even
a number of older ones too, are engaged in the struggle to right the
wrongs in medicine. And their efforts—our collective efforts—may
eventually pay off.

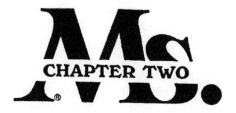

CHAPTER TWO

PUBERTY, MENSTRUATION and ADOLESCENCE

Puberty is the process of physical sexual maturation. In girls, this takes place over a three-to-five-year period, usually between the ages of eight and seventeen, and climaxes when the regular cycle of menstruation is established.

If a girl is completely unprepared for puberty, it may frighten her; when she gets her first period, she may think some terrible internal disorder is causing her to bleed. Even the best-prepared girl may be a little overawed by the enormous changes in her body, so certain basic, positive ideas should be communicated to her from the beginning.

Every healthy young woman in the world menstruates. Nothing is more usual, more routine, more normal. Menstruation is not a curse; it should never be labeled as such, or by any other euphemistic name; it is not to be hidden shamefully from the other members of the family.

The menstrual cycle is a vital indicator of a woman's good health. It tells her as much about her physical well-being as the level of her appetite or the level of her blood pressure.

Menstruation is not a disease. It should never be treated as a disease, or its routine discomforts dealt with as though they were disease symptoms.

With puberty come the years of *adolescence,* when the girl matures psychologically and socially. It is a tumultuous, emotional time and a lot of fun; its strains on both parents and daughter will be much lessened if everybody deals with its physical aspects forthrightly.

Sex can be discussed separately or together with menstruation. A girl needs to know everything she can about puberty and the menstrual cycle, regardless of whether she has started consciously thinking about sexuality. However, with the great peer pressure toward early sexual relationships, puberty is a logical time to begin discussions of sexuality and contraception, if not before. In addition, the years of puberty and adolescence are years of intense sexual drive, so discussions of sexuality are not only appropriate—they are vital. No mother can hope to keep her girl isolated from the explosion of explicit sex at the corner newsstand, in everyday book stores, in all the media. There is pressure on young people—real social pressure—to be grown-up sexually when they are still kids at heart.

If a parent can take the pressure off a little—by giving her child a sense of self-respect, a sense of the responsibility of sex—that may help to give a girl some extra time to grow up, and at the risk of sounding old-fashioned, to postpone sex until she's ready to enjoy it.

If you can convince your girl to set her *own* sexual agenda—and not allow it to be set for her by some sweet but clearly rapacious teen-age boy—then she is well on her way to being a free woman all her life, a woman who will always be in control of her own sexuality.

PUBERTY

1. External signs of puberty

Several key outward changes signify that a girl is maturing sexually:
a. Breasts begin to develop;
b. Pubic and axillary (underarm) hair begins to grow;
c. There is a spurt in height and weight;
d. The pelvic bones widen;
At the end of this process, e., the menstrual period begins.

This is the usual order of the outward changes during puberty. However, *there is nothing at all abnormal if changes occur simultaneously or in a different order, as long as they all occur.* The exception to this is that the menstrual period does not usually start until most of the other development is complete.

2. Breast development in puberty

A girl may normally start developing breasts as early as seven to eight years of age.

Initially, only the nipple protrudes from the chest wall.

Then glandular tissue begins to grow under the nipple. This is a *breast bud.*

Sometimes one breast bud develops before the other. Since it is usually firm, this bud has occasionally been mistaken for a tumor and removed by aggressive surgeons. Don't be misguided! Uneven breast development is not unusual at all; but breast tumors are extremely rare in pubescent girls. Get a second opinion if surgery is recommended.

3. Breast soreness during puberty

Breast buds may feel sore because they are composed of gland tissue responsive to the concentrations of estrogen in the blood, which begin to rise during puberty, prior to menarche—(me-NAR-ke), the onset of menstruation.

The discomfort is mild, and girls can be assured that it will pass. Sometimes young girls, curious about their new breasts, will touch or rub them repeatedly, making the breast bud sore. This too is nothing to worry about. Only if there is redness or discharge from the nipple should medical advice be sought.

4. When to start wearing a brassiere

Brassieres are of dubious value except for heavy-breasted women. So there's no good reason at all for young girls to wear them. Young girls sometimes like to emphasize the fact that their breasts are growing by wearing a "bra"—in fact, fancy bra and panty sets, imitating the underwear of mature women, are now a fad among many youngsters who are still completely flat-chested.

Try to encourage your girl not to wear a bra before it makes sense but don't put her down by saying there's no reason to do so. If you honestly feel that she faces some psychological disadvantage by going braless, by all means let her have her desire. Peer pressure is a powerful force when you're growing up. And bras are never a powerful force for good or ill, at any stage.

5. Pubic hair growth

The first pubic hair usually appears at about the same time the nipples begin to protrude. First a few strands of hair appear on the outer lips of the vagina; these gradually grow more numerous until they cover the pubic area. Later the hair grows sideways toward the upper thighs. At the time of menarche, hair growth is not complete and usually needs another year for full development. The woman's pubic hair thus grows in a typical triangle pattern, with a sharp upper border. Occasionally a light growth of hair will extend up to the navel.

6. Underarm hair growth

The hair in the axillary (underarm) regions appears about the same time as that in the pubic area. This is in response to the same hormonal process, the increased production of androgen by the adrenal glands. Small amounts of hair around the breasts is also normal.

7. Growth spurt in puberty

By the time menarche occurs, 90 per cent of a girl's pubescent growth spurt has usually taken place. The average height gain for American girls after the first period is an additional 2¼ inches. Because growth is steady and continues until menstruation, well-nourished girls who menstruate later are usually taller.

OPINION: The use of high doses of estrogen to stop the growth of tall girls is a practice to be condemned! Only in extraordinary circumstances should a young girl be exposed to the risks of estrogen (See p. 291) and certainly not when the goal is only to make her a few inches shorter.

Simultaneously with the spurt in height, girls experiencing puberty usually gain weight as well. By age seven or eight, girls are generally more plump—and taller—than boys. However, parents should carefully distinguish pubescent weight gain from general obesity. An overweight child has developed a greater *total* number of fat storage cells. A child growing plump at the onset of puberty is only experiencing an increase in the fat content of the cells she already has and a change in the *distribution* of fat on her body.

As a rule, children who are fat before puberty experience earlier menarche. This lends support to the idea that sexual development depends partly upon the achievement of a "critical mass"—a certain weight per unit of height. (Ref. 1) This and many other theories about what causes the onset of puberty are all unproven.

8. Changing body shape
Total body fat increases during puberty, and the bones of the pelvis grow and widen. Together, these developments create a redistribution of body fat onto the thighs and hips. The resulting figure change is more or less pronounced, depending on the individual. If it isn't very pronounced at all, there's nothing to worry about; a quick look back at the female figures on the family tree will usually provide ample explanation.

9. When the first menstrual period occurs
The average age for menarche in the United States is 12.6 years—but the *normal* age is nine to seventeen years. Over the past century, the average age for menarche has decreased three to four months each decade, probably the result of improved nutrition and hygiene.

10. Factors influencing the age of first menstruation
a. *Nutrition:* a poorly fed girl will usually menstruate later.
b. *Light:* blind girls menstruate earlier.
c. *Climate:* not a factor.
d. *Race:* not a factor.
e. *Altitude:* girls living at high altitudes will usually menstruate later.
f. *Heredity:* this is probably the most important factor of all—if other conditions are equal. Even though the average age of menarche is decreasing, mothers who experienced menarche late in their generation

will generally have daughters who experience menarche late within the range for *their* generation.

g. *General physical health:* severe illness during puberty—such as diabetes or rheumatic fever—tends to delay menarche.

h. *General mental health:* when a girl is under great strain during puberty—due to mental illness or a severe shock such as the death of someone close to her—menarche may be delayed. (Ref. 2)

11. Irregular menses are normal during puberty

Young girls tend to menstruate irregularly at first, and it normally takes two or three years for the monthly cycle to establish its lifelong pattern.

The irregularity is due to the fact that, although the young girl's ovaries are not yet releasing eggs, they are producing high levels of *estrogen,* the hormone that controls a woman's physical development and secondary sexual characteristics. The estrogen is building the endometrium (en-do-ME-tree-um)—the lining of the uterus that is periodically eliminated during menstruation. However, no ovulation—egg release—is occurring to govern *the time span* at which this elimination occurs.

Estrogen production without ovulation leads to irregular menstrual bleeding.

The same situation often occurs in older women, who have ceased ovulating but whose bodies are still producing estrogen or who are receiving estrogen by medication. (See ※45–48 below for abnormalities of bleeding)

12. Other changes of puberty

The onset of puberty creates changes in the internal organs of a woman's body.

The uterus gets bigger and changes shape.

The vagina begins to elongate, and a watery discharge appears.

The small inner lips of the vagina—*labia minora* (LA-bia)—begin to grow.

The pelvic bones grow and change shape.

Body cells increase their fat content.

The body's metabolism changes, requiring additional calories and protein. (These nutritional needs are greatest just before menarche and coincide with the body's growth spurt.)

Sweat glands in the underarm area enlarge.

13. Growth of the uterus

Under the influence of estrogen during early puberty, the uterus enlarges and changes shape. The fundus, or upper part of the organ, grows larger and continues to change shape until young adulthood, when it has become round (or pear-shaped).

14. Growth of the vagina

The vagina begins to grow longer during puberty and its lining thickens. The labia minora—the inner lips of the vagina which are very small before puberty—begin to grow and protrude between the labia majora, the larger outer lips of the vagina.

15. Vaginal discharge before menarche

A discharge of vaginal cells may occur as menarche approaches—it is usually thin and watery, whitish or pale yellow. The discharge is a sign of normal growth and good health; only if it is accompanied by severe itching or irritation should medical advice be sought. A slight, yellowish stain on underwear is normal. Cotton panties are advisable.

16. Pelvic bone growth

The bones of the pelvis change their shape early in puberty, laying the skeletal foundation for a new distribution of fat and muscle over the hips and thighs.

17. Growth of sweat glands

Sweat glands in the underarm area enlarge during puberty, leading to an increase in perspiration and odor. Now is the time for a girl to start washing her underarms at least once daily and familiarizing herself with powders, deodorants, antiperspirants. (See p. 235)

MENSTRUATION AND THE HORMONES THAT GOVERN IT

18. What is happening when you menstruate?

Every month, the lining of the uterus (the endometrium) grows thicker, enriched by blood and other nutrients brought to it by chemical and hormonal reactions in your body. Unless and until you decide to become pregnant, your body simply does not need all the cells that have built up inside your uterus, and, therefore your body eliminates them—at regular monthly intervals—in the bleeding that appears as menstruation.

This process is a sign of general good health in all women.

19. How to calculate your menstrual cycle

Count the days of your menstrual cycle from the first day of bleeding, ending it on the day before resumption of bleeding. If you started menstrual bleeding on the first of September and started again on the thirtieth of September, then your cycle was twenty-nine days long—September 1 through 29.

20. When is a menstrual cycle "regular"?

A *normal* menstrual cycle is twenty-one to thirty-five days long (twenty-eight days is the average). A *normal* menstrual flow is one to seven days long. A certain pattern in the length of period and cycle usually establishes itself for each individual woman in the first few years of menstruation. However, a variation of several days either way is common from time to time and does not mean that the period is "irregular," nor does it imply ill health.

21. How much bleeding is normal?

The amount of blood loss during a menstrual period varies greatly from woman to woman, *but is usually about the same with each period for an individual woman.* The normal range can require, on the light side, one or two tampons or pads per day, to (on the heavy side) eight to ten tampons or pads per day. The flow should not be so heavy as to gush down a woman's legs. Any marked increase or decrease in flow should be medically evaluated. The amount of blood loss during menstruation is *not* an indicator of fertility.

22. What is a hormone?

A hormone is a chemical substance produced by one part of your body, which enters the blood stream and causes changes in other parts of your body. It is a product of the endocrine or chemical-glandular system. The word comes from the Greek—to rouse or set in motion—and that's exactly what a hormone does. Hormones set in motion the whole process of sexual maturation, and govern the menstrual cycle.

23. Hormones that make the menstrual cycle work

Six hormones work together in a chain reaction that governs the menstrual cycle.

a. *Estrogen* (ESS-tro-jen), produced primarily by the ovaries, controls much of a woman's growth and physical sexual development.

b. *Progesterone* (pro-GESS-ter-own), produced by the ovaries, alternates with estrogen for dominant effect during the menstrual cycle.

c. *FSH-RF* are the initials for *Follicle Stimulating Hormone-Releasing Factor.* It is produced by the hypothalamus (hipe-oh-THAL-amus).

d. *FSH* is the *Follicle Stimulating Hormone* which FSH-RF activates. It is produced by the pituitary gland (pi-TOO-it-ary) and triggers the growth of follicles—groups of cells surrounding eggs in the ovaries—which then produce estrogen and progesterone.

e. *LH-RF* are the initials for *Luteinizing Hormone-Releasing Factor,* produced by the hypothalamus.

f. *LH, Luteinizing Hormone,* produced by the pituitary, is released by LH-RF and triggers ovulation—the release of the egg from the ovarian follicle and the ovary—then changing the broken follicle to a *corpus luteum* (LOOT-ee-um) or yellow body. (Luteinizing means yellowing; lutein is a yellow pigment, another form of which gives an egg yolk its color.)

24. The ovaries

The word "ovary" comes from the Latin word *ova,* meaning egg. It is your two ovaries that contain the eggs or germ cells. When a girl is born, each ovary contains 100,000–400,000 eggs. This number progressively decreases throughout a woman's life until menopause, when very few remain. The ovaries also produce estrogen and progesterone.

25. The ovarian follicles and corpus luteum

Ovarian follicles are clusters of cells surrounding the eggs in each ovary. The cells of the follicles are the major producers of estrogen and progesterone. After ovulation, the follicle becomes the corpus luteum and produces higher levels of estrogen and progesterone.

26. What is ovulation?

Ovulation is the process, usually at mid-cycle, by which an ovarian follicle breaks and releases an egg from the ovary into one of the Fallopian tubes.

27. The Fallopian tubes

The Fallopian tubes receive the egg that is released during ovulation. They are connected to the uterus, and when and if the egg is fertilized by a sperm, it is carried along these tubes to the uterus itself.

(The reason Fallopian is written with a capital letter is that the tubes are named for Gabriello Fallopio, a sixteenth-century Italian anatomist who discovered them. He also did some basic work on bone typing and analyzed how our sense of taste works, and is credited with inventing the first condom.)

28. The hypothalamus

The hypothalamus is a glandular and nerve center located in the center of the brain, directly above the pituitary gland. Besides producing

FSH-RF and LH-RF, the hypothalamus is thought to be the major control center for hunger, thirst, sleepiness, sexual appetite, and all the other endocrine systems besides the reproductive system.

Because of its location, the hypothalamus is greatly affected by signals from other parts of the brain. For example, it is very sensitive to general illness and mental stress and often passes these negative signals on through the hormone chain to affect the menstrual cycle itself. *It is for this reason that irregularities in the menstrual cycle may accompany a disorder that has nothing to do with a woman's reproductive system.*

29. The pituitary

The pituitary gland is located at the end of a stalk, just below the hypothalamus, at the base of the brain. It is very important in its role of producing all the "stimulating" hormones for all the glands of the body—in addition to FSH and LH, thyroid-stimulating hormone (TSH) and adrenocorticotropic hormone (ACTH). The pituitary also produces prolactin, important in milk production and oxytocin, important in milk letdown and uterine contractions. (See p. 158)

30. How the hormone chain reaction works in the menstrual cycle (This example assumes a twenty-eight-day cycle.)

DAY ONE — On the first day of menstrual bleeding, estrogen and progesterone are at their lowest levels in the blood stream. The hypothalamus reacts to these low levels by producing FSH-RF, which triggers production of FSH. FSH stimulates development of *several* ovarian follicles, which then begin producing estrogen at increased rates.

THROUGH DAY 14 — Ovarian follicles continue producing estrogen for about fourteen days until the hormone reaches a high level in the blood stream. This high level causes the hypothalamus to produce a spurt of LH-RF, the hormone that triggers production of LH. LH stimulates ovulation, causing *one* (occasionally more) eggs to be released by the ovary. (No one really knows why only one egg is released and the other follicles just degenerate and disappear.)

DAYS 15 AND 16 — The egg pops out of the ovary and is picked up by the fimbria, the fringe at the end of the Fallopian tube. For twelve to thirty-six hours, while the egg is in the Fallopian tube, it is available for fertilization. When it is not fertilized, it disintegrates with *no symptoms or ill-effects*.

THROUGH DAY 28   Meanwhile, the action of LH is changing the ruptured ovarian follicle into the corpus luteum or "yellow body." This yellow body produces increasing levels of estrogen and progesterone for the next eight to ten days, with progesterone usually becoming dominant. The yellow body degenerates after this time and the blood levels of estrogen and progesterone decline unless pregnancy occurs.

DAY ONE   When estrogen and progesterone reach low enough levels in the blood stream, the lining of the uterus (endometrium)—which has thickened in response to the hormonal chain reaction—is sloughed off. Menstruation begins again. The cycle repeats itself.

31. How estrogen and progesterone affect the endometrium

Estrogen stimulates the growth of the endometrium, the lining of the uterus.

After ovulation, in the second half of the menstrual cycle, progesterone dominates and thickens the endometrium even more.

Near the end of the cycle, estrogen and progesterone levels decrease. The endometrium cells stop multiplying and degenerate. The uterus sloughs off the unneeded cells along with some blood, resulting in menstruation.

32. How estrogen and progesterone affect the glands of the endometrium

Before ovulation, the glands of the endometrium—viewed by the microscope—appear to be straight. After ovulation, progesterone makes the glands appear long and twisting. The change probably makes a more hospitable place for the fertilized egg to implant.

The change in the shape of glands is useful in the evaluation of an endometrial biopsy, taken in the work-up of an infertile couple (see Infertility, Chapter Four). The pathologist will be able to detect whether the woman has ovulated if the biopsy is taken in the second half of the cycle.

33. How estrogen and progesterone affect the Fallopian tubes

Inside the Fallopian tubes are cilia (SIL-ee-a)—wavy, hairlike projections—which, if they have the opportunity, help to push the sperm and egg together and then move the fertilized egg on into the uterus. (To give you an idea what cilia look like, the word derives from a Latin word meaning eyelashes.)

Around the time of ovulation, estrogen and progesterone work to increase the number of cilia and their movement in the tubes.

Estrogen and progesterone also cause increased mucus production and stronger muscle contractions in the tubes—both aids to the sperm in reaching the egg. Strong contractions of the Fallopian tubes at mid-cycle may be the cause of the severe cramping that some women get in the lower sides of the abdomen. This pain is called *mittelschmerz* (German for "pain in the middle"). (See pp. 326–27)

In addition, the muscular contractions of the Fallopian tubes and the ligaments that support the ovaries bring the tubes closer to the ovaries. This means that when ovulation occurs, the Fallopian tube is in a better geographical position to catch the egg.

34. How estrogen and progesterone affect the cervix

The cervix is the lower part of the uterus that extends into the vagina. Glands in the cervix normally secrete mucus to lubricate the vagina, to protect the endometrium from infection and to facilitate passage of sperm into the uterus at the right time for fertilization.

The amount of mucus is smallest right after menstruation ends.

But as estrogen levels rise, the cervical glands secrete more and more mucus.

At mid-cycle, the time of ovulation, mucus becomes sticky and so abundant that you may notice it as a vaginal discharge. This sort of mucus has a texture and chemical make-up (alkaline Ph) most welcoming to sperm. (See Chapter Three, ✕138, the cervical mucus method in rhythm birth control.)

Later on in the cycle, progesterone makes the cervical mucus thicker and more impenetrable to sperm, changing it chemically to an acid Ph.

35. The ferning test, a simple lab procedure, can indicate much about a woman's hormonal status

Estrogen causes an increase in the salt content of the cervical mucus during the first half of the cycle. If a smear of this mucus is taken and analyzed, before ovulation, when estrogen levels are high, a *ferning* pattern will appear as the smear dries. The ferning is caused by crystallization of the salt. This is a very simple test.

After ovulation, the rising influence of progesterone causes a decrease in salt content. The dried smear shows a cellular pattern.

By checking how the salt pattern develops, the gynecologist can tell you if ovulation has occurred. But an endometrial biopsy is a better way of informing a woman whether the corpus luteum is functioning properly.

36. How estrogen and progesterone affect the vagina

Estrogen helps the cells lining the vagina to multiply and the cell layers to become thicker. This causes an increase in watery discharge (which includes cervical and vaginal secretions and cells) in the early part of the cycle and before menarche.

Progesterone slows the increase in these cell layers and, as a result, fewer are sloughed off. The amount of discharge toward the end of the menstrual cycle is less than in the earlier weeks.

37. A vaginal smear can indicate a great deal about a woman's hormonal status

There are three kinds of cells in the vaginal lining: basal cells (the deepest layer), intermediate cells (the middle layer), and superficial cells (the outermost layer).

Since estrogen causes an increase in the number of superficial cells, these should predominate in a smear taken during the first half of the cycle.

Since progesterone reduces the number of superficial cells, intermediate cells should predominate in a smear taken during the second half of the cycle.

If there is anything awry in the normal ebb and flow of these hormones during the menstrual cycle, the cell balance in the smear will show it.

This test may be done during an infertility work-up or around the time of menopause to evaluate the amount of estrogen still present in the body. It is also done to evaluate children with premature sexual development.

38. How estrogen and progesterone affect the breasts

In the early part of the cycle, estrogen causes an increase in the number of glands and ducts in the breasts. These are mostly milk carriers—although they don't normally function as such until after a delivery.

Progesterone, in the second half of the cycle, has a much more marked effect, causing the swelling of breast glandular tissue and congestion of blood vessels in the breast.

39. Mild breast tenderness is normal before menstruation

Sometimes progesterone and estrogen cause breast tenderness and swelling toward the end of the cycle. The veins in your breasts may appear more prominent at this time, because progesterone is triggering congestion of blood vessels.

The discomfort is usually mild, *a normal sign* of the forthcoming period. Nothing is wrong if it *doesn't* occur.

Severe tenderness may happen as part of premenstrual syndrome. (See p. 327)

40. Menstrual protection: pads or tampons?

There is no intrinsic advantage to one type of protection over another: individual comfort should be the deciding factor. Most girls who are still virginal prefer pads, indicating difficulty in wearing tampons. A young girl should start with the smallest kinds of tampons and put lots of water-soluble lubricating jelly on the tip so it slides in easily. When a tampon expands, it is sometimes hard to remove. Again, a lubricating jelly can be used or a girl can remove it in the bathtub; it slips out easily when wet. The only times when tampons are a must is for swimming, horseback riding, and prolonged bicycle riding.

41. Regular bathing should continue during menstruation

A girl should be encouraged to continue bathing, showering, and washing her hair during her menstrual period just as she would usually. The same goes for swimming and other athletic activities.

42. Managing a menstrual period during school hours

A teen-age girl may hate to go to school during the first few days of menstruation because the simple act of changing a pad or tampon is made so difficult by school rules and schedules. A note from parents or doctor requesting extra bathroom privileges during menstruation will help.

If a girl takes medication for menstrual discomfort, her mother or father should tell the school authorities that she is carrying the medication with their knowledge and approval. A doctor's note may be required.

43. Menstrual extraction

Menstrual extraction is a medical procedure by which the cells of the endometrium, which would ordinarily be sloughed off over a period of days, are extracted all at one time. It is also used for very early abortions. (See pp. 192–93)

It is not recommended as a routine procedure.

Women should not perform the procedure on themselves. They cannot be sure of performing it under sterile conditions, and therefore risk infection of the uterus or Fallopian tubes.

44. Dysmenorrhea (dis-men-or-REE-ah)

Menstrual cramps, a common problem in teen-agers, do not usually begin until the second or third year of menstruation, when the young woman begins to ovulate. In many cases, mild to moderate pain-killers bring complete relief. In more severe cases, medical help may be needed. (See Chapter Eleven for complete discussion of dysmenorrhea)

45. Irregular menses after menarche are normal

As mentioned before, the first year or two of menses may not be accompanied by ovulation. This means that the levels of estrogen are high in the body, and changes in this one hormone causes the bleeding which occurs. However, the absence of the high levels of progesterone, which are normally present before menstruation, tends to make the periods irregular. The most usual pattern is to skip several months in between periods. If the length of flow is normal (one to seven days), this irregularity is of no concern during the first few years of menstruation. There are some patterns of menstruation which are not normal during puberty, and these are discussed below.

46. Excessively lengthy menstrual periods after menarche

Once in a while, a girl who has just begun menstruating will experience periods which come infrequently, but last two to three weeks at a time. This usually signifies that she is not ovulating. In some girls this amount of bleeding can cause anemia (see pp. 368–69), but for most, this pattern is just a severe nuisance. A frequent treatment is progesterone tablets, taken five–seven days each month for several months. The girl will get her period in the few days after stopping the progesterone each month. This progesterone therapy will not affect the hypothalamus significantly, nor will it cause ovulation. It will, however, affect the source of the trouble—too much estrogen working in the endometrium.

47. Frequent menses after menarche

In some girls who are not yet ovulating, periods come too frequently —say, every two or three weeks—in addition to lasting too long. (See above) This is not only a nuisance; it can also lead to anemia.

Progesterone tablets over a two-to-three-week period can be given to stop the bleeding. Thereafter they can be given for several days every month to regulate menstrual flow. Again, this treatment will not significantly affect the hypothalamus but it will control the bleeding from the endometrium. Some physicians prescribe low-dose combination birth-control pills, if progesterone alone does not work. This is not recommended because it *does* affect the hypothalamus. If the treatment is suggested by several physicians, it may be tried—but *only for very short periods of time.*

48. Amenorrhea—prolonged absence of menses

Occasionally, girls who are not yet ovulating miss their periods for very long spans of time—say, six to twelve months. This is called amenorrhea (ah-men-o-REE-a).

If a girl was menstruating irregularly, the amenorrhea has less significance. It is probably related to the menstrual cycle itself and not to another more serious disease process. If a girl was previously *irregular* but misses her period for four to six months, she should receive a physical (*not just a gynecological!*) examination.

If a girl had *regular* menses previous to the amenorrhea, an examination is a must. Certain causes must be checked for:

a. Pregnancy

b. Serious illness such as diabetes or thyroid disease

c. Extreme weight loss. If a girl has been on a crash diet and lost a lot of weight quickly, she may also lose her periods. (The most extreme example of this is *anorexia nervosa*—see below. But it can happen just from crazy dieting, when the girl is not anorexic at all but simply ill-advised about nutrition.)

d. Extreme weight gain. If the cause is just overeating, then the amenorrhea should not last long. If another disease process has caused her to weight gain, this must be treated with concern.

e. Severe emotional stress. (Life can sometimes be awful or terrific enough to make you miss a period.)

49. Premature puberty

When a girl experiences the changes of puberty before age seven, she must be examined for other problems such as possible tumors on the ovaries, on the pituitary gland, or hypothyroidism—underactive thyroid gland. In most cases, nothing is wrong. The girl is just ahead for her generation.

50. Premature breast growth

If a little girl is developing breasts at a very early age, with no other signs of puberty, she should be examined for other problems. Usually, there are none, and the rest of puberty will proceed normally at a later time.

51. Premature pubic-hair growth

Pubic-hair growth, before other signs of puberty, occurs most often in children with known neurological problems—for example, nervous disorders such as cerebral palsy or seizures. If neurological damage was not previously apparent, then premature pubic-hair growth is *not* a sign of it. As with premature breast growth, puberty usually occurs normally at a later date.

52. Delayed puberty

If the various other stages of puberty are progressing, there is no need to worry if menarche has not occurred before the sixteenth birthday. But if menarche does not occur within the next year, or if the other changes of puberty do not occur, then disease must be suspected.

a. When *no* changes of puberty occur, there may be some congenital abnormality present such as *Turner's Syndrome.* A girl born with Turner's Syndrome has very tiny ovaries or none at all: therefore estrogen and progesterone are not being produced in sufficient quantities. The disorder is named for Henry H. Turner, a pioneer American endocrinologist, who discovered it in the 1930s.

In such cases, estrogen and progesterone therapy can be used to develop breasts, pubic hair, and other female sexual characteristics, including menstrual periods, so that a woman with Turner's Syndrome can lead a normal life. However, since there is no ovulation, she will not be fertile.

b. When puberty seems to be occurring normally, but there is no menarche, an examination can usually determine the cause. There may be a condition present such as *imperforate hymen* in which the hymen —the membrane that covers the vaginal opening in little girls—must be broken surgically to allow menstrual blood to flow out.

Some physical abnormality about the uterus may impede menarche. If the cause is not gynecological, then another disease process may be involved. So with this, *as with all deviations in the menstrual cycle,* a general physical as well as a gynecological examination is in order.

ADOLESCENCE

Strictly speaking, adolescence is that period of time when young people (usually in their teens) establish an identity separate and distinct from their parents. It is a tumultuous time, made more so by the soaring sexual and emotional demands of puberty. Parents usually have problems during the adolescence of their children; they have to put up with a lot of rejection (as their ideas are challenged) and fear (as their children go off on their own). It is often very difficult for a parent to distinguish between normal adolescent behavior and real pathologic abnormality. Keep in mind that this time of exploration and experimentation is necessary; that it will probably pass: when you are being driven to despair by your teen-agers, remember your own youth and think with sympathy of your own mother.

53. It is "normal" today for boys and girls to experience sexual intercourse during adolescence

Parents may not like it, but society at large condones and encourages early sex. *You will have to fight* to keep your child virginal until she is old enough to enjoy sex. You may lose the battle. RECOMMENDATION: Fight anyway.

54. Temporary homosexual attachments are normal during adolescence

Boys and girls often form passionate attachments to older role models of the same sex in early adolescence, a normal manifestation of the break with parental identification. Girls often have very close friends from whom they are inseparable at this time, with whom they share all their intimacies, sometimes including bodily touching and mutual exploration. This is normal too. Don't make a girl feel guilty about it.

55. Don't wait for your girl to become sexually active to tell her about reproduction, sex, and venereal disease

Children should be told the facts of life as soon as they start asking about them. As your child approaches puberty, discuss all aspects of sex with her; open communication between parent and child is vital at this time. Studies have shown that teens engaging in sex have less accurate knowledge about vital sexual topics than those who are not. So in this case, knowledge may actually serve as a healthy, intelligent deterrent. *Support sex education in the schools.*

56. Sexual arousal and vaginal discharge are normal in adolescence

Excessive watery discharge from the vagina is a normal result of estrogen influence on the vaginal mucosa at puberty. But it also may be due to fantasies and sexual arousal. (Boys have wet dreams; girls do as well.) If the vagina is not irritated, don't be alarmed. Suggest cotton underpants to your daughter; they are more absorbent. You will have an easier time getting her to wear them if you wear them yourself (they're the best kind of underwear for grown women too).

57. Masturbation and self-exploration are normal in adolescence

Unless masturbation is obsessive, it is a completely healthy way for a girl to learn about her body.

58. Discipline is a comfort no adolescent should be without

Discipline, whether in the form of curfews which bring children home by a certain time, or instructions to girls *and* boys that they behave with courtesy and decency to all people, must not stop with adolescence. It is an ongoing reminder to a child that her parents love her and care about what kind of person she turns out to be. Besides, parental discipline is the mother of self-discipline, a priceless tool for coping throughout life.

59. Encourage your girl in athletics

At one time, the only physical activity acceptable for girls in high school was cheerleading; thankfully, those days seem to be over. An adolescent girl should be encouraged to take part in sports, *whether she is good at them or not,* because they build her general health and accustom her to competition. The emotional lessons learned on the baseball field or the volleyball court spill over to relationships later in life, so that as an adult the girl is less inclined to accept passive, non-competitive roles. Likewise, boys who see girls participating actively in athletics are more likely to grow into men who are unafraid of strong, equal female partners.

60. Recommendation: the first gynecological examination should occur around age sixteen

If a girl has become sexually active before this age, she should see a gynecologist at that time. OPINION: Your own gynecologist may not be the right person for this task; check around for doctors in your area who *specialize* in adolescent gynecology.

Do not accompany your daughter into the examination room, unless she is very young and is seeing the gynecologist upon recommendation of a pediatrician for a specific health problem. Leave her alone with the doctor after the examination as well, so that they can talk in privacy, and she will feel free to ask anything she wants.

61. What can be gained by a gynecological examination for adolescents

a. Dysmenorrhea may bother adolescents. An examination and discussion which shows a girl that it is normal and nothing to worry about will be reassuring.

b. If a girl is sexually active, she should be tested for venereal disease and cervical cancer.

c. If she is pregnant, the gynecologist will find this out.

d. It may be necessary for a girl to discuss a method of birth control with the doctor.

62. A rectal examination by a pediatrician is an alternative to the gynecological examination

If your daughter doesn't want to see a gynecologist, and you yourself have severe doubts about subjecting her to the examination, ask your pediatrician to perform a rectal examination. This is sometimes less disturbing to girls when performed by the doctor whom they know very well. By inserting a finger into the rectum, the doctor can feel the uterus and the ovaries and detect any cyst or other abnormality which might be present.

63. Don't expect to find out from a gynecologist whether a girl is sexually active

The hymen, the thin membrane covering the opening to the cervix, can stretch and disappear because of many things besides sexual intercourse (i.e., tampons), so the gynecologist cannot be sure about your girl's sex life from its absence.

64. Adolescent pregnancy

Pregnancy among teen-agers is on the rise as social mores change to allow greater sexual contact among young people. In addition, the age of puberty is decreasing—so the age of fertility starts earlier.

WARNING: *If your daughter becomes pregnant, don't try to counsel her entirely by yourself.* Talk with the people at Planned Parenthood or other family-planning agencies, who are neither as hurt nor as angry nor as frightened as you are, who know all the options, and who can recommend good counselors, an invaluable assistance at this time.

65. The options in adolescent pregnancy

a. If the father is known, and the youngsters want to get married, they can do so with your permission. *But if they are very young, this is probably a bad idea.*

b. The girl can have the baby and bring him up with her parents' help. Federal funds for teen-age pregnancies have been cut back now, so this may be hard on the family financially. *Try to keep your girl in school.* The social stigma of being an unwed teen-age mother is fast declining; even though you may find it horrifying that your daughter is going through her junior year with a big belly, the kids in school and the teachers have probably witnessed this before and may notice it less than you would have thought.

c. Very often, girls who drop out of school because they become pregnant never finish their education. This is a tragedy; it penalizes the girl forever for something she did when she was very young. Check in your locality for child care centers that are associated with schools; there are very few and the need is often greater than their capacity.

d. The baby may be given up for adoption immediately after birth. Don't push this option without the wholehearted agreement of your daughter. *Do not choose it without counseling.*

e. While the mother finishes school, the child may be placed in *temporary* foster care. If the baby is retrieved by her mother permanently by the time she is a toddler, the break with the foster parents may be uneventful.

f. If the pregnancy is discovered early enough, the option of abortion should be discussed. *Do not make the decision for abortion without counseling.* An abortion is one thing for a mature woman who knows her own mind. It is quite another thing for a young girl who may have terrible fears about her future fertility, and great qualms about the operation once it is over.

g. There is no reason that the father and his parents should not share in the decision as to how the pregnancy is handled, and its attendant costs. If your girl is violently against involving them, do not press it.

h. Teen-age pregnancy is often a self-repeating phenomenon, especially if a girl is made to feel guilty and dirty by her parents and friends, and even more so if she drops out of school. So try to see adolescent pregnancy for what it is: something that can happen to anyone, something which has *not* happened to *you,* but to a young woman you love, whose whole life is before her.

66. Medical aspects of adolescent pregnancy
Teen-agers who decide to have their babies experience a higher incidence of
a. Anemia
b. High blood pressure
c. Prematurity
d. Caesarean-section delivery

67. Adolescent mothers often do not get good prenatal care
Very often, a teen-ager who thinks she is pregnant will not know where to turn. She may tell her boy friend before she tells her mother; he may not know where to turn either. If a girl hides her pregnancy until it is well advanced, passing the critical first trimester without prenatal care or advice, she creates unnecessary hazards to her baby. In addition, clinics and physicians are often completely unprepared to cope with the emotional complexities of the adolescent personality;

they may look down on the girl, condemn her; she may feel uncomfortable with them and neglect to show up for her appointments. If she goes into labor without having had the advantages of routine prenatal attention, the risk of complication grows. Make sure that the pregnant teen-agers you know get good prenatal care.

68. Opinion: Venereal disease is a major hazard of teen-age sexual activity, so tell your girl to insist that her sexual partners use condoms

More than 50 per cent of the cases of venereal disease in America occur in people under twenty-five. Tell this to your daughter. If she decides to sleep with any man, tell her to insist that he use a condom. Tell your boys to use them as well. (Foams and jellies have some VD-protective effect too. Acquaint your children with them.) Other forms of birth control may protect a girl against pregnancy, but they will not protect her against venereal disease.

69. Good nutrition is essential for adolescents

Obviously, it is essential for everyone—but adolescents, so concerned with their bodies, seem to love crash diets and fad diets that at best do no harm. Eating poorly is another way that teen-agers have of breaking the parental hold. Parents should be forewarned that a diet of hamburgers, soda, and french fries is inadequate. If they cannot control what their children eat outside the home, they should at least be rigid about the rules of nutrition inside the home. Don't let your daughter out of the house without watching her eat a good breakfast with a vitamin supplement. It may be the only meal in the day that you control.

70. Neurotic dieting: anorexia nervosa (an-oh-RECK-see-a nair-VOH-sa)

Teen-age girls diet a lot, because they want to be beautiful; so do teen-age boys. However, there is one condition—anorexia nervosa—when the dieting is obsessive, when a girl feels that she must lose more and more weight, stops eating almost entirely, and *still* thinks she is fat. She keeps on in this pattern until she is concentration-camp thin and her body begins to break down and die. Literally, she is starving herself to death for deep-rooted psychological reasons that are still incompletely understood. Fortunately, anorexia nervosa is rare; it primarily affects teen-age girls, but boys can get it too.

71. Symptoms of anorexia nervosa

a. A teen-ager who is on a crash diet will complain of feeling hungry all the time; the anorexic will maintain, no matter that she has virtually stopped eating anything at all, that she feels full and fine. Sometimes she will eat a lot and then vomit. Or she will take laxatives to force elimination of the food.

b. Crash dieters start to eat again eventually, when they've lost enough weight to be satisfied with themselves. The anorexic is never satisfied; she always maintains that she must get thinner, even when she is down to skin and bones.

c. A crash dieter may lose her period, because the hypothalamus is affected by weight loss. (See ✗48 above) This usually worries a girl enough to set her eating properly again. But the anorexic is not scared by the loss of her period; she may even welcome this sign that she has withdrawn from maturity.

ANY ONE OF THESE SYMPTOMS SHOULD TAKE THE GIRL AND HER PARENTS TO A PHYSICIAN IMMEDIATELY.

72. Treatment of anorexia nervosa

Treatment is frequently extended hospitalization and psychotherapy. If the condition is caught early, it is easier to cure. Families of anorexics may expect to be involved in the therapy, because the roots of this problem are often found in family interpersonal relationships.

73. Acne: a very common problem of adolescents

Adolescence is accompanied by an increase in the male hormones— androgens—from the adrenal glands, which cause the growth of pubic and underarm hair and increase the oil secretions in the skin pores. This sudden spurt in oil secretions may cause acne in teen-agers. Pimples or lesions called blackheads and whiteheads break out on the face, the chest, and the back. No one really knows why one teen-ager has only a few pimples while another may be broken out all over. There are two principles in acne treatment:

a. To render it as mild as possible during the adolescent years;

b. To make sure it will leave no scars in the future.

74. Blackheads: the least serious acne lesion

Sometimes a skin pore is blocked by a collection of oils. The tip of the oil collection, exposed to the air, turns black; the rest of the oil in the pore remains whitish. This is called a blackhead. It will not usually leave a scar unless picked or squeezed with dirty fingers and thus become infected. Gentle squeezing *with very clean hands* to release the oil from the pore is probably no danger; or the teen-ager can use a comedo extractor (any bump on the face is called a comedo).

75. Whiteheads: more serious acne lesions

A whitehead forms just like a blackhead except that the pore has no opening to the outside air. The oil cannot drain; cysts form underneath the skin; a dot of white pus will indicate infection. The area around a whitehead may be painful, for it is the tip of a small infection, not as with a blackhead, the tip of a blocked pore. Whiteheads should not be squeezed or picked, for this can lead to scarring.

76. Recommended treatment for mild acne

a. Don't pick at the pimples. This may lead to infection and scarring.

b. Wash hair two or three times a week, to keep it from becoming oily. Oily hair can aggravate acne, especially on the forehead. Avoid hair creams, sprays, grease.

c. Wash the face two or three times a day. Don't scrub hard. Press a hot washcloth over the affected area, then lather gently with an acne soap containing resorcinol, salicylic acid, or benzoyl peroxide.

d. Try going over your face with an ice cube after washing; the cold will help to keep the pores tight and closed.

e. Avoid greasy skin lotions or cosmetics.

f. To cover up the acne, use the special cosmetics that have been developed for this purpose.

g. Astringents like witch hazel or alcohol may be useful in cleaning excess oil from the face.

h. Sunbathing or the use of a sun lamp may help—*in small doses only*. However, people with sun-sensitive skin should avoid this. Immoderate and constant exposure has been shown to cause skin cancer.

i. Don't rub the acne lesions or put excess pressure on them. For example, don't lean your chin or your face continually on your hand.

j. Stay away from foods known to aggravate acne—chocolate, nuts, iodized salt, bromides, and colas. Some dermatologists feel acne sufferers should avoid milk as well. If after three to four weeks of avoiding these foods, the acne is not improved, then you can conclude that diet is simply not a principal cause of the lesions.

77. For treatment of severe acne, consult a dermatologist

Don't try to treat severe acne alone if you can secure the advice of a dematologist, who is especially trained in skin care.

78. Antibotics as a treatment for severe acne

a. If skin infection is present, the doctor may prescribe a broad-spectrum antibiotic such as tetracycline. Usually the dosage is 250–500 mg three times daily for several weeks. Thereafter, the dosage tapers off to one to two capsules per day for several months. This treatment fights the skin bacteria thought to cause infection in whiteheads.

Remember! Antibiotics can cause monilia vaginitis. (See Chapter Eleven) So if vaginal itching occurs while you are on the medication, call your doctor.

b. Dermatologists may prescribe an antibiotic cream, to be applied directly to the skin.

79. Vitamin A acid as a treatment for severe acne

Probably the most popular treatment today, Vitamin A acid can be applied as a solution or in presoaked swabs. It works by breaking down the keratin, the fatty substance produced in the pores.

Apply the Vitamin A acid when the face is dry, lightly and once a day at first, to see how much can be tolerated. During the first three weeks of treatment, the acne may appear to worsen. Skin may redden, cystic areas enlarge. Thereafter expect improvement. Continue the daily treatment for six to eight weeks, then decrease the applications to two to three times per week. A compound related to Vitamin A which seems to be effective by mouth is currently being tested. (Ref. 3) Watch for reports.

80. Side effects of Vitamin A acid

a. There may be no side effects at all. b. People using Vitamin A (Retin-A) may become highly sensitive to the sun and sun lamps; some skin tumors have even been reported. c. Some people become highly sensitive to soap. *As a general rule,* avoid sunbathing and excess face washing while under treatment. d. Loss of skin pigment may occur, but this reverses itself when treatment stops.

81. Surgery as a treatment for severe acne

A dermatologist may lance very large cysts or whiteheads in the office, making a tiny cut right over the lesion so the pus can escape.

82. Cryotherapy as a treatment for severe acne

Cryotherapy or cryoslush therapy is the application of a mixture of dry ice (cryo- is from the Greek *kryos* meaning ice cold) and acetone to affected skin areas with gauze once a week. It makes the outer layers of skin peel off and may help severe acne. This treatment should only be given by a dermatologist.

83. Warning: Do not accept X-ray or ultra-violet light therapy for acne. Both may cause cancer

84. Opinion: Estrogen and steroids should not be used routinely for acne treatment in adolescents

When women began taking birth-control pills, it was noted that as a result many no longer suffered from acne. This is because the estrogen in the pills counteracts the androgens which build up oily skin secretions. Using this knowledge, dermatologists will sometimes recommend estrogen treatment for young women suffering from bad acne. Likewise, corticosteroids, taken orally and applied in cream form, have been used. *All of these hormones are very strong agents, with potential for adverse effects on other parts of the body, so they should not be used routinely or for long periods of time.*

85. Some unavoidable elements which aggravate acne

Acne can be aggravated by a. hot, humid weather; b. strenuous sports, which cause an increase in adrenal hormone production; and c. emotional stress.

There is sometimes no way to avoid emotional stress or hot, humid weather; and sports are too important for general health to give up. There is also no way to avoid adolescence, and the parent and teenager trying to cope with these remarkable years should remember that they will fade away, like acne, with remarkable haste.

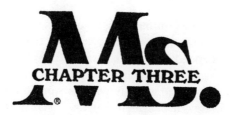

CHAPTER THREE

BIRTH CONTROL

No single scientific breakthrough has altered our lives so momentously as the discovery and mass use of safe, effective contraceptive methods. These discoveries ended an epidemic of death and chronic illness from unpreventable pregnancy that had always ravaged the women of the world. In days still not completely gone, a woman literally had babies until she died. Margaret Sanger, the great American pioneer of family planning, was the sixth child of a woman who bore eleven children and died at forty-eight. This was *not* an exceptional case.

Against such a background, birth control was really the first liberator of women. All our other efforts at liberation are its spinoffs.

When a woman chooses to practice birth control, she is not just making a decision about her personal life and her health—she is making a judgment about what is best for her economy, her political system, her soul, and the very destiny of her species. That's why people fight so furiously about whether and how women should limit their families. That's why virtually every government in the world today has, written or unwritten, a "family policy." That's why the individual's freedom to decide on birth control is so important.

Make yourself familiar with as many methods as possible; one type may be good now, but tomorrow, a backup or an alternative method may be required.

Never let anyone else decide what kind of birth control is best for you—not your lover, not your neighbor, not your consciousness-raising group, not your doctor, not even this book. Some doctors prefer contraceptives that they are required to prescribe; many doctors have a particular method they think is best for most of their patients most of the time; magazines and media resound with the opinions of the individuals who think the pill is terrible for everyone, or the foams are terrible for everyone. Listen to all this advice, the way you would listen to a candidate for office. But when you cast your ballot, cast it according to what *you* think is best for *you*.

Birth control is never to be taken for granted.

For even if a woman never avails herself of it, without the *choice* of doing so, she would not be a free woman.

ORAL CONTRACEPTIVES

1. History of oral contraceptives

Since the beginning of recorded history, men and women have been taking potions to render themselves temporarily sterile. Most of these—until the pill—were ineffective. A few, like arsenic, mercury, and strychnine, could render the taker sterile by rendering the taker dead.

In 1927, two physiologists in Germany, Bernhard Zondek and Selmar Aschheim, discovered that when the urine of pregnant women was injected into lab animals, the animals went into heat. The Zondek-Aschheim test became an early test for pregnancy; it was also a breakthrough necessary for the discovery of the estrogens, female hormones, by Adolf Butenandt in Germany and Edward Doisy in St. Louis. In the early 1930s, the Schering-Kahlbaum Co. in Germany, and Parke-Davis in the United States, began manufacturing hormones from animal sources, an expensive process. Further research in St. Louis showed that administration of hormones could prevent conception in lab animals. Soon it was discovered that cholesterol was the basic substance on which all hormones were built, and this led to the discovery of the androgens, male hormones. In 1937, diosgenin, a chemical used to synthesize androgen, estrogen, and progesterone, was discovered in large quantities in a Mexican yam. This made it much more feasible and inexpensive to produce hormones for clinical use.

The discovery of the hormones opened up new possibilities for controlling many sexual and reproductive functions. In the 1940s, it was learned that estrogen and progesterone could inhibit ovulation in women, a breakthrough which led eventually to development of the pill.

2. The original "pill" experiments

In the 1950s, G. D. Searle and Co. began work on the synthesis (production in a laboratory) of steroids, a large group of chemical substances that includes hormones, vitamins, and other bodily substances. (Cholesterol, cortisone, and the sex hormones are all steroids.) In 1952, Norethynodrel, the progestogen in the Enovid pill, was synthesized, along with another progestogen, Norethindrone. (See ✗12 below) In 1956, John Rock, Celso-Ramón García, and Gregory Pincus began experiments in Puerto Rico and Haiti with Enovid 10 mg, reporting on 8,133 menstrual cycles in 519 women. There had been small field trials among private patients in Boston before these larger tests.

In 1960, the FDA (Food and Drug Administration) approved Enovid 10 for use in this country, restricting it to only two years' constant use at a time. (This restriction is no longer in effect.) The United States became the first country to approve use of the pill; American companies were the first to market it. (Ref. 1)

3. Statistical context of the pill

Today, an estimated 10 to 15 million American women take the pill; there are about 50 million women using it throughout the world; approximately 20 to 25 per cent of American women between fifteen and forty-four now use the pill.

4. Warning: If you are taking the pill, relate that fact to any doctor you see for any reason

Like pregnancy, the pill has some effect on virtually all the body systems. Studies indicate that more than 100 laboratory tests show significant changes in women on the pill. (Ref. 2) This means that the pill can affect *many* aspects of a woman's health, and since so many millions of women use it, *any as yet undiscovered health hazard from the pill is potentially disastrous.* Therefore, any woman taking the pill must relate that fact to any doctor she sees for any reason. For example, since the pill can affect your eyes, the eye doctor should be told if you are taking the pill—even if your visit is just to check your glasses.

5. Recommendation: Avoid the pill unless you absolutely cannot allow the possibility of pregnancy

Even though it is the most effective form of birth control, the pill—whether the combined pill or the minipill—carries with it a very wide range of known and potential side effects (see below). In addition, there *may* be cumulative effects for women who take the pill over many years, that are now only suspected.

Only if it is absolutely unthinkable for you to become pregnant—and only if you are unwilling to consider the abortion option—should you choose the pill over other methods of birth control. (This recommendation is, of course, predicated on the assumption that abortion *is* an option available to women.)

If you must take the pill, do not take it for longer than five years without a break. (See below)

6. Two different types of pills are currently on the market: combined pills (with estrogen and progestogen) and minipills (with progestogen alone)

Until recently, sequential pills were also available, but have now been removed from the market because of evidence of increased endometrial cancer among users. (See below)

(Table 1 on pp. 89–91 shows the brands of pills currently available.)

7. Limitations on the pill

a. The pill may be obtained only by prescription from a licensed pharmacist or family planning clinic.

b. The FDA has seen to it that the quantities of estrogen and progestogen in the pill have been constantly lowered over the years. In 1970, the FDA advised that physicians should prescribe the *lowest effective* dose of estrogen and a number of very low-dose pills are now available.

c. There is now no limit on the number of years the pill may be taken (but recent studies suggest there should be a break at regular intervals—at least every five years). Women who have taken the pill for more than five years have a higher death rate even after stopping than those who never took the pill. (Ref. 3)

8. The combined pill

The combined pill is most widely used in this country. Each pill contains an estrogen and a progestogen. All pills in the package are identical. The exception to that is the twenty-eight-day package, which contains seven inert pills (without active hormonal ingredients).

9. Estrogenic compounds used in the combined pills

There are two of these—*mestranol* and *ethinyl estradiol.*

For most practical purposes—including evaluation of side effects—there is little difference between these two estrogens. Some tests show ethinyl estradiol to be more potent than mestranol; others find it about equivalent in strength. (See Table 1)

10. Progestogenic compounds used in the combined pills

There are five of these (listed in order of potency, the strongest first): *norgestrel, ethynodiol diacetate, norethindrone acetate, norethindrone, norethynodrel.* (Ref. 1) The reason there are so many progestogens is basically that each company developed its own. All except norgestrel come from the Mexican yam (barbasco root). Norgestrel is synthesized completely in the laboratory. (See Table 1)

11. How the combined pills prevent pregnancy

a. They block ovulation.

The hormones block the release of FSH-RF (Follicle Stimulating Hormone-Releasing Factor) from the hypothalamus, and therefore the follicles in the ovary do not mature completely. In addition, hormones in the pill stop the release of LH-RF (Luteinizing Hormone-Releasing Factor) so that there is no spurt of Luteinizing Hormone at mid-cycle and therefore no ovulation. (See Chapter Two, Menstruation)

b. They change the cervical mucus so that it is thick and relatively impenetrable by sperm—replacing the stringy, watery mucus that is normal at mid-cycle and easily penetrated by sperm.

c. They keep the endometrium (the lining of the uterus) thin, so that implantation of a fertilized egg is much less likely. Because the combined pill keeps the endometrium thin, women who are taking it tend to have lighter menstrual flows.

d. They may slow down the rate at which the egg passes along the Fallopian tube, preventing implantation.

e. They prevent *capacitation* of the sperm—that is, the ability, given to the sperm by substances within a woman's body, to fertilize the egg.

Capacitation is a process still incompletely understood. It was only discovered in 1951, when tests on rabbits showed that the sperm when it enters the vagina is *not* capable of fertilizing the egg. Therefore, substances in the uterus and the tubes (probably *not* hormones) must activate the enzymes in the head of the sperm, and this is called capacitation. These enzymes have to be activated before the sperm can pass through the outer coatings of the egg and fertilize it. Progestogen slows this process, which usually takes from one to six hours to complete, but does not completely block it. This is one of the major hurdles that Steptoe and Edwards had to overcome in their in vitro fertilization work. (See pp. 113–14)

12. If taken correctly, the combined pills are almost 100 per cent effective in preventing pregnancy

Even if some pills are missed and ovulation occurs, the other four factors are at work. The pills with less than 50 mcg estrogen are a fraction less certain to prevent pregnancy—but still more than 99 per cent effective. (Below 35 mcg the risk is higher—effectiveness drops to 97–98 per cent.) The benefits of reducing the estrogen in the pills and avoiding the side effects *may* justify running the highly remote risk that the pill will not work (see below).

13. Warning: Sequential pills have been removed from the market because they are associated with cancer. Do not take them

Sequential pills were on the market for many years and were originally favored because they were believed to copy the natural hormone cycle—estrogen dominance followed by progesterone dominance. However, the dosage of estrogen in the pill was higher than that in most of the combined pills, and the progestogen was relatively weak. Probably in the same way that high doses of replacement estrogen during menopause have been associated with endometrial cancer (see p. 290), the sequential pills have been found to be associated with endometrial hyperplasia and cancer in younger women. (Ref. 4)

WARNING: *If you are on the sequential pills (C-quens, Nor-quens, Ortho-Novum SQ, or Oracon) switch to another birth-control method.* Recent studies have shown that this same problem *may* arise in women on the combined pills, but as yet this remains to be confirmed. The risk seems to be *much* less. (Ref. 5)

14. The minipill

The minipill was first marketed in 1973. It contains no estrogen, only progestogen. There are two kinds of minipills (see Table 1 below), one containing norethindrone, one containing norgestrel.

15. Advantages of the minipill

Because the minipill contains no estrogen, it is felt to be free from the major side effects that sometimes result from estrogen action in the pill (see below) and which have caused the major controversies over the combined and sequential pills.

16. Disadvantages of the minipill

a. The minipills are estimated to be only 97 per cent effective (about the same as the IUD). This is because they do not block ovulation so completely as combined pills.

b. There is a high incidence of breakthrough bleeding with the minipill, the factor which most women who discontinue it cite in doing so.

17. A backup method should be used during the first six months on the minipill

Since women who become pregnant while taking the minipill usually do so during the first six months of use, a backup method—ideally a spermicide or condom—should be used at this time.

18. When to start taking birth-control pills

The pill (all kinds) can be started on Sunday or Day 5 of the cycle. It can be started the day of an abortion, or three to four days after childbirth if the mother is not breast-feeding. When started at these times, the pill is effective immediately and requires no backup birth control. The minipill (see ⚹17 above) is an exception. (Recently there have been warnings to wait two weeks after a delivery—watch for news.)

19. Sunday-starting pills

Some brands are meant to be started the Sunday after a menstrual period, an abortion, or childbirth. When starting after a period, however, count the days from day one of bleeding to Sunday. If there are more than five days in between, then a backup method should be used for the first two weeks of the cycle. If a menstrual period starts on Sunday, start the pill that same day.

20. Twenty-day and twenty-one-day pills

When using the twenty-day and twenty-one-day pills, take one a day until the pack is finished, wait eight or seven days, respectively, without taking pills, then start a new pack. Since all pills are now recommended to be taken on twenty-eight-day cycles, you would always be starting a new pack every twenty-ninth day, on the same weekday each month.

21. Twenty-eight-day pills

It's somewhat easier to take the twenty-eight-day pills because you don't have to remember *not* to take them. Just take them every day, with no breaks between packs.

22. Minipills: thirty-five-day pills

The minipills come in packages of thirty-five pills which are taken continuously with no break between packs, starting at the times discussed above. Most women become regulated and bleed only once a month or less often, although they take the pills continuously.

23. Pills should be taken at the same time each day

The best time is after eating, for this prevents nausea, one of the most frequent complaints of women on the pill.

24. What to do if pills are missed

If one pill is missed, it should be taken the next day or as soon as the fact that it was missed is noticed.

If two or three pills are missed in sequence, then pills should be taken twice daily for two or three days—until the missing pills have been worked back into the cycle.

If more than one pill is missed, a backup method should be used *until the next period,* because ovulation might occur later in the cycle. This is even more likely on the low-dose pills (less than 50 mcg of estrogen), so that *a backup method should be used with even one missed pill.*

Sometimes, if one or more pills are missed, the menstrual period will begin. In these cases, the pills should be discontinued and a new pack started on the fifth day of bleeding, or Sunday, using a backup method for the first two weeks of the cycle.

WARNING: Severe diarrhea or vomiting (as in a viral illness) may cause the body to absorb the pill poorly. Use a backup method for the remainder of the pack if this occurs.

25. When to use a backup method with the pill
  a. When one or more low-dose pills have been missed
  b. When two or more combined pills have been missed
  c. During the first six months on the minipill
  d. After a gastrointestinal illness (vomiting, diarrhea)
  e. When you are taking any medications listed in ✕53 below.

26. Menstruation while taking the pill
Menstruation is reorganized by the pill. The hormone effects of the pill allow bleeding to occur only at regulated time which can always be anticipated. A woman bleeds as a reaction to her withdrawal from the pill (during the seven or eight days she does not take them, with the twenty- to twenty-one-day types or during the inert pills in the twenty-eight-day type). This kind of controlled menstruation is called "withdrawal bleeding."

The absence of estrogen in the minipill means that you cannot anticipate when bleeding will occur, an inconvenience which may be aggravating but *not a danger or an indicator of ill health.*

27. Decreased menstrual flow while taking the pill is normal
Many women think that decreased menstrual flow while taking the pill indicates that something is wrong. *This is not true.* The menstrual flow should be only the amount of blood and endometrium that builds up each month. (See Chapter Two.) When a woman takes the combined pills, there is less endometrium buildup and consequently less menstrual flow. *Even if bleeding lasts only a day, a few hours, or is limited to spotting, that is sufficient.* Scanty periods occur most frequently when progestogen-dominant pills are used. If for any reason, even a

psychological one, additional menstrual flow is desired, then estrogen-dominant pills can be taken instead. However, high-dose estrogen pills have other problems. (See below)

28. Breakthrough bleeding

Breakthrough bleeding is usually a light blood flow that surprises the pill-taker by occurring while she is on the active pills and not at the time allotted for menstrual flow during the cycle. *It is a harmless side effect. It does not indicate ill health.*

With low-dose pills, breakthrough bleeding is very common in the first one or two cycles. If it amounts only to spotting, then no particular action is indicated. If the bleeding is heavy and bothersome into the second or third cycle, then a woman may surmise that she needs a slightly higher-dose pill and should try a different type.

Occasionally, a woman will experience breakthrough bleeding once or twice a year; this is nothing to worry about.

When changing to another pill because of breakthrough bleeding, a pill with more estrogen should be used if the bleeding has occurred early in the cycle; a pill with more progestogen should be used if bleeding has occurred late in the cycle.

Some women experience breakthrough bleeding on all types and doses of pills and must switch to another method of contraception. *This is not an indication of ill health,* merely one of many signs that tell a woman she cannot tolerate the pill.

29. Heavy breakthrough bleeding

If breakthrough bleeding involves a heavy flow, then pills should be stopped and a new pack started on the fifth day of bleeding. Use a backup method. (See ⚡24 above) If the bleeding is *very* heavy or persistent, or associated with severe pain or fever, consult a physician.

30. Dysmenorrhea during breakthrough bleeding

Breakthrough bleeding sometimes involves dysmenorrhea. The pain should not be severe, and should not last very long; if it is severe or continuous, consult a physician.

31. Conditions which the pill can help

a. *Heavy menstrual flow that causes anemia:* Menstrual flow is usually lighter among women on the pill.

b. *Dysmenorrhea* is less frequent and less severe among women on the pill. (See p. 324)

c. *Premenstrual syndrome* is rare among women on the pill. (See p. 327)

d. *Acne* is known to improve in women using estrogen-dominant pills, so much so that some physicians will sometimes prescribe the pills for short periods of time as treatment for acne even when no birth control is desired. (See p. 33)

e. *Ovarian cysts:* Women on the pill experience a definite decrease in functional ovarian cysts. (See p. 340)

All of the above benefits occur because women who are taking the pill do not experience the hormonal changes inherent in an unregulated menstrual cycle, thereby avoiding the discomforts associated with menstruation.

CONSIDER THE RISKS CAREFULLY (SEE ✻36–51) BEFORE ACCEPTING THE PILL AS THERAPY FOR THESE CONDITIONS.

32. Minor side effects indicating a pill change or discontinuation is in order

Some minor side effects of the pill indicate that the woman is taking the wrong dose pill for her body, and should change to another type.

a. *Breast tenderness:* This is a normal sign of adjustment to a new hormonal cycle in the first two to three months of pills. If it continues or is severe, consult a physician and change to another type of pill. *Breast tenderness while taking the pill is not a sign of cancer.* If the pain is mild, a bra with better support and some over-the-counter analgesics should relieve it.

b. *Change in breast size:* Some women on the pill report a decrease, some an increase in breast size. Neither is cause for worry. If the change involves a bra size or more, consult a doctor and stop the pills.

c. *Weight gain* is a common complaint among women on the pill; it is thought to be related to the progestogen component. Tests on large numbers of women show little or no weight gain on the average is associated with pill usage, but many women *know* better. So if a woman feels she has gained, or that the fat distribution on her body has changed for the worse, she should switch to a different form of birth control.

d. *Monilia infection of the vagina* (see p. 301), sometimes is aggravated by the progestogens in the pill, which increase the glycogen or cell sugar in the cells of the vagina. If these infections recur frequently, try a new pill with lowered progestogen. Many women experience changes in the *amount* of vaginal discharge (either more or less than usual) because of the pill. Unless this really bothers you, it is nothing to worry about.

e. If *headache* occurs repeatedly while taking the pill, try another pill with lower estrogen. If headache occurs while taking the inert pills, or while off the pills, try a compound with lower progestogen. WARNING: If migraine headaches appear or are aggravated by the pill, it should be discontinued. If there is any doubt as to whether the headache is migraine, make sure; check with a physician; frequent migraine is an absolute contraindication for the pills. (See ✗36 below) If any weakness, dizziness, or blurring of vision occur with the headache, see a physician immediately. (See ✗42 below)

f. *Loss of menstrual period:* If no pills have been missed and the period does not occur, the pills should be continued for one more month. If no menstrual period occurs during the second month, this probably indicates that the endometrium-suppressing component in the pill is too strong and the woman should switch to another type of pill. (If no pills have been missed, loss of, the period is not necessarily a sign of pregnancy. However, if you've missed two periods, *or* if you have any other signs of pregnancy, have a pregnancy test—just in case.)

g. *Mood changes:* As with the menstrual cycle generally, hormonal changes may cause changes in mood which appear as psychological but are essentially endocrine. Studies on psychologic changes among women on the pill show a variety of differing results: no changes; deep depression; improvement in depression; loss of libido or sexual drive. (Ref. 1, 6) Vitamins B-6 and B-12 may offset some of these changes.

Be your own judge. If you are experiencing some change in temperament, if you're feeling *very* bad, the pill may be aggravating a pre-existing condition. Stop the pill and seek further professional advice if the problem persists.

h. Some women on the pill need to take vitamin supplements. (See p. 253)

33. Hair loss
If a woman taking the pill experiences hair loss, she should discontinue using it and see if hair growth begins again. If it does not, investigate other causes and treatments.

34. Skin changes
Aside from the beneficial effect on acne, several unpleasant skin changes are often associated with pill-taking.

a. Some women experience a greater sensitivity to sun, more frequent burning. It is always wise to limit exposure to the sun (see p. 246) and even more so if taking the pill.

b. Moles frequently become darker when the pill is taken. This may be a harmless pill effect; to make sure, check with a doctor.

c. Pre-existing skin conditions, such as rosacea—a red rash on the chest and face—and eczema—a rash on the neck and in the creases of the elbows and knees—can be aggravated by the pill.

d. Chloasma (mask of pregnancy) is a brownish discoloration on the cheeks, forehead, and nose which is deepened by exposure to the sun. (This is very strange since the word chloasma comes from the Greek word meaning to become green.) Very rarely, the pill can cause chloasma; if it does, use another form of birth control.

e. Acne may appear for the first time or become severe during the few months *after stopping* the pill. Treat it as you would treat other acne. (See p. 31) This problem usually does not last more than six months.

35. Delay in return of menses after stopping the pill
After discontinuation of the pill, the first period is usually delayed a few weeks, as the body readjusts to a new cycle. This is usually not a cause for concern unless this time is very prolonged. (See #48 below)

36. Who should not take the pill?
Generally accepted, absolute contraindications to the pill include women who:

a. have a history of blood-clotting disorders (phlebitis, embolus, heart attack, stroke);

b. have severe or frequent migraine headaches;

c. have hypertension;

d. have hyperlipidemia (increased fat in the blood);

e. are smokers (especially over age thirty);

f. are over age forty;

g. have sickle-cell anemia and related diseases which predispose to blood-clotting problems;

h. have liver abnormalities or dysfunction as shown by blood tests (recent history of jaundice, hepatitis, mononucleosis, and idiopathic jaundice of pregnancy);

i. have large fibroid tumors of the uterus;

j. have had cancer of the breast or uterus;

k. are breast-feeding;

l. have grossly irregular menstrual periods.

OPINION: *The following conditions should also serve as strong contraindications to the use of the pill.* They include women who:

a. have *severe* chronic diseases such as heart disease, kidney disease, and asthma;

b. have diabetes, or a strong family history of diabetes;

c. were exposed to DES and/or related compounds before birth;

d. have epilepsy;

e. have severe varicose veins;

f. have cystic disease of the breast or a family history of breast cancer (see p. 358);

g. have eye problems such as optic neuritis, glaucoma;

h. suffer from severe depression;

i. are severely overweight;

j. have a history of Sydenham's chorea (sometimes associated with rheumatic fever, see p. 52).

Of course, any woman who experiences disquieting bodily changes after going on the pill should immediately consider another method of birth control.

37. Thromboembolic diseases (clotting disorders); the major proven negative side effects of the pill

The clotting factors in blood give blood its ability to thicken, to clot. They are essential to the healing process. If we did not have them, we might bleed to death from scratches.

However, an *increase* in clotting factors may cause *thrombosis* (thromm-BO-siss)—a thickening or coagulation of the blood inside the veins or arteries. Thrombosis is a very serious health matter, for when it occurs, the flow of blood through the body is obstructed and the system of circulation which nourishes each part of the body is threatened.

Tests in Britain and the United States (Ref. 1, 7) have shown that in a few women, the estrogen content of the pill somehow increases the number of clotting factors in the blood, increasing the danger of thromboembolic disease. *Therefore, any history of thromboembolic disease is an absolute contraindication for the pill.* There are several types of thromboembolic disease of major concern:

a. Superficial thromboses

b. Deep-vein thrombophlebitis

c. Stroke

d. Heart attack

38. Symptoms of thromboembolic disorders: See a doctor immediately

a. Severe headaches

b. Blurring or loss of vision (especially if it is in one eye only)

c. Sensation of lights flashing

d. Swelling and pain in the legs

e. Severe chest pain; coughing blood

f. Acute shortness of breath

g. Numbness of the side of the face or in one arm

39. Superficial thromboses

These are clots in the outermost veins of the legs. The symptom is a hot red painful area over a vein. The treatment is bed rest, heat; the affected leg should be elevated. Generally, superficial clots are not serious—*but a physician should always be consulted.* If there is any possibility of deeper clots, heparin, a blood-thinning medication may be prescribed. The pill must be stopped immediately on recognizing the symptom, but *that will not in itself cure the condition. Further care is needed.* This and the following disorders occur in women not on the pill as well, so all women should be aware of the symptoms.

40. Deep-vein thrombophlebitis

This is less common than superficial thrombosis but more serious. Here, the clot forms in the veins deep inside the muscles of the legs and the pelvic area. When it occurs, it carries a risk that the clot will break out of the area and travel through the circulatory system to the lung, causing a pulmonary embolus (M-bo-liss) (a blood clot in the lung) which is very dangerous, sometimes fatal.

The symptoms of deep-vein thrombophlebitis are severe pain, redness and a hot feeling in the leg—usually in the calf muscle. Any woman with any of these symptoms should seek emergency medical care. If the diagnosis is confirmed, the treatment is bed rest in the hospital along with blood-thinning medicine.

41. Varicose veins

This common disorder of women (see p. 383) may be aggravated by the pill. If the varicose veins are mild, then the woman can take the pill. If she notices any increase in the severity of her condition, she should go off the pill.

If the varicose veins are severe, the woman should not take the pill. The condition is related to *stasis* of the blood inside the vein—a tendency of the blood to idle, to flow sluggishly. The more pronounced the stasis, the more severe the varicosity, and vice versa—and the more likely it is that the condition could be a prelude to a clotting disorder. So, if you have severe varicose veins, don't use the pill.

42. Stroke

A stroke is caused by a blood clot or hemorrhage in the brain, and occurs more frequently in pill-takers than in other women. The incidence is also much higher in women who take the pill and are over thirty-five, who have taken it for five years or more, have migraine headaches or hypertension, or who are smokers. A stroke is potentially fatal, or paralyzing. The symptoms are weakness on one side of the body, numbness, blurry vision, a sensation of seeing bright lights, head-ache, or seizures. *If you have any of these symptoms, stop the pill and see a doctor fast.* In women under age thirty-five who don't smoke, the risk is only slightly greater than for non-pill takers. (Ref. 3)

43. Heart attack

A heart attack is caused by a clot in the arteries leading to the heart. Conditions which predispose to heart attack are heavy smoking, hyper-lipidemia (high blood fats), hypertension, and use of oral contra-ceptives. When these factors are sorted out, it seems that *smoking* has a dominant role, and compounds the risk of the pill. (Ref. 7, 8) The symptoms of heart attack are severe chest pain, pain in the left arm, and shortness of breath. Any of these should take you to a doctor im-mediately. *The FDA has strongly urged smokers not to take the pill.*

44. How to minimize the risk of thromboembolic disease as a result of pill-taking

In some cases, there is no obvious predisposing factor toward throm-boembolic disease other than taking the birth-control pill. However, other pre-existing conditions can cause a greater chance of these disor-ders. Follow these suggestions:

a. Stop smoking. Smoking is much worse for your health than pill taking.

b. Do not take the pill if you are over forty years old.

c. Do not take the pill if you have hypertension.

d. Do not take the pill if you have migraine headaches. (These are associated with disturbance of the blood flow to the brain.)

e. Do not take the pill if you have hyperlipidemia (high-per-lip-ih-DEEM-ia: increased blood cholesterol and other fats). Many fat peo-ple and some thin ones have this trouble: *only a blood test can detect it.* Women over thirty who are on the pill should get blood tests for blood cholesterol and fats. (See p. 258)

f. Use a pill containing 50 mcg or less of estrogen.

g. Do not take the pill if you have severe varicose veins, any previ-ous history of blood clots, heart attacks, or coronary artery disease.

h. Stop the pill if you are about to have major surgery (any opera-tion which will require recuperation in bed for a long period of time). Don't start the pill again until you are completely recovered. Surgery carries a concomitant risk of clotting trouble, which the pill might ag-gravate.

45. Liver tumors and related problems

There have been reports of a number of liver tumors, called adenomas, occurring more often in women on the pill than in other women. (Ref. 7, 9) Although these tumors are usually benign, they have caused serious problems with bleeding into the abdomen. These are fortunately very rare (about five hundred having been reported), for they are very difficult to diagnose.

RECOMMENDATION: They also seem to occur mainly in women who have been on the pill for longer than five years. All the more reason to take periodic breaks from oral contraception.

In other women, the progestogen in the pill may aggravate pre-existing liver dysfunction. In some women, it may slow the elimination of waste products by the liver, allowing bilirubin (a red bile pigment) to build up, causing jaundice. (When deposited in the skin, in jaundice, bilirubin shows up yellow.) *This change is reversible upon stopping the pill.*

Anyone who has had hepatitis or a recent history of mononucleosis should have a test to see that liver function is normal before starting the pill. Alcoholic women or drug-dependent women should not take the pill without liver tests. Idiopathic jaundice of pregnancy is an absolute contraindication to the pill, for the pill generally causes it to recur.

A related disease is the increase in gallstones among women on the pill (about twice normal). (Ref. 1) The progestogen in the pill may cause decreased excretion of cholesterol from the gall bladder, resulting in stones.

46. Other serious side effects of the pill: hypertension, urinary tract infections, eye problems

a. *Hypertension* (high blood pressure): Several studies show a definite increase in high blood pressure among women taking the pill. (Ref. 10, 11) The effect is more pronounced in older women, and obese women, who *generally* show higher rates of high blood pressure anyway.

To minimize the risk of hypertension while taking the pill, make sure a blood pressure check is done three months after starting the pill and every six months thereafter. Severe headaches or persistent dizziness at any time may be signs of high blood pressure which should be checked.

b. *Urinary tract infections:* There are some reports of an increase in the incidence of urinary tract infections among women on the pill.

These are treatable (see p. 319) but if they recur, change to another form of birth control.

c. *Eye problems:* Contact-lens wearers have experienced difficulty with the pill because it sometimes causes swelling of the cornea. Other reports suggest that some changes in the retina and optic nerve *may* be caused by the pill; these have not been proved. If any unusual changes in vision or pain in the eyes occur, an examination should be obtained whether the woman is on the pill or not. *Always tell your eye doctor if you are taking the pill.*

47. Many medical problems may be aggravated by the pill

The pill affects so many body systems, that it should be avoided if at all possible by women who have a disease or a tendency toward a disease.

a. *Diabetes:* The pill decreases the tolerance of some women for carbohydrates—e.g., sugar—increasing the risk of diabetes or making diabetes more difficult to control. Women who show a predisposition toward diabetes through blood-sugar tests, or because of personal or family history, should try to avoid the pill. If a woman with such a history does take the pill, she should have glucose tolerance tests yearly. Urine sugars should be checked each time she has an examination.

b. *Severe kidney disease* may be aggravated by the pill. The severity must be judged by blood and urine tests.

c. *Heart disease:* If a woman has severe heart disease with shortness of breath and edema of the ankles, she should avoid the pill. Women with mild or asymptomatic heart disease who feel they must take the pill should only use a low-dose variety. (Ref. 12)

d. *Sydenham's chorea* (usually associated with rheumatic fever) is a nervous disorder affecting the muscles of the face, neck, and limbs. It used to be called St. Vitus Dance. It is rare but may recur when the woman is on the pill. (See pp. 379–80)

e. *Fibroid tumors* (see p. 337): The pill may protect some women against fibroid tumors of the uterus, but may *increase* the growth of fibroids in others. Women who do have fibroids should use low-dose pills and should have an examination every three months to make sure the fibroids are not getting bigger. Women who already have *large* fibroids should *not* use the pill.

f. *Epilepsy* may be more difficult to control in women on the pill. If a woman takes barbiturates, phenytoin or primadone, for treatment of epilepsy, the pill may be rendered less effective: so use a backup method, such as foam. (See ✕53 below)

g. *DES exposure:* There is some early evidence that oral contraceptives may cause changes in the adenosis present in the vaginas of women exposed prenatally to DES. (Ref. 13) Because the *original* changes were associated with estrogens, the pill should be avoided by these women. (See p. 367)

48. Prolonged amenorrhea and infertility following pill use

About 3 per cent of women who use oral contraceptives experience prolonged cessation (up to two years) of ovulation and menstruation after stopping. This problem is accompanied by a milky discharge from the breasts in one third of the cases. About half the women who develop this problem were not ovulating regularly when they started the pill. For this reason, the pill should not be used by women with irregular cycles (by this we mean women who get their period every two to three months or at wider intervals, not women who vary only slightly in their days). The treatment of this problem may be difficult, for there is a disturbance in the hypothalamus and pituitary relationship. (See p. 18) If a woman has drainage from the breasts (galactorrhea) in addition to the loss of periods, she should have studies of prolactin levels (see p. 158) and sometimes skull X rays, to rule out a coincidental pituitary tumor which might cause similar symptoms in a small number of these patients. (Ref. 14, 15) In these latter cases, consult a *gynecologic endocrinologist.*

49. The pill and cancer

Probably the biggest worry concerning the pill is as a possible cause or promoter of cancer. (See p. 345 for more extensive discussion of hormones and cancer.) At present, this worry seems justified in regard to the endometrial cancer associated with the sequentials. (Ref. 4) Combined pills and minipills are composed differently from sequentials, however, having a progestogen dominance in most cases. Studies have shown no increase in cervical cancer among women on the pill. (Ref. 16) Watch for more studies on gynecologic cancers.

LOOK AHEAD: The answer on breast cancer will probably not be forthcoming for many years. Initial studies show *lower* rates of *benign* breast disease in pill users: this may be a good sign if these benign diseases are precursors to cancer. However, cancer researchers are generally convinced that female hormones stimulate the growth of pre-existing cancer of the breast (acting as promoters) and strongly urge that women who are at high risk for breast cancer *not* take the pill. (Ref. 17) There is no hard data on this problem; watch the newspapers for new research; now, you have to judge for yourself and make a risk-benefit decision.

50. The effect of the pill on the fetus

If a woman becomes pregnant while using the pill—usually because she has missed several days without any alternative protection—and then continues taking the pill without knowing she is pregnant, there may be some adverse effect on the fetus. Some studies indicate an increase in limb abnormalities and heart defects among babies whose mothers continued to take the pill before they realized they were pregnant. (Ref. 7)

51. Warning: Wait at least three months after going off the pill before becoming pregnant

Women who become pregnant before three months may have an increased risk of spontaneous abortion, and the fetuses thus aborted sometimes show severe chromosomal abnormalities. (See p. 167) Children born after a woman has stopped the pill have shown no increase in congenital defects. However, an increase in twins has been reported by some researchers.

52. Do not take the pill while breast-feeding

If the pill is started early after a pregnancy, it may inhibit the production of milk. Furthermore, the hormones in the pill can pass into the mother's milk and may have some yet unknown effect on the child. The ability to become pregnant is naturally diminished during lactation, so another, usually less-effective contraceptive method will be very effective now. (See p. 159)

53. Certain drugs may decrease the effectiveness of the pill

In addition to the anti-epilepsy drugs mentioned in ⅍47 above, other commonly used drugs *may* decrease the pill's effectiveness. These are phenylbutazone (used for arthritis) and the following antibiotics: ampicillin, neomycin, penicillin V, chloramphenicol, nitrofurantoin, and isoniazide. Rifampin (used to treat tuberculosis), is *proven* to have this effect. (Ref. 18) If the additional drugs are taken for only short periods, use a backup method such as foam during that cycle. If long-term therapy is needed, check out the advisability of a higher-dose pill or another method or combination of methods.

54. How to evaluate reports on side effects of the pill

A woman must carefully read all published reports in the press and listen to TV discussions of the pros and cons of the method and then make up her own mind. The huge dilemma is that the pill is the most effective and most convenient method of contraception available—*but* it has the potential for being the most dangerous to the woman's health.

If you are considering stopping the pill, decide on an alternative method of birth control *first*.

LONG-ACTING HORMONAL CONTRACEPTIVES

Since 1963, various tests have been conducted with hormonal contraceptives to develop a dosage which would be effective for long periods of time, eliminating the necessity for daily application.

A pill which need be taken only once a month, or a shot which need be given only once in three or six months, is particularly attractive to population planners in underdeveloped countries. In poorer lands, where physicians are so few, and drug supplies and distribution so limited, many families find themselves cut off from medical care for many months by many miles. The side effects of the long-acting contraceptives, which have thus far kept them off the American market, often are less worrisome to underdeveloped nations, where deaths from childbearing are so frequent. Research on drugs is now being conducted in many countries. Most long-acting hormonal contraceptives for women are progestogens, for estrogens are less effective and are associated with major side effects.

55. Depo-Provera, a long-acting progestogen

Depo-Provera is the most widely used of the long-acting hormonal contraceptives; however, it is only used now in countries other than the United States. It is 99 per cent effective. Depo-Provera is an injectable; usually a woman will receive a shot once every three months. The highly sustained doses of Depo-Provera (medroxyprogesterone acetate) block ovulation and in addition change the cervical mucus, thin the endometrium and alter the motility of the tube. (Ref. 19)

56. Depo-Provera cannot be used for birth control in the United States

Currently the FDA only approves Depo-Provera for use in treating cancer of the endometrium.

57. Side effects of Depo-Provera

a. The injectable contraceptives—especially Depo-Provera—have been implicated in a higher incidence of early cancer of the cervix. This is the main reason that the FDA has withheld approval. More careful and complete testing is now being done to confirm or disprove the drug's connection to cancer.

b. Menstrual irregularities—especially temporary loss of menses—is associated with Depo-Provera usage. For undernourished women in poor countries, loss of menses may be a blessing—for blood loss, including menstruation, is very hard on a body already weakened by malnutrition.

c. Permanent loss of menses is a frequent side effect in Depo-Provera use. For this reason, in other countries the method is generally recommended only to older women whose families are complete.

d. Minor side effects include mild weight gain, nausea, dysmenorrhea, and decreased libido. However, none of these effects are as pronounced as they are with some forms of the pill.

e. If Depo-Provera is unwittingly administered during pregnancy, some tests suggest it may cause malformations of the fetal heart and limbs. (Ref. 20)

f. Tests in beagles show that Depo-Provera causes a dramatic increase in breast nodules. However, a study in women shows no increase in breast tumors of any sort. (Ref. 19)

58. Look ahead: Other sustained-release progestogens for birth control are now being researched

a. Subdermal pellets, implanted under the skin and having an effectiveness against pregnancy of three to five years, are now being tested.

b. Cervical rings which contain time-release progestogen are now being tested. These would be insertable into the vagina like a diaphragm each month after the menstrual period, and left in place until the next period begins.

THE IUD

Between 3 and 4 million women in the United States, and many millions more throughout the world, use the IUD. The types of IUDs currently in use were developed during the 1960s, when the seriousness of the population explosion became apparent. In poorer countries, where the population crush is most acute, where hospital care is minimal and the attention of a physician or paramedic is almost impossible to secure, and endless childbearing is still a health hazard of incredible proportions, the IUD is ideal. It is cheap. It requires little care after insertion and it requires nothing of men, who may or may not agree with birth control.

59. History of the IUD

In the mid-1880s, stem pessaries were developed to help women with displaced wombs. A T-shaped device was inserted in the womb; its top fit over the cervix; its stem jutted into the womb, giving what was then thought to be helpful support. Later on the same device was used to treat severe dysmenorrhea, also with doubtful benefits. Infection was a serious and frequent side effect of this device. The most important effect, unanticipated, was that women who used it conceived less frequently. This led to the first experiments with an intrauterine device (IUD) to prevent pregnancy.

Scientists thought that if the entire device could be located inside the uterus, the risk of infection would diminish. The first such device was created in the early twentieth century. It was made of silkworm gut and bronze. It was associated with a number of infections, and the medical community was so skeptical about it that it was not widely used. In the 1930s Ernst Graefenberg, a German gynecologist, developed another type. His was a ring, a silver wire wound with silkworm gut. A similar device was developed simultaneously by Dr. Ota in Japan. (Ref. 21) Still, there was no great interest in the IUD until the 1960s, when the population explosion was acknowledged as a serious matter.

60. Types of IUD

Several IUDs are currently approved for use in this country; they should only be inserted by trained medical personnel. They are

a. the Lippes Loop (named for the Buffalo physician who developed it);

b. the Saf-T-Coil;

c. the Copper 7 (a similar Copper T device may soon appear); and

d. the Progestasert (a T-shaped device with slow-release progesterone in the tail).

61. How the IUD works

a. The actual mechanism by which the Lippes Loop and the Saf-T-Coil work is still not completely understood. They are made of a type of plastic. Probably, the presence in the uterus creates an inflammation (not an infection) in the uterine lining. This local inflammation may destroy the sperm as they pass through the uterus (Ref. 22) or may inhibit the implantation of the fertilized egg in the uterus. Some will argue that the IUD is thus creating repeated abortions—but since it has not been proven that fertilization actually occurs routinely in women using the IUD, this interpretation is debatable.

b. The Copper 7 (Cu7, for short) works by its presence *and* its substance. It is made of plastic covered by copper wire. It causes an inflammation in the endometrium, like the other IUDs. In addition, the copper wire competes with other metal ions that figure in the enzyme metabolism of the endometrium, preventing this metabolism; either killing the sperm or preventing implantation. (Ref. 23)

c. The Progestasert has the added effect of the progesterone on the endometrium, and probably on the cervical mucus and Fallopian tubes (very similar to the minipills). (See above)

62. An IUD is 97–98 per cent effective in preventing pregnancy

No one of the devices has a better record than any other. *For near 100 per cent effectiveness, a backup method such as foam should be used at mid-cycle.*

63. How long can the IUD be used?

The plastic IUDs can be used continuously, for as long as there are no side effects and no expulsion occurs or is required. This can be as long as several years.

The Cu7 must be replaced every three years, because by that time the copper becomes oxidized and the safety of the device decreases. The Progestasert must be changed every year, because the progesterone supply runs out.

All IUDs should be removed within six months after menopause.

64. Is there any danger from the copper or the progesterone?

Copper is a naturally occurring element in the body; women using the Cu7 do not appear to experience any increase in copper levels. (Ref. 23) The amount of copper released into the body by this device is less than the average intake of copper from food. So there is *probably* no danger to a woman from the copper itself.

The effects of the progesterone would be similar to the minipill except much more localized. Decreased and sometimes irregular menstrual flow is frequently reported.

65. When the IUD should be inserted

The IUD should be inserted immediately after an early abortion, during a menstrual period, or during the first week after the menstrual period. After a late abortion or the delivery of a child, it should not be inserted for six to eight weeks.

These times should always be adhered to, in order to minimize the risk of perforation of the uterus, which is the most serious complication of IUD insertion. (See below)

66. How the IUD is inserted

The IUD must be inserted under aseptic conditions, only by a physician or qualified nurse.

The cervix and upper vagina are cleansed with a septic solution; sterile instruments and gloves must be used.

At the time of insertion, a woman should receive instructions in how to feel for the string attached to the IUD that hangs down through the cervix into the vagina (not outside the vagina). She should be able to feel this string if the IUD is properly in place. If she cannot feel the string, or if she feels any part of the device besides the string, the insertion should be checked right away.

The FDA mandates that a booklet explaining the IUD and its potential side effects be read by women before inserting. Ask for it and read it.

67. Normal discomfort during insertion of the IUD

When the IUD is inserted, it is normal to feel severe menstrual cramps which stop almost immediately, and normal thereafter to feel a dull ache, which also soon goes away.

It is also normal not to feel any discomfort at all.

68. Routine care of the IUD after insertion

A woman should have an examination after her first period after the IUD has been inserted. For the first three months, she should use a backup birth-control method (foam, condom, or pill if she's already on them), because the device is more frequently expelled during the first three months, if it is expelled at all. Also, during the first few months the woman may not be used to examining herself, so she may miss an expulsion. Most physicians and clinics see the patient again after two or three months, to check for undetected expulsion. The device should be checked at least once a year thereafter.

It is important to make sure you can feel the string, *and only the string,* two or three times during the first week after insertion, before sexual intercourse and after each menstrual period. Sometimes it is easier to reach the string if you are squatting or sitting on the toilet, bearing down.

69. Normal side effects after insertion of the IUD

a. It is perfectly normal not to experience any side effects at all.

b. There may be cramps sporadically during the first few weeks after the IUD is inserted, and then for two days or less before each period.

c. Some bleeding or spotting between periods may occur during the first two months of use.

d. The first three periods after insertion may be heavy; thereafter, periods usually decrease.

e. There may be a mucous discharge the first one or two months after insertion. This is normal while the endometrium sets up the inflammation that is the basic birth-control mechanism of the IUD. The discharge is *not* normal if it is heavy and foul-smelling; this would be a sign of possible infection, and should be checked immediately.

70. About 70 per cent of the women who have the IUD inserted continue using it one year later

That means that 30 per cent find they cannot continue to use it. Therefore, when deciding to use an IUD, be as prepared for failure as for success. Use a backup method (a spermicide, for example) for at least the first three months. The major reasons for discontinuation usually occur during the first year of use; the incidence of problems with the IUD declines steeply after that. During the first year, about 5 per cent of the IUDs inserted are expelled; about 23 per cent of women using it stop because of pain, bleeding, infection, or other problems; 2–3 per cent become pregnant. All IUDs have about the same continuance statistics. Choose carefully. *The skill of the inserter is very important in determining the success of the device,* so if you decide on an IUD, make sure you have it inserted by a gynecologist, or by a physician or nurse who has done a large number of insertions. (Ref. 24)

71. Serious side effects of the IUD
a. Uterine and tubal infection
b. Increased bleeding
c. Severe and chronic cramping
d. Perforation of the uterus

72. If uterine or tubal infection does not respond immediately to treatment, the IUD should be removed

Uterine and tubal infections from the IUD usually occur in the first several months after insertion and should be treated with antibiotics. The main symptom is a constant, often foul-smelling vaginal discharge, perhaps pain and fever as well. If the infection does not improve *immediately* (within a few days) the IUD should be removed and treatment for the infection continued.

73. The IUD may threaten the future fertility of women who use it

Recent reports by several groups of researchers show that women wearing IUDs have a risk of pelvic infection three to five times greater than the average woman. These infections may lead to damage to the

Fallopian tubes and possible infertility. (See p. 97) The FDA has recently issued warnings about these risks and women should take the warnings seriously. (Ref. 25, 26)

The problem of infections has plagued IUD users for a century now.

74. IUD users should take an iron supplement to prevent anemia

Women using the IUD lose on the average *twice as much* blood each menstrual period as non-users. Therefore, IUD users should always take an iron supplement to prevent anemia. (See p. 368) (Ref. 27)

Heavier flows during the period are caused by:

a. the chronic inflammation in the uterus that makes bleeding start a day or two earlier than usual; and

b. an increase in the amount of prostaglandins released, causing prolonged bleeding and more serious menstrual cramps than usual. (See p. 326)

75. If anemia occurs, and persists, have the IUD removed

A yearly blood count will indicate whether a woman is anemic. If iron added to her diet does not improve her condition quickly, she should consider that 'her IUD may be a factor. Even if the IUD is not *causing* the condition, it should be removed, for it is almost surely *aggravating* it. Some women find that switching from the plastic to the Cu7 or progesterone devices helps.

76. Overlong strings on the IUD

If the strings on the IUD are too long, they may irritate a man during intercourse. In addition, they may cause cramping in a woman during intercourse. See a doctor if this occurs; the doctor can cut the strings shorter, a painless office procedure. If discomfort continues, the device should be removed and another form of birth control used instead. The Cu7 is inserted in such a way that shortly after insertion, the strings become longer. Unless this makes you uncomfortable—or if you can feel the tip of the device—don't worry about it. The strings can be shortened later.

77. If severe cramps are chronic, the IUD should be removed

If the IUD user finds herself suffering from severe or intolerable cramps, she should have it removed. The cramps are probably not a sign of ill health. However, there are enough types of birth control so that suffering from cramps with the IUD is simply not necessary.

78. Perforated uterus: the most serious side effect of the IUD

In some women, if the IUD is placed incorrectly, or if the uterus is particularly soft (e.g., just after a pregnancy), the IUD can work its way through the wall of the uterus into the abdominal cavity. This is perforation.

Various studies estimate that perforation occurs in between 1 in 400 and 1 in 1,000 women. (Ref. 24) Usually, perforation happens or starts happening at the time of insertion; it may take some time for the perforation to occur as the improperly placed IUD works its way through the uterus.

If perforation occurs, the hole in the uterus usually heals itself, but the device must be removed either with a small laparotomy or laparoscopy. (See p. 84)

79. If the string of the IUD cannot be felt, see a doctor

This may be a sign of perforation in progress. Usually it has just curled up inside the cervix out of reach and nothing is wrong.

Maybe the IUD has been expelled without a woman's knowledge. in which case she is unprotected against pregnancy.

But just in case the IUD is not exactly where it should be in the uterus, have an examination.

80. What to do if the IUD strings "disappear"

If the examining physician cannot see or feel the string, the cervix is usually probed to see if the string has curled out of sight. (This is usually what has happened.)

If the string is not there, the device *must* be found—either it has been expelled from the body, or it is in the correct place in the uterus (but the string has curled inside) or it has perforated the uterus. The best method to localize the IUD is an ultrasound. (See p. 186) It bounces sound waves off the device, giving a reading on its location, and the radiologist can tell whether the IUD and the uterus are in the same place. If ultrasound is not available, simple X ray will suffice, as long as another IUD or uterine probe is placed in the uterus at the same time to see whether the device and the uterus are in the same place. The IUDs all contain some barium sulfate, so they show up on X ray. If the IUD is not seen on the X ray, then it has been expelled without the woman's knowledge. If it is not in the uterus, then it is in the abdomen and must be removed as soon as possible, probably by laparoscopy.

81. Good news: There is no evidence that the IUD causes cancer

82. Women with copper-containing devices should not receive diathermy

Diathermy (or microwave therapy) is a deep-heat treatment used by some physical therapists and rehabilitation therapists for muscle problems and sometimes for backaches and pelvic pain. The metal in the devices may become very hot and cause damage to the uterus.

83. Warning: If you are allergic to copper, don't use the copper-containing IUD

84. Recommendation: If the IUD is in place and pregnancy occurs, have the device removed immediately

Several deaths have been reported among women who have had the IUD left in place after they became pregnant and who developed septic or infected pregnancies as a result, usually in the fourth to sixth months. (Ref. 28)

If a woman does not intend to continue the pregnancy, the IUD can be removed at the time of abortion. If she decides to terminate the pregnancy, the woman should do so as soon as possible, before the beginning of the fourth month. (See Chapter Six, Abortion) Although the Dalkon Shield (see ⚡85) was the most dangerous IUD, all the other devices have been implicated in septic pregnancies too.

85. The Dalkon Shield controversy

The Dalkon Shield is a crab-shaped IUD that was used for several years in the late sixties and early seventies. It has been removed from the market and *any woman with the device remaining in place should have it removed*. The Dalkon Shield caused multiple problems with pelvic infections and infected pregnancies most likely because its string was composed of many small filaments (rather than the single string of the other manufactured devices) and this seems to have encouraged the passage of bacteria into the uterus. (Ref. 28)

It was the trouble with the Dalkon Shield, among other troubles, that prompted recent congressional legislation setting up regulations for the testing and design of medical devices. (Ref. 29) Prior to this legislation, the FDA did not regulate medical devices such as IUDs, unless there was an active ingredient in them such as copper. Therefore, the copper- and progesterone-containing devices have been tested more extensively than the plastic devices were before they were placed on the market. The plastic devices have the advantage of longer-use data.

86. Ectopic pregnancy and the IUD

About 5 per cent of the pregnancies which occur with the IUD in place are ectopic or tubal pregnancies. (See p. 167) The symptoms of a tubal pregnancy are abdominal pain, irregular menstruation and at times shoulder pain from blood being in the abdomen. The progesterone-containing devices have been implicated in higher instances of ectopic pregnancy. The FDA is studying this now; watch the papers for their conclusions.

87. Who should not use the IUD?

a. *Women with fibroid tumors* large enough to distort the endometrial cavity should not use the IUD.

b. *Women with a recent history of pelvic infection or tubal infection* shouldn't use the IUD because insertion of the device could cause a flare-up of the problem. If a woman knows she has tubal damage, she should not use the IUD. If a woman has recently had gonorrhea, she should have *at least two negative cultures* after treatment before the IUD is inserted. RECOMMENDATION: *Ideally, all women should have gonorrhea cultures before a device is inserted.*

c. *Women who are pregnant should not have a device inserted;* this is why the device should be inserted during a period. If inserted into a pregnant uterus, the risk of perforation and infection are high.

d. *Women who have severe menstrual cramps and heavy bleeding* should consider another method. The IUD will generally make these problems worse (with the exception of Progestasert). If a woman has iron-deficiency anemia, she would be wise to use another method.

e. *Women who have never been pregnant* have more difficulty with the IUD. They have more pain on insertion, higher expulsion rates, and usually heavier menstrual flow. If you must have an IUD and have never had a child, choose the smaller copper and progesterone-containing devices.

DIAPHRAGM

The diaphragm is a round rubber dome with a relatively firm edge. It is inserted into the vagina, hooks behind the pubic bone, and springs back into shape inside, covering the cervix. It has virtually no serious side effects.

The diaphragm should not be considered a method of birth control in and of itself. It should *always* be paired with a spermicidal cream or jelly. It should be thought of not just as a physical barrier to the sperm, but as a kind of plate which holds in place the medication to kill the sperm.

88. History of the diaphragm

The vulcanization of rubber in 1844 made the development of the diaphragm possible. The first device was developed by Dr. Wilhelm Mensinga, a Dutch anatomy professor, in the 1870s. It was called "The Dutch Cap." (All methods of birth control had euphemistic names in those days since it was considered immoral and often illegal to discuss their actual uses.)

News of the discovery and instructions as to how to employ it were energetically repressed. The Comstock Law of 1873 prohibited using the mails to describe birth control. Anthony Comstock originated the law; he was a dry-goods salesman and chief special agent for the New York Society for the Suppression of Vice. For over half a century he stood between the American public and family planning. Ironically, Comstock was born in 1844, when rubber was vulcanized and birth control became a feasible alternative for the masses. He died in 1915, when Margaret Sanger, the pioneer of American family planning, launched her campaign to familiarize everyone with the diaphragm. (Ref. 30)

Until the sixties, when the pill and the IUD became available, the diaphragm was the most popular method of birth control among women. Now it is regaining popularity, as the side effects of IUDs and the pill have become well known.

89. A diaphragm may be acquired only by prescription

It can be prescribed only by a physician or family planning clinic. Spermicidal jelly or cream may be bought in a drugstore without prescription.

90. How the diaphragm is fitted

The diaphragm must be fitted by a physician or nurse practitioner.

An examination determines the size required by the individual woman; it should be the largest size that does not give the woman discomfort. A woman should not be aware of the diaphragm within her body. If she can feel it, then it is the wrong size. If the diaphragm is too large, it may become painful, especially during the six hours it must be left in place after intercourse. If it is too small, it moves excessively during intercourse—and does not reliably protect the user against pregnancy. RECOMMENDATION: Have the size rechecked after a week to make sure the fit is proper. Many physicians will suggest this. If yours doesn't, you should ask for it.

91. A virginal woman may find it difficult to have a diaphragm fitted

She may prefer that condoms be used by the man the first several times she has intercourse. If she uses a diaphragm, then she should have it rechecked for fit several months after she has become sexually active.

92. When should a diaphragm be refitted?

a. After childbirth or an abortion.

b. After weight loss or gain (of twenty pounds or more).

c. At the time of the annual examination.

93. It is easy to use a diaphragm correctly

And it *must* be used correctly if it is to give, as it can, excellent protection against pregnancy.

a. Squeeze the diaphragm into an oblong and insert it into the vagina until it hooks behind the pubic bone and snaps in place over the cervix.

Usually the diaphragm is inserted with the dome down; if a woman finds it takes up too much room in the vagina that way, she can insert it with the dome up. For women who have difficulty inserting the diaphragm, inserters are available. These have the additional advantage of not being so messy to use when the diaphragm is covered with spermicide.

b. Practice inserting the device the first time it is fitted, before leaving the doctor's office, so that the physician or nurse can check that you know how to insert it properly.

c. Before inserting the diaphragm, fill it with water or stretch it before a light to check that there are no holes or cracks in it.

d. Spermicidal cream or jelly must be placed in the center of the diaphragm on the side which will be closest to the cervix and all around the rim before insertion. *Every time intercourse occurs, a new application of cream, jelly, or foam must be made into the vagina!* The diaphragm should *not* be removed if intercourse has taken place during the previous six hours; rather, it should be left in place and the cream or jelly inserted with the applicator that accompanies the package.

e. The diaphragm can be inserted up to two hours before intercourse, but *not longer than that* without adding additional jelly—it can also be placed immediately before intercourse.

f. *The diaphragm must be left in place six hours or more after intercourse,* to give the spermicide time to work.

g. When removing the diaphragm put your index finger over the top edge and separate the diaphragm from the vagina. Wash it with warm water and mild soap, let it dry and dust it with a little cornstarch. This keeps the rubber dry and prolongs the life of the diaphragm; most last for a couple of years.

94. Creams and jellies to use with the diaphragm

Most women find the creams or jellies easier to use than the foam, which makes the diaphragm cumbersome on first insertion. For repeated applications, foam is just as easy as creams and jellies. (See Table 2 below)

Many women use foam *in addition* to the diaphragm and cream, and this makes the method even more effective.

95. Urinary urgency during intercourse with the diaphragm

Some women complain that the diaphragm gives them the feeling that they have to urinate during intercourse. This is because the device is irritating the urethra. You can avoid the feeling by always remembering to empty your bladder before intercourse. If the sensation persists, the size of the diaphragm may be wrong and should be checked. Some women get cystitis (see p. 316) repeatedly with a diaphragm and just have to use another contraceptive method.

96. Difficulty in urinating with the diaphragm in place

Some women find it difficult to urinate or to defecate with the diaphragm in place. It may help to insert a finger into the vagina and hold the device in place. If a woman finds it continuously difficult to urinate while wearing the diaphragm, the size may be too large; she should have it checked.

97. Many men can feel the diaphragm during intercourse

Some are annoyed by it, or claim it deters sexual drive. If this occurs, have the diaphragm checked for size; neither the man nor the woman should feel irritated by the diaphragm if it fits properly. Sometimes the man's reaction is simply psychological; try and convince him that if you can get used to it, he can too.

98. Psychological blocks about the diaphragm should be overcome

If a woman does not like the idea of the diaphragm, of touching herself repeatedly during insertion, then she should try hard to overcome the feeling. Young girls particularly express this feeling—and they should be told that it will pass in time, that sex without pregnancy is worth the very small cares that must be taken to make the diaphragm effective. The more "convenient" alternatives, such as the pill, are often preferred by young women for this reason. *They should be aware of all the contraindications to the pill before choosing it over the side-effect-free diaphragm, or foam and condoms.*

99. Effectiveness of the diaphragm

If the diaphragm fails to prevent pregnancy, that is almost always because it has not been used properly—usually because the spermicide has not been reapplied properly and in great enough quantity before intercourse or the diaphragm has not been left in place for a full six hours after intercourse.

When used properly, it is estimated that the diaphragm fails 2–3 times per 100 woman years. (If a woman used the device for 100 years, she would become pregnant while using it only 2 or 3 times.) (Ref. 31)

If improper use is taken into consideration, the diaphragm is estimated to fail 16 times per 100 woman years. (Ref. 32)

Many women find that the diaphragm slips out of place when the woman is in the superior position during lovemaking. In this case, proper application of the spermicide becomes even more important, or another contraceptive method may be preferable.

100. Watch for news: the collagen sponge diaphragm

The collagen sponge diaphragm is a new type of device now undergoing widespread clinical trials. Its advantage is that it is soft and easy to use. Some of these diaphragms are pretreated with spermicide, so it may not be necessary to use additional jellies, creams, or foam. Watch the newspapers and the media for further news on this innovation.

101. The cervical cap may be coming back

The cervical cap is an old method, similar to the diaphragm, except that it fits over the cervix rather than into the top part of the vagina. In Britain, interest in cervical caps has been renewed and experiments with it are under way. No long-term effectiveness studies are available yet; watch the news for these. If the news is good, this method may become increasingly popular in the United States.

VAGINAL CHEMICAL CONTRACEPTION
(Foams, Creams, and Jellies)

Like the diaphragms and condoms, the vaginal chemical contraceptives are "barrier" forms of birth control—they create a barrier between the sperm and the egg.

102. History of vaginal chemical contraceptives

For centuries, women have been looking for substances that would turn back or kill the sperm without interfering with intercourse. Egyptian women in the nineteenth century B.C. used plugs of crocodile dung; Indian women used elephant dung. (Ref. 30) In the Middle Ages, rock salt was placed in the vagina—and in fact, salt is a fairly effective spermicide. In 1885, the first contraceptive suppositories were manufactured from cocoa butter (the medium) and quinine (the active ingredient). Women tried to prevent conception by inserting vaginal sponges, soaked with acid substances—for example, citric acid in lemon juice. (Ref. 33)

No one paid much attention to the development of really effective vaginal chemical contraception until use of the diaphragm became widespread. In the twenties and thirties, acid and antibacterial substances were used in the hope that they would be as effective against sperm as against bacteria.

WARNING: *In the forties and fifties, phenyl mercuric acetate was introduced into these products;* an excellent spermicide, it has been removed recently because it has been shown to cause fetal damage in animals. (Ref. 34) *Check the label of all products you use to make sure there are no old tubes on the shelves containing mercury.*

In the late fifties, products containing *detergents* were introduced— obviously, not the washing products, but a large number of surface active agents that are very effective spermicides.

103. Contraceptive jellies

The jellies are water-soluble; they tend to become very watery at body temperature. A woman who wants a vaginal lubricant as well as a spermicide may prefer them; for other women, the jellies may be too messy.

104. Contraceptive creams

These are in a water-insoluble base. Some women feel that they tend to be drying or that they do not distribute as well in the vagina as jellies or foam when used without a diaphragm. However, when they are used with a diaphragm—*which is the way they should be used*—they adhere more firmly to the device.

105. Contraceptive foams

The foams are packaged in aerosol cans—the detergent itself is the foaming agent and they come out of the can on the same principle as shaving cream or whipped topping.

The advantage of the foams is that they distribute better in the vagina and, without a diaphragm, may have more of a barrier effect for the sperm.

106. Contraceptive suppositories

A suppository is generally a bullet-shaped wedge which is inserted into the vagina and then dissolves, distributing its active ingredients. This must be inserted at least 10 or 15 minutes before intercourse. Contraceptive suppositories have been touted recently with claims of very high effectiveness. But there is no evidence that the suppositories are any more effective than other foams or jellies.

107. Side effects of vaginal chemical contraceptives

So far, no major side effects have been found—and the minor ones occur rarely. These include irritations, *not* infections, either in men or in women. No treatment is necessary usually. Just switch to another product. If chronic irritation persists, see a physician.

108. How effective are vaginal chemical contraceptives?

When not used with a diaphragm, the chemical contraceptives are not completely effective. The foams are probably most effective; failure rates with the foam alone are very low when it is applied religiously before intercourse. Some of the creams are also effective alone with *some* women. RECOMMENDATION: *The best general rule is to use the vaginal chemical contraceptives always in conjunction with a diaphragm, or as an auxiliary method with the IUD or condom.*

Overall failure rates for foams, jellies, and creams when used alone are four to eight times per 100 woman years, if the woman always uses the product correctly. The rates of failure taking into account user mistakes are 20–30 per 100 woman years for the foam, and much higher for jellies and creams. (Ref. 33)

109. How to use vaginal chemical contraceptives

a. Women who have just given birth and women who have had many children should use *two applications* of the product rather than one.

b. When using these products with a diaphragm, make sure they are reapplied before each intercourse.

c. Do not douche or remove the contraceptive by bathing for at least six hours after intercourse.

d. Women who are traveling may avail themselves of various smaller packages, including a prefillable container which can be carried for seven days before use, and a small, six-dose container which can be carried in a purse.

110. It is possible that vaginal chemical contraceptives may prevent V.D.

Studies are being conducted to check reports that vaginal contraceptives may have a preventive effect against gonorrhea and syphilis.

The theory is that if they destroy the one-celled sperm, they *may* well do the same to the bacteria that cause V.D. (Ref. 35)

111. Warning: Douching with any substance now available is not a reliable form of birth control

The sperm pass into the uterus in less than a minute. Thus, no douche can work fast enough to prevent pregnancy. *No woman who is serious about preventing unwanted pregnancy should use this method alone.*

POSTCOITAL CONTRACEPTION: THE MORNING-AFTER PILLS

112. How the morning-after pill works

Several drugs are effective in preventing pregnancy when taken for five to ten days after intercourse. All high-dose estrogen products, they alter the endometrium and motility of the Fallopian tubes so that implantation cannot occur. These pills must be started within seventy-two hours after intercourse in order to be effective; the earlier the better.

Because of the very high doses of the estrogen needed for this preventive effect, all of these drugs have a high incidence of side effects such as nausea, vomiting, headache, and breast tenderness. Long-term side effects are not yet known. If you have to take them, do so in divided doses, with meals, and have medication on hand to treat nausea. These drugs do not act to bring on a period immediately, and, in fact, the period may be a week late depending on the time during the cycle that a woman took the pills. A woman who uses this method should remember that it only works for one particular incident; she can still become pregnant later in the cycle if she does not use contraception.

113. Recommendation: Avoid DES—diethylstilbestrol—if you must take a morning-after pill. Other estrogen compounds are as effective and probably safer

When taken within seventy-two hours after unprotected intercourse, DES is virtually 100 per cent effective in preventing pregnancy. But we do not consider it safe for women to use, given that there are alternatives.

114. DES: vaginal cancer and breast cancer

DES and related compounds have been strongly associated with abnormalities in the children of women who took it in early pregnancy. (See p. 366) In addition, DES may also be associated with an increased risk of breast cancer. So it is best to avoid it.

115. Other estrogens are effective as postcoital contraceptives and are probably safer than DES

These include ethinyl estradiol (5 mg. per day for 5 days) and conjugated estrogens (10 mg per day for 10 days or 30 mg per day for 5 days). (Ref. 36, 37) *As with DES, these should be used for emergencies only!* Reports of congenital defects from hormones taken in pregnancy should make one worry about these powerful drugs.

116. Insertion of CuT as postcoital check on pregnancy

It is reported that if a Copper T (not yet on the market) is inserted one to five days after intercourse, it is 100 per cent effective against pregnancy. Of course, just as the woman using hormones can anticipate the side effects of a heavy dose of estrogen, the woman using the CuT (under circumstances in which she may possibly become pregnant) is risking the side effects of the IUD. (Ref. 38) The Copper 7 presumably acts in the same way as the Copper T. This method is not widely used. Many physicians will not insert an IUD unless a woman is menstruating.

117. Recommendation: Menstrual extraction is a safe, alternative form of postcoital contraception

If a woman who has been placed in an emergency birth-control situation finds that her period is late, she can consider menstrual extraction. (See pp. 192–93) The cost will be higher, however, and this precedure is not available in all parts of the country.

CONDOMS AND OTHER MALE METHODS OF CONTRACEPTION

The condom is an excellent method of contraception. It is relatively cheap, convenient, and without side effects. Before the appearance of the pill and IUD, it was widely used by the men of this country. Since it requires complete participation by the male, it is relatively unreliable in those areas of the world where the population explosion is acute, where pregnancy is a grave danger to a woman's health, and male chauvinist attitudes prevail. In the United States, this is less true, but still often true. Many physicians prefer female methods of birth control simply because these generally require a doctor's prescription. A condom can be bought over-the-counter.

Certainly it is vital for the mother of sons to make sure her boys are familiar with condoms, as a primary lesson toward making them sexually responsible people.

118. History of the condom

The condom is a pliable casing which fits over the penis and prevents the sperm from entering the vagina. It was originally conceived not as a method of birth control but as a device to prevent venereal disease and other infectious diseases. Primitive peoples who otherwise wore very little often wore condoms to protect the man against infectious tropical diseases. In the Middle Ages, workers in slaughterhouses found that animal intestines could be used as condoms. Fallopius, discoverer of the Fallopian tubes, advised men to wear linen condoms in a publication of 1564. The most effective proponent of the device, however, was Casanova, the legendary Italian lover of the eighteenth century who used the animal-intestine condoms for his own protection. At this time, condoms were widely sold in brothels to protect customers against the almost certain venereal disease of prostitutes. For centuries, authorities responsible for the health of men—from ordinary fathers to the United States Army—have recommended the device. (Ref. 39) Indeed it did protect both men and women against venereal disease; and since use of the condom began to decline in the sixties, with the advent of the pill and the IUD, there has been an epidemic rise of venereal disease in the United States, complicated by the fact that strains of gonorrhea brought back from Vietnam have proved resistant to penicillin. (See p. 310)

119. When to ask a man to use a condom

a. A woman who is otherwise unprotected against pregnancy should be forthright in asking a man to use a condom.

b. A woman who may otherwise be protected against pregnancy but who has some doubt about the health of the man she is with should ask him to use a condom.

120. Condoms available in the United States

Condoms are sold in almost any drugstore, without a prescription. Most are mass-produced of thin latex rubber; standards for tensile strength and to guard against holes are controlled by the FDA and the Government Services Administration (GSA). Some condoms made of lamb intestine are sold here; the standards for testing are not so rigid with these, and they are not recommended.

121. Effectiveness of condoms

Any rubber condom available in the United States is safe and very effective for birth control. A recent report from England put the failure rate at 4 failures per 100 woman years. (Ref. 40) If, in addition, the woman uses a spermicide, the combination should be almost 100 per cent effective.

122. Important: There are virtually no side effects from condoms, for men or women

123. The few disadvantages of the condom are procedural

A man does not have to have an erection to put on a condom—but many men find it much easier to do so. If this is the case, just putting on the condom requires an interruption in lovemaking which is very annoying to some people. Sometimes a woman can put it on, which helps. Some couples report that it decreases sexual sensation. Whether this is actual or a psychological reaction is impossible to prove.

124. Condoms are useful in preventing premature ejaculation

Some men ejaculate too quickly for their own and their partner's satisfaction; this usually is an emotional—sometimes a physical—condition. For such men, condoms tend to be helpful in maintaining an erection longer. (See p. 394)

125. The pill for men

It is well known that androgens, estrogens, or progestogens can be used to limit sperm production by the testicles; therefore, it is entirely possible that a hormonal compound pill could be produced for men.

126. Why the development of the male pill is moving slowly; the value of hindsight

Researchers today have the advantage of hindsight on side effects of the pill. If there have been so many side effects for women, surely there would be as many or more side effects for men. For example, progestogens and estrogens can cause decreased *libido* (sex drive) and cause breast enlargement; testosterone may cause increased incidence of heart attacks and cancer of the prostate. It has taken the scientific community years to minimize the risk of pill side effects in women, and many women have been adversely affected in the meantime. This in itself is enough to deter a similar outlay of time, money, and risk in developing a male pill. There are other factors involved as well:

a. The original pill development was for women because it was assumed that women were more interested in birth control than men (since women had to bear and care for the babies) and that women would therefore be more reliable, conscientious users of the pill. Although many Americans may reject this assumption, it certainly holds true for most people in the world; *only a very few women can trust men to protect them against pregnancy.* Obviously, it is unfair for women to have to bear the whole responsibility in this matter—a woman should insist that the men in her life participate and cooperate.

However, before governments donate huge amounts of money for research in this particular area, they need the assurance that it will be a widely used method, once developed. This may not be the case, *especially in developing countries.*

b. Finally, we must recognize that men control all the funding agencies which might contribute to this research, and may be feeling a bit apprehensive about the whole area of research. (Ref. 41)

127. A progestogen-androgen pill for men

Recently, a pill compounding progestogen and androgen was tried on fifty-one men; the sperm count went way down without the more serious side effects. Although this line of research is promising, it does not seem likely that it will be followed by the large and costly field trials necessary for perfection of the pill. (Ref. 42) *Watch for news.* Recent press reports from China claim that they have an effective and safe male pill.

128. Other methods of male contraception

a. *Withdrawal* of the penis before ejaculation is probably the oldest and most widely used method of contraception in the world. It is a difficult and distressing method, and should be used only in birth-control emergencies. The man must be able to recognize when he is going to ejaculate and withdraw before that. However, even this is not completely safe, because before ejaculation, the lining of the man's urethra contracts along with the vas and seminal vesicles and the contents of the urethra go into the vagina. Sperm are frequently present in these drops of fluid, so pregnancy may result.

Other problems with the method are the fact that intercourse cannot occur again until the man urinates, which may be up to several hours. Also under these circumstances a woman may not achieve orgasm and may thus be short-changed sexually, by a method that may leave her pregnant in the end—20–30 failures per 100 woman years. Ultimately, withdrawal places a great strain on both partners which is unjustified when there are so many other methods of birth control.

b. *Heat and ultrasound to decrease sperm count*

Under some carefully controlled experimental conditions, heat and ultrasound waves applied to the testicles before intercourse have been shown to cause *reversible* decreases in sperm count, thereby decreasing the chance of pregnancy. Whether these methods are applicable to widespread use remains to be proved. (Ref. 43, 44)

RHYTHM

The rhythm method of birth control depends on the rhythmic cycles of fertility and sterility within a woman's menstrual cycle, and allows her to protect herself somewhat against unwanted pregnancy by having sexual relations only during her non-fertile period.

Of course, the great difficulty lies in determining exactly *when* the non-fertile period occurs. For this reason, rhythm is not a reliably effective method of preventing pregnancy for large numbers of women.

129. History of the rhythm method

The cyclical nature of fertility has been understood for thousands of years—yet it was understood *wrongly* until 1930.

Soranus of Ephesus, a Greek physician who lived in the second century A.D., suggested that the most fertile days of the cycle were the two days immediately after menstrual bleeding ended. He believed that pregnancy occurred when the sperm implanted itself in the uterus, that menstruation prevented this implantation and that, therefore, the best time for implantation—the most fertile time—was just after menstrual bleeding ended.

The trouble with Soranus' theory was that he simply did not know of the existence of eggs; he thought the sperm did all the work. So as far as he and his cohorts for the next sixteen centuries were concerned, a woman's body produced nothing that was necessary to conception except the locale.

In 1827, the eggs of the female were discovered. However, for a long time scientists believed that menstruation produced ovulation in women as it does in animals, and so continued to say that the most fertile period was immediately after menstruation.

Only in the 1930s was the time of ovulation—the most fertile time— correctly placed at the middle of the menstrual cycle. This new knowledge for the first time made rhythm a viable method of birth control. (Ref. 45)

130. Basic methods of rhythm

There are three basic methods of rhythm, of testing when ovulation occurs and a woman is fertile: the calendar method, the temperature method, and the cervical mucus method. These can be used separately or in combination. Many couples use rhythm in conjunction with mechanical contraception.

131. Why rhythm is not reliably effective

Sperm usually live in the female reproductive tract for at least three, sometimes five or six days. Therefore, people practicing rhythm must correctly calculate the time of ovulation so that they can cease having unprotected sexual intercourse *at least three days before ovulation occurs*. Virtually no woman can rely on complete regularity in her menstrual cycle, so any judgment as to when ovulation will occur is fraught with risk. (See p. 16)

132. When rhythm is most effective

a. Rhythm is most effective as birth control among women who are *extremely* regular in their menstrual cycles. Even for them, it is not as effective in preventing pregnancy as other forms of contraception.

b. Rhythm is most effective when used with mechanical birth-control devices, such as diaphragms or condoms. (Rhythm without a diaphragm is like a diaphragm without spermicide—very, very risky.)

133. The calendar method

With the calendar method of rhythm, a woman must record the dates of six to twelve successive menstrual periods, and from these, calculate the range of possible ovulation days. Then she adds three or four days at each end of the range, and abstains from sexual intercourse during that entire time.

For example:

For one year, a woman has menstrual cycles from twenty-seven to thirty days long, counting from the first day of menstrual bleeding to the next onset of bleeding.

She can calculate, therefore, that ovulation will probably occur on days thirteen, fourteen, fifteen, or sixteen of her menstrual cycle. She adds four to each end of the ovulatory period. And she abstains from sexual intercourse (or uses a mechanical method) on days nine through twenty of *each* cycle. (Ovulation is most likely to occur thirteen to fifteen days *before* the next period.)

134. Difficulties with the calendar method

The calendar method becomes unreliable when a woman experiences menstrual irregularity, and especially when she experiences a shorter cycle, wherein the "risk days" are more numerous than she had anticipated. *These eventualities are not predictable.*

135. The temperature method

The appearance of progesterone in the second half of the menstrual cycle often causes a slight rise in the basal body temperature of a woman. The temperature method of rhythm works by the woman recording her temperature until she detects the rise (sometimes preceded by a slight drop), at which time her ovulatory period is probably over; and she can return to sexual intercourse shortly thereafter.

A woman takes her temperature each morning while she is still in bed, after five or more hours of sleep. She uses a regular thermometer or a basal body thermometer; she can take her temperature rectally or orally. When progesterone becomes dominant, her temperature will rise between 0.5 and 1.0 degrees. She waits for this temperature rise to repeat itself *three days in a row*. Then she can probably safely return to unprotected sexual intercourse.

136. Difficulties with the temperature method

If all other conditions are controlled, the temperature method has a failure rate of only 2–6 times per 100 woman years. (Ref. 45) However, body temperature is indicative of so many other factors in a woman's health that the margin for error in ascertaining when the "safe" days have arrived is relatively great.

a. The temperature method requires that couples abstain from sexual intercourse until *after* ovulation—for roughly the first twenty days of the cycle. This leaves relatively little time for sexual intercourse unless mechanical methods are used as well.

b. Often the rise in temperature is not abrupt and is difficult to detect.

c. Ovulation *can* occasionally occur without a rise in temperature, foiling the method completely.

d. Any external factor—a common cold, a bad night's sleep—can be enough to throw off the temperature method.

137. Combining the calendar and the temperature methods

Since many couples find it difficult to abstain from sexual intercourse during the days of probable risk both before and after ovulation, the temperature and calendar methods may be combined with good effect. The calendar method determines when the earliest possible ovulation can occur, allowing couples some safe days beforehand. The temperature method determines when ovulation is probably over, allowing couples some safe days afterward.

138. The cervical mucus method
A more recent proposal for rhythm is the cervical mucus method, which depends on a woman recognizing the changes in her cervical mucus that normally occur during the menstrual cycle.

The cervical mucus goes through five phases:

Phase 1: right after menstruation. At this time, there is very little cervical mucus. A woman will find her vagina and cervix rather dry.

Phase 2: prior to ovulation. At this time, a woman will detect a cloudy, white, sticky mucus.

Phase 3: around ovulation. At this time, a woman will notice a feeling of wetness, usually for three or four days.

Phase 4: after ovulation. There will be a decrease in the amount of mucus, and that which is detected will be cloudy and sticky.

Phase 5: before menstruation. At this time, a woman will notice that the cervical mucus is thin and watery, clear.

The unsafe period is roughly from the beginning of Phase 2 through the first four days of Phase 4. (Ref. 45, 46)

139. Difficulties with the cervical mucus method
a. The entire method is predicated on the woman being able to recognize the changes in her cervical mucus. *But an estimated 30 per cent of women do not have a regular mucus flow,* which means that they cannot detect the changes as they occur.

b. Like body temperature, the cervical mucus is responsive to many outside factors. For example, a minor case of vaginitis can alter the mucus completely, foiling the method. Thus the failure rate is very high —an estimated 25 times in 100 woman years. (Ref. 45)

140. Experiments in rhythm
Other means of predicting the time when ovulation begins have been tried in recent years, *without success.* These include testing for sugar in the saliva and chloride in the cervical mucus by means of specially treated paper strips.

Look ahead: Recent reports of a new device called an *Ovulimeter* seem to hold promise. This is a tamponlike device which is placed in the vagina and by a chemical change, depending on the state of the cervical mucus, can determine the phase of the cycle. Initial studies are promising; long-term studies are in progress.

141. The rhythm method and fetal abnormalities

The assumption that the rhythm method has no side effects has been challenged recently by some highly suggestive evidence that *conceptions occurring when rhythm is used are subject to higher rates of fetal abnormality—miscarriage and mental retardation.*

It is theorized that this may be due to the "overripeness" of the egg. Since failures in the rhythm method often occur at the very end of the ovulatory period, an egg fertilized at this time has been in the tube for a relatively long while. There is no definite proof that this causes higher fetal abnormality rates—but the evidence to that effect is disturbing. (Ref. 45)

142. Look ahead: antifertility vaccines—the "ideal" contraceptive

The ideal contraceptive agent would be a shot, with no side effects, which can be given periodically to prevent pregnancy. Large-scale studies of such a vaccine are now being conducted in India, but it will take *many years* to know whether this is successful. The vaccine is basically a shot of human chorionic gonadotropin—HCG—a hormone produced by the placenta in early pregnancy. The body produces antibodies against HCG and reacts against early pregnancies. The potential is great; the efficacy remains to be proved. (Ref. 47)

VOLUNTARY STERILIZATION

143. Recommendation: Tubal surgery (cutting, clipping, or cauterizing) is the most acceptable sterilization procedure for most women

A woman who of her own free will wishes to end her childbearing days through permanent sterilization should consider surgery on her Fallopian tubes. There are several rather simple operations by which the tubes are cut and sealed off so that the sperm and egg do not meet.

144. Recommendation: Other methods of sterilization should be shunned by healthy women

Hysterectomy—surgical removal of the uterus and sometimes the ovaries—and *oophorectomy*—surgical removal of the ovaries alone—are major operations, involving much risk, pain, and bleeding, and a long recovery, *all of which is absolutely unnecessary for simple voluntary sterilization in a healthy woman.* (See p. 333)

High-dose radiation applied to the pelvic area will also sterilize a woman. *Except as treatment for cancer, it is to be totally condemned.*

145. History of female sterilization

Voluntary sterilization is a brand-new phenomenon.

For almost all of recorded history, a woman who was unable to bear children felt herself cursed. She would never seek sterility therefore; and sterilization was generally something that men mandated for a woman who had no way of resisting.

In the fourth century B.C., the Greek physician Hippocrates, known as the Father of Medicine, recommended sterilization of women to prevent inherited insanity. Some Middle Eastern peoples, eager to protect men from dishonor by women who might sleep with someone not duly authorized, created methods of "temporary" sterilization whereby the lips of the vagina were sewn together, or a ring was placed through the labia. During the Crusades, departing European warriors would have their wives locked into metal and leather girdles known as "chastity belts" to which the only key remained in the possession of someone more trusted than the wife.

Eventually, the world progressed so that sterilization was recognized as a procedure more related to the health of the woman than the honor of the man. The first tubal ligation was performed in this country in 1880 by Dr. S. S. Lungren, at the same time as a Caesarean section delivery. (Ref. 48) For the next eighty years, tubal ligation was almost always performed immediately postpartum—by physicians who were convinced the woman's health would be endangered by further childbearing.

146. Voluntary sterilization: a new idea

Only within the last ten years has the idea of truly voluntary sterilization gained acceptance in this country. Up until that time most hospitals had calculated formulas (e.g., twenty-five years of age and five children, thirty with four children, etc.) into which a woman had to fit before they would permit her to be sterilized for other than severe medical reasons. The idea that men and women can make all their own decisions in this regard is part of the new trend in American medicine that the will of the *patient* should control the destiny of the patient.

147. Routine legal procedures before sterilization

Because of the recent scandals of forced sterilization in some young women, the federal government and most states now require long, detailed consent forms for both male and female sterilizations. They also require a waiting period from three to thirty days from the time of signature until the time when the procedure can be performed. This, of course, protects a woman from being coerced into accepting sterilization at time of abortion or delivery and gives her time to go home and think it over. However, long waiting periods may be obstructive in some cases. For instance, when a woman finds herself pregnant and would like to have a tubal ligation at the same time as abortion, this is forbidden under the new guidelines for federally funded sterilizations.

Most states no longer require the signature of spouse, but the hospital will have a standard medical permission form for the patient to sign.

148. Make sure you are not pregnant when you go for tubal sterilization

It is a terrible shock indeed for a woman who thinks she cannot become pregnant to become so after tubal sterilization. So take every possible precaution to guarantee that you are not pregnant at the time of the operation. Have a pregnancy test—*even if you just completed what appeared to be a normal period.* Some doctors suggest a D & C (dilatation and curettage) be performed at the time of the sterilization to guarantee that any pre-existing pregnancy will be ended. This is a simple operation (see p. 330) that does not add substantially to recovery time.

149. Methods of performing tubal sterilization

There are various methods of entering the abdomen to look at the tubes and to operate on them:

    a. Laparotomy
    b. Laparoscopy
    c. Colpotomy
    d. Culdoscopy

150. Laparotomy: an old method that is coming back

Laparotomy means that an incision is made in the abdominal wall and the tubes are *directly* visualized as they are operated on. The size of the scar determines the recovery period needed. If performed immediately after delivery, a very small scar below the navel is all that is needed. If performed when the woman has not recently been pregnant, a larger incision will usually be needed and this will be placed at the top of the pubic hairline.

There is now a procedure called *mini-laparotomy,* which many physicians are using, which needs only a small incision (one to two inches). For mini-lap, cannula is placed in the uterus so that the tubes can be brought up to the abdominal wall and grasped with a clamp. Then the tubes are tied and cut as with an ordinary tubal ligation.

151. Methods of tying the tubes by laparotomy

a. Once the belly has been opened, there are various procedures which can be done on the tubes. The most common is the *Pomeroy tubal ligation* (named for Ralph H. Pomeroy, who practiced at Kings County Hospital in the early 1900s) in which a loop of the midsection of the tube is elevated, tied and cut. A section is removed and sent to the pathologist. This is the most easily performed method, and can be done with a very small incision in the belly. The failure rate is 1/200 to 1/500.

b. The Irving method of tubal sterilization (named for F. C. Irving, a Boston gynecologist who used this method in the 1930s and later) involves burying the cut ends of the tube into the tissue around the tube. This method is essentially 100 per cent effective but has the disadvantage of needing a larger scar, and a longer operating time.

c. A *fimbriectomy* is the removal of the entire distal end of the tube, including the fimbria (the fringed ends). This is also a simple fast procedure which is very effective. The failure rate for this operation is about one per cent. Its major disadvantage is irreversibility. If a woman at a later date would like to try to have the tubal sterilization reversed (see p. 110) it is impossible with a fimbriectomy. Of course one should never undergo a tubal sterilization with the thought that one might want it reversed, but life circumstances do change.

152. Routine procedures before laparotomy

a. The hospital should perform routine lab tests several days before the surgery. These include blood tests, urinalysis, and a chest X ray, if the woman has not had one recently.

b. The woman will be asked not to eat or drink anything for eight hours before the operation.

c. The abdomen will be shaved, and then scrubbed in the operating room.

d. A catheter will usually be placed to keep the bladder from interfering with the surgery, but this is removed immediately after the procedure.

153. Routine procedures after laparotomy

The recovery and postoperative pain are directly related to the size of the surgical scar. If performed immediately after delivery, the area is sore but does not require any extra days in the hospital than the usual three to four postpartum. If a laparotomy is performed, the woman will have to stay one to five days depending on the size of the scar. In some places, the mini-lap is being performed as an outpatient procedure, but this is difficult except on thin women, when a very small incision can be used.

As with all surgical procedures, there are risks of infection in the wound or excess bleeding but these are very minimal in tubal sterilization procedures. The only restricted activity would be on heavy lifting for the three to four weeks after surgery.

154. Laparoscopy

A laparoscope is an instrument, known for almost seventy years, which allows a physician to see the Fallopian tubes. Until recently, it was used only as a diagnostic instrument to examine the contents of the abdomen in case of disease, and to determine what, if anything, was blocking the tube and preventing conception. (See p. 105) Now it is also being used to extract eggs from women in the very new test-tube fertilization. (See p. 113)

As a method of sterilization, laparoscopy became popular in the early 1970s—for it is fast and relatively easy, requires little recovery time, and leaves only one or two tiny scars which are usually buried in the folds of the navel and lower abdomen (depending on the type of equipment).

In laparoscopy, a general anesthesia is usually given; regular operating-room conditions prevail. A small needle is placed into the abdomen just below the navel. Two to three liters of CO_2 are allowed into the abdomen through this needle, expanding the abdomen. The hole through which this needle is placed is now enlarged somewhat by a trocar, a sharp, triangular tube. The laparoscope is inserted through this enlarged hole (which is still small); it visualizes the tubes; another instrument which cauterizes (electrically burns) the tubes is passed into the abdomen, either through the scope itself or through another small incision. The tubes are cauterized for a length of 3–4 millimeters, and the ends sealed shut.

The whole procedure takes less than an hour in the operating room and requires the woman to spend a maximum of two nights in the hospital. Sometimes, it can be done on an outpatient basis. The woman is left with several stitches in her navel which are removed after the wound has healed, about one week later. Some stitches absorb by themselves.

155. Procedures before laparoscopy

These are essentially the same as before laparotomy. (See ⌗152 above)

156. What to expect after laparoscopy

a. Mild abdominal pain that should not last longer than a day or two.

b. Some shoulder pain, a result of the CO_2 that was injected into the abdomen. It can be fairly severe—mild analgesics will control it.

c. A woman should be up on her feet the day after the procedure, but should try to take it easy for a day or two.

d. The two or three stitches may cause mild discomfort; they usually dissolve themselves or are removed in about five to seven days.

e. There should be no fever, bleeding, or severe pain after the operation. If there is, see a doctor immediately.

f. There will usually be no noticeable scar.

157. Make sure your doctor is experienced

If your doctor performs a tubal sterilization by laparoscopy only once or twice a year, go to another doctor for your procedure. Skill is absolutely critical in avoiding the few major complications associated with laparoscopy. This is not so critical in performing laparotomy.

158. Possible complications of laparoscopy

a. Burns of the skin and internal organs, particularly the bladder, stomach, or bowel. New instruments have considerably reduced the risk of this side effect—which occurs in less than 1 per cent of cases.

b. Bleeding from the tube or other organs sometimes occurs during the operation. It usually can be easily controlled, but may require a large incision.

c. Pelvic infection may occur—it is always a risk with any abdominal surgery.

d. The total incidence of major complications (burns, tubal bleeding, pelvic infection) from laparoscopy is 0.7 per cent. (Ref. 49)

e. The failure rate is somewhat higher than with laparotomy, varying from 0.1–2 per cent. As more and more physicians are becoming more experienced with the device, the complications and failures will decrease.

f. Recent reports from England have suggested that after tubal sterilization by cautery, there may be an increase in irregular menstrual bleeding. This awaits confirmation in this country. (Ref. 50)

159. Who should not have laparoscopy?

a. Women with heart or lung disease

b. Women with pelvic infection or scarring

c. Women with hernia from the umbilicus

d. Women with abdominal scars which may limit the pathways of necessary incisions

e. Severely obese women

For women with these contraindications, one of the other tubal sterilization procedures is preferable.

160. Laparoscopy with tubal clips or rings: an alternative to cautery

Since the most severe adverse side effect of laparoscopy with cauterization of the tubes is auxiliary burning of the bowel or other pelvic organs, some physicians recommend the use of tubal clips or rings to do the same job as cauterization.

The clips or silicone rings are placed over the midsection of the tubes, using specially adapted laparoscopy equipment.

While the clips are relatively safe compared to the cautery method, the failure rate is slightly higher. Early data on the silicone rings (Fallope rings) show a better success rate. (Ref. 49)

161. Tubal ligation through the vagina: colpotomy and culdoscopy

The Fallopian tubes may be visualized by making an incision in the top of the vagina, between the uterus and the rectum. The tubes can be grasped with instruments and either a Pomeroy procedure or fimbriectomy can be performed.

Although colpotomy incision is a simple procedure in most cases, bleeding may be heavier and the incidence of infection is higher, since the vagina is a relatively non-sterile place to operate through. Postoperative discomforts are minor—there is no abdominal scar. Intercourse and douching must be avoided for four to six weeks, to give the vagina a chance to heal. (Ref. 51)

A culdoscope is an instrument similar to the laparoscope except that it is inserted, as with a colpotomy incision (see above) into the top of the vagina. The tubes are caught, pulled out through the vagina, tied and cut. The procedure has the same advantages and disadvantages of the vaginal colpotomy.

162. Experimental methods of tubal sterilization

Several researchers are experimenting with various procedures using a hysteroscope (an instrument for visualizing the inner surface of the uterus through the cervix). These methods involve inserting plugs into the Fallopian tubes or injecting caustic substances which cause the tubes to seal off. These methods are still highly experimental, but if perfected, would offer simple office procedures for sterilization. Early studies have shown *very* high failure rates. (Ref. 52)

163. Tubal sterilizations are neither 100 per cent effective nor 100 per cent reversible

None of the procedures described above is 100 per cent effective *even if performed correctly*. There are many reports of tubes developing new channels or coming "untied." (For some reason, the risk of this is somewhat greater if sterilization is performed right after a pregnancy—either delivery or abortion.) However, the vast majority of women who have surgical sterilization will never again become pregnant (99 per cent at least). One should always approach sterilization with that in mind.

Although some physicians occasionally claim that one or another sterilization procedure is reversible, it is not something that a woman should count on. Sterilization is for keeps, and although we can never fully anticipate our lives, it should only be sought by women who are mature and completely convinced that they will never want another child and, even if they change their minds at a later date, will be willing to accept the fact of their sterility.

164. Vasectomy: the recommended method of voluntary sterilization for men

In recent years, as men have finally come to see that birth control is their responsibility too, vasectomy (vas-ECK-toe-me) has become increasingly popular. It is a much simpler procedure than any form of tubal sterilization. Although it has been available for many years, it has been passionately resisted because men are generally traumatized about any surgery on the genitals, because most physicians are men, and because women too are very frightened about possible emasculation. As public information has increased, the general fear of all groups has subsided. An estimated 750,000 vasectomies were performed in the United States in 1970, with about 500,000 each additional year thereafter. (Ref. 53) In other countries, like India, where the population crush is desperate, millions and millions of men have had vasectomies, encouraged by birth-control carnivals and free gifts and enormous public relations campaigns.

For a mature American man who knows his own mind, who is content that he has brought enough children into the world and wants no more, vasectomy is an ideal form of birth control.

165. The vasectomy procedure

The vas is a muscular tube inside the scrotum that carries the sperm. If it is cut, the sperm count eventually drops to zero, leaving the man sterile. In the vasectomy procedure, the patient comes to a doctor's office—usually not a hospital. The pubic and genital hair is shaved. The genital area is cleansed with a septic solution and local anesthesia is given. Either one incision is made down the center of the scrotum or two incisions are made, one on each side. The vas is isolated and clipped, or tied and cauterized. The incisions are small. The patient can walk out of the office an hour later, with little discomfort.

166. Routine care after vasectomy

Normal activities can be resumed a few hours after the procedure. Heavy lifting should be avoided. Some doctors suggest that there should be no intercourse for five to ten days afterward.

167. A man is not immediately sterile after vasectomy

Sperm that are already in the vas is capable of fertilizing the egg for some time after vasectomy. It may take up to six months until all the sperm are gone. Therefore, for eight to twelve weeks, semen samples should be checked for sperm and again every two weeks thereafter. When two consecutive sperm checks come up negative, then the man is considered sterile, but until this point, another method of birth control must be used.

168. Who should not have a vasectomy

The only medical contraindications to vasectomy are local infection of the genital area or previous scarring that may complicate the incisions and healing. Of course, a young man who may one day want to have some or more children should think very carefully about having this procedure.

169. Complications of vasectomy

Hematoma (he-ma-TOE-ma—blood collecting under the skin) and infection occur in less than 4 per cent of vasectomies; these are the major complications and can be avoided by using an experienced physician working under sterile conditions. Men develop antisperm antibodies after vasectomy and the notion that these would cause everything from thrombophlebitis to arthritis has created considerable hysteria. *There is no scientific evidence at all to substantiate these reports at this time.* (Ref. 53, 54)

170. Will vasectomy affect potency?

No. Vasectomy affects no known male function. Erection and ejaculation occur nomally as before—except that there are no sperm in the semen. Psychological changes may affect potency, however.

171. Vasectomy should not be considered reversible

Although some vasectomies have been reversed and the man rendered fertile again, this is a chancy supposition. *No man having a vasectomy should anticipate that the operation will be reversible.* Like tubal sterilization, vasectomy is for keeps. Also, as in tubal sterilization, there is a failure rate of approximately one per cent. (Ref. 53)

172. The use of sperm banks to store sperm before vasectomy

Some sperm banks offer deep-freeze service for storage of sperm.

Theoretically, a man could store up some sperm, then have a vasectomy, and if he ever wanted another child, use the sperm in the bank for artificial insemination of the mother. In reality, the sperm seem to lose their ability to fertilize after a few years, so this is not too practical. There are also reports of accidents occurring with the freezing units, destroying the sperm altogether. *Again, don't have a vasectomy with the idea that you may want more children: technology is just not that far along.*

173. Abstinence: an alternative for free people

Because birth control is today so readily available, and so reliable, many women feel they no longer have an excuse to say "no" to sexual intercourse. A woman may sleep with men she neither knows well nor likes much just because saying "no" is unfashionable.

Nothing prevents sexual fulfillment more thoroughly than sex under pressure. *Social pressure is not a valid reason to have sex.* Sex is for individual people, not social trends. It should be an emotional event, not the fulfillment of a social obligation.

Young women who repeatedly have sexual intercourse with men they do not care about during their early years of sexual activity are giving up the liberation that birth control gave them.

So consider abstinence.

It keeps you from getting pregnant.

But just as important, it can keep you from becoming uninterested in sex; it can keep you free.

TABLE 1

ORAL CONTRACEPTIVES AVAILABLE IN THE
UNITED STATES—May 1979

TRADEMARK	ESTROGEN	PROGESTIN	DRUG COMPANY
Brevicon (21 & 28)	Ethinyl Estradiol 35 mcg	Norethindrone 0.5 mg	Syntex
Demulen (21 & 28)	Ethinyl Estradiol 50 mcg	Ethynodiol diacetate 1.0 mg	Searle
Enovid-E (20, 21 & 28)	Mestranol 100 mcg	Norethynodrel 2.5 mg	Searle
Enovid 5 mg (20d)	Mestranol 75 mcg	Norethynodrel 5.0 mg	Searle
Loestrin 1/20 (21 & Fe)	Ethinyl Estradiol 20 mcg	Norethindrone acetate 1.0 mg	Parke-Davis
Loestrin 1.5 /30 (21 & Fe)	Ethinyl Estradiol 30 mcg	Norethindrone acetate 1.5 mg	Parke-Davis

TRADEMARK	ESTROGEN	PROGESTIN	DRUG COMPANY
Lo/ovral (21 & 28)	Ethinyl Estradiol 30 mcg	Norgestrel 0.3 mg	Wyeth
Modicon (21 & 28)	Ethinyl Estradiol 35 mcg	Norethindrone 0.5 mg	Ortho
Norinyl 1/50 (21 & 28)	Mestranol 50 mcg	Norethindrone 1.0 mg	Syntex
Norinyl 1/80 (21 & 28)	Mestranol 80 mcg	Norethindrone 1.0 mg	Syntex
Norinyl-1 (21 & 28)	Mestranol 50 mcg	Norethindrone 1.0 mg	Syntex
Norinyl-2 (21 & 28)	Mestranol 100 mcg	Norethindrone 2 mg	Syntex
Norlestrin 1 mg (21, 28 & Fe)	Ethinyl Estradiol 50 mcg	Norethindrone acetate 1.0 mg	Parke-Davis
Norlestrin 2.5 mg (21 & Fe)	Ethinyl Estradiol 50 mcg	Norethindrone acetate 2.5 mg	Parke-Davis
Ortho-Novum 1/50 (21 & 28)	Mestranol 50 mcg	Norethindrone 1.0 mg	Ortho
Ortho-Novum 1/80 (21 & 28)	Mestranol 80 mcg	Norethindrone 1.0 mg	Ortho
Ortho-Novum 2 mg (20)	Mestranol 100 mcg	Norethindrone 2.0 mg	Ortho
Ortho-Novum 10 (20d)	Mestranol 60 mcg	Norethindrone 10.0 mg	Ortho
Ovcon-50 (21 & 28)	Ethinyl Estradiol 50 mcg	Norethindrone 1 mg	Mead Johnson
Ovcon-35 (21 & 28)	Ethinyl Estradiol 35 mcg	Norethindrone 0.4 mg	Mead Johnson
Ovral (21 & 28)	Ethinyl Estradiol 50 mcg	Norgestrel 0.5 mg	Wyeth
Ovulen (21 & 28)	Mestranol 100 mcg	Ethynodiol diacetate 1.0 mg	Searle
* Zorane 1/20	Ethinyl Estradiol 20 mcg	Norethindrone acetate 1.0 mg	Lederle
* Zorane 1.5/30	Ethinyl Estradiol 30 mcg	Norethindrone acetate 1.5 mg	Lederle
* Zorane 1/50	Ethinyl Estradiol 50 mcg	Norethindrone acetate 1.0 mg	Lederle

*(Production of Zorane Products Discontinued 1/1/79)

MINIPILLS—PROGESTERONE ONLY

Micronor	Norethindrone 0.35 mg	Ortho
NOR QD	Norethindrone 0.35 mg	Syntex
Ovrette	Norgestrel 0.075 mg	Wyeth

TABLE 2
VAGINAL CONTRACEPTIVE PRODUCTS*

BRANDS	MANUFACTURER
Foams:	
Dalkon Foam	A. H. Robbins Co.
Delfen Foam	Ortho Pharmaceutical
Emko Foam	Emko Co.
Jellies and Creams:	
Conceptrol	Ortho Pharmaceutical
Delfen	Ortho Pharmaceutical
Finesse	Schmid Labs
Immolin	Schmid Labs
Koromex	Holland Rantos
Lorophyn	Norwich Pharmacal Co.
Orthogynol	Ortho Pharmaceutical
Preceptin	Ortho Pharmaceutical
Ramses	Schmid Labs
Suppositories:	
Lorophyn	Norwich Pharmacal Co.
Encare Oval	Eaton-Merz

* List may not be complete, but includes the most widely used brands.

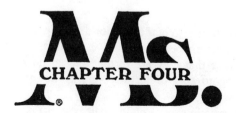

CHAPTER FOUR

INFERTILITY

It takes two to be fertile. Whether or not a couple can have a child is a vague, abstract concern before a child is wanted. If they are healthy, they usually assume that they are fertile, and spend early years of sexual activity trying to *control* fertility—trying *not* to become mothers and fathers.

But when two people want a child, their concern is no longer abstract but deeply personal. They become—for some of the rarest moments in life—completely committed to each other—each other's health, each other's ancestors, each other's continuation. If people with that kind of commitment are unable to have a child together, they face an emotional, a historical, crisis that can break the strongest heart and shake the strongest relationship.

Between 10 and 15 per cent of the American couples who want children face difficulty in having them. At one time, little help was available. If investigations into the woman's fertility provided no answers, the matter was often dropped. Today, since it has been recognized that men are equally responsible for the fertility of a couple, the possible causes —and possible cures—for infertility have more than doubled. The infertile couple can try many possible solutions before abandoning hope of having children naturally. And even after infertility has proven an insurmountable problem, there are solutions—from the adoption agencies and artificial insemination, for example—that can still give some couples, who want them so desperately, the joys, and agonies, of parenthood.

1. Why are women infertile?
   Because of:
   a. Hormonal imbalance and menstrual irregularity
   b. Ovarian abnormality, or corpus luteum abnormality
   c. Tubal abnormality
   d. Uterine abnormality
   e. Cervical mucus abnormality
   f. Habitual abortion

2. Why are men infertile?

Because of:

a. Low sperm production, which can be caused by:
  1. Hormonal imbalance
  2. Genital abnormalities
  3. Autoimmunity (antisperm antibodies)
b. Block in the transport of sperm from the testicles to the vagina
c. Sexual dysfunction—impotence or premature ejaculation.

3. Why are couples infertile?

In about five sixths of all cases, the problem of infertility can be traced to one of the partners. However, several causes of infertility affect *couples,* and such problems are especially hard to solve because, generally, they pertain to the *immunology of conception,* about which little is known at present. Somehow, the woman's body rejects the sperm, most often at one of three critical junctures:

a. If the cervical mucus and the sperm are not compatible
b. If capacitation (see p. 40) does not occur properly as the sperm pass through the uterus
c. If incompatibility occurs during the actual fertilization process in the tubes.

In all of these processes, the *positive interaction* of the two partners is absolutely essential to fertility.

CAUSES OF INFERTILITY IN WOMEN

4. Hormonal imbalance as a cause of infertility in women

Any hitch in the menstrual cycle may be enough to prevent fertility. (See p. 15)

If the hypothalamus does not produce FSH-RF or LH-RF, then the pituitary is not stimulated to release FSH or LH. Too much or too little estrogen or progestogen production can alter fertility as well.

Since the menstrual cycle is very sensitive to problems affecting the woman's *general* health (a sensitivity mediated by the hypothalamus), anything affecting general health can affect fertility. For example, a serious illness and a high fever can alter the cycle; when the illness is cured, the cycle may return to normal and fertility be restored. A severe psychological shock may alter the cycle and cause infertility; when the trauma is ended, fertility may be restored.

5. Ovarian abnormality as a cause of infertility

If a woman cannot ovulate, she cannot become pregnant. Therefore, any disease of the ovary which prevents ovulation causes infertility.

a. *Congenital abnormalities* in which a woman is born without ovaries or with malformed ovaries, prevent fertility absolutely. Most of these causes will be detected before or at puberty.

An example is Turner's Syndrome, in which a girl is born without one X chromosome which is essential for complete female development. (See p. 25)

b. *Polycystic ovaries,* the Stein-Leventhal Syndrome, is a more common condition in which the ovaries develop a thick coating that prevents ovulation. Many small follicle cysts develop, and the ovaries enlarge. The syndrome may be related to an imbalance between the hormones from the ovaries and those from the adrenal gland, or it may be caused by abnormality in the hypothalamus.

Women suffering from infertility due to polycystic ovaries frequently begin to ovulate in response to Clomid or as a result of surgery in which a wedge of ovary is removed. (See ⸭38 and 40 below)

c. *Infections of the ovaries by gonorrhea or mumps can cause infertility.* (See pp. 312–13)

6. Abnormality of the corpus luteum as a cause of infertility

In some women, the second half of the menstrual cycle (from ovulation to menstruation) is abnormally short, because the corpus luteum begins to degenerate after four to five days rather than after the normal eight to ten days. This is called luteal insufficiency. The normal amounts of progesterone and estrogen are not produced, leaving the endometrium inadequately prepared for implantation of the fertilized egg. Luteal insufficiency can also cause recurrent abortion. (See ⸭10 below)

Progesterone therapy is a frequently suggested treatment which may possibly help—but it has its limitations. (See ⸭39 below)

7. Tubal abnormality as a cause of infertility in women

After ovulation, the egg must be picked up by the fimbriated (or fringed) end of the Fallopian tube. Then the egg must move freely along the tube to the ampulla, a wider portion of the tube which is lined with secretory cells. It is here that fertilization of the egg by the sperm takes place. After fertilization, the fertilized egg must move down the tube at just the proper speed to arrive in the uterus at just the proper time for implantation.

The Fallopian tube is a muscular organ; its *motility* (mo-TILL-ity) is the power that muscles have to move spontaneously. Scarring or blockage will prevent the muscle from moving spontaneously, carrying the egg to the womb. *Therefore, the motility of the tube is crucial to fertility.*

Similarly, any scarring or blockage of the fimbriated end of the tube which prevents the egg from being picked up in the first place can cause infertility.

Abnormalities in the tubes can be caused by:

a. *Pelvic infection* that blocks or scars the tube, usually caused by gonorrhea, or by infection from an IUD, or by infection after abortion or delivery. A *ruptured appendix* may also cause damage to the pelvic organs if pus is discharged into the pelvic area. (See pp. 60, 314)

b. *Endometriosis*—a condition in which some endometrial tissue gets out into the pelvic cavity—may cause infertility by disturbing the motility of the tube. (See p. 342)

8. Uterine abnormality as a cause of infertility among women

Once fertilization occurs, and the fertilized egg (conceptus—con-SEPP-tus) is released into the uterus, the uterus must be in good enough shape to receive it for implantation. If something has gone wrong in the hormonal cycle, if the egg arrives too soon or too late, if the lining of the uterus is not ready for implantation, or a physiological defect in the lining of the uterus makes implantation impossible, the conceptus will not take hold and infertility may result.

For example, scarring from previous disease or injury that makes the endometrium rough or alters the even blood supply to it, can prevent implantation.

a. An infection or inflammation, for example from venereal disease or tuberculosis, can prevent implantation, causing infertility.

b. Fibroid tumors may distort the shape of the uterine cavity so that implantation is difficult. Malformation, such as a double uterus or a uterus with a septum can have the same effect. (These abnormalities are more likely to cause habitual abortion, usually in the mid-trimester of pregnancy.) (See ⚲10 below)

9. Abnormality of the cervical mucus as a cause of infertility

The sperm cannot penetrate the cervix unless the cervical mucus is at a proper thinness, with a welcoming chemical balance.

a. Infection or inflammation of the cervix can cause the mucus to be filled with white blood cells that keep the sperm out, causing infertility.

b. Hormonal imbalance may leave the cervical mucus too thick for the sperm to penetrate, causing infertility.

c. Sometimes the cervical mucus is the site of an immunological reaction between individuals that prevents fertility. This is an interaction between the partners. (See ✕3 above, ✕17, ✕46 below)

10. Habitual abortion as a cause of infertility in women

In this rather special form of infertility, the woman has no difficulty in conceiving but repeatedly (more than twice) loses the pregnancy. There are several possible causes:

a. genetic abnormality of the fetus (if this is suspected, both partners should be evaluated genetically. See Chapter Seven)

b. medical problems of the mother, such as thyroid disease or severe heart disease

c. an abnormality of the uterus, such as a fibroid tumor or a deformed cavity with a septum (usually causing late abortions)

d. corpus luteum insufficiency

e. exposure to environmental pollution (for example, anesthetic gases in operating rooms and fumes from lead and plastics factories may cause increased spontaneous-abortion rates)

f. infections such as mycoplasma and toxoplasmosis

Good news! These infections can now be detected in a culture taken from the cervix, or by blood tests. (See p. 306)

About *80 per cent* (!) of women who have suffered from habitual abortion eventually have normal pregnancies.

CAUSES OF INFERTILITY IN MEN

11. Abnormal sperm production due to hormonal imbalance: a cause of infertility in men

Hormone production in men is guided through the hypothalamus and pituitary just as in women—but it is a more constant, non-cyclical process. Millions of sperm are produced each day. FSH and LH must be present together, all the time, for adequate sperm production to occur. Diseases of the hypothalamus or pituitary, such as brain tumors, can block production of FSH and LH, cause the testicles to atrophy and become incapable of producing sperm, thus leading to infertility.

12. Abnormalities of the testicles causing low sperm production and infertility

a. Some men have congenital absence or deformity of the testicles which renders them infertile. As with Turner's Syndrome in women (see ⚥5a above), such a condition is usually noticed early in life and is usually accompanied by other deficiencies in masculine development. Hormone treatments can normalize the man's life—but infertility will probably persist.

b. *Undescended testicles:* Sometimes, a testicle will not grow in the scrotum but will remain up in the abdominal cavity. This condition, usually detected in young boys, can be corrected by surgery.

Unless the testicle is moved into the scrotum, it will not produce sperm. This is because the testicles in the scrotum have *a slightly lower temperature* than the rest of the body.

13. Body temperature is critical to sperm production

Conditions which elevate the temperature of the environment in which sperm are produced will *inhibit* sperm production and may lead to infertility. Men with varicosities in the spermatic vein may have a low sperm count because of the increased blood flow and increased heat to the testicles. This condition can often be corrected by surgery, rendering the man more fertile. For the same reason, men who wear jock straps all the time tend to show lower sperm counts than those who don't. (In fact, some researchers have suggested applying heat to the scrotal area as a means of birth control.) (See p. 76)

14. Other causes of decreased sperm count

a. Certain infections—*mumps* is a prime example—can render a man permanently sterile by stopping sperm production. Mumps causes sterility only when it infects the testicles. Other acute infections, such as gonorrhea, can cause temporary sterility.

b. Various medications—*corticosteroids* particularly—may inhibit sperm production.

c. Exposure to some industrial chemicals—notably those used in some *pesticides*—can cause decreased sperm count. For this reason, pesticide manufacturers have suggested that only older people who have completed their families should work with these chemicals. RECOMMENDATION: Pesticides should be a danger to bugs, not to people. Get involved in the fight to reform the technology of this and other industries whose products hurt the environment.

d. *Marijuana* can lower sperm count when it is used in high doses.

e. Sperm production usually decreases with age—*but this is by no means a reliable event*. It depends on individual make-up, and should never be assumed in decisions about birth control.

f. Some men have an autoimmune reaction to their own sperm. Antisperm antibodies circulate in their blood, preventing the production of strong sperm in sufficient quantities for fertility. Why does the body go to war against itself in this way? The answer is unclear.

Frequently, men suffering from sperm autoimmunity have had previous infection or obstruction of the vas deferens (see ⋕15 below), which caused the sperm to leak into the tissue around the genitals and set up an immune response in the blood stream. Since research into the immunology of conception is only now coming into its own, this remains the most baffling source of male infertility. Every breakthrough in such far-flung fields as organ transplants and the immunological reactions that accompany them brings us closer to a solution to the autoimmunity problem.

15. Abnormality in transport of the sperm from testicles to the woman's vagina as a cause of infertility

Sperm have to travel a long way from the site of production in the testicles to the ejaculation through the man's urethra; *any obstruction* along the path can cause infertility.

After production in the testicles, mature sperm are stored in the *epididymis* (ep-ih-DID-dee-mus), eighteen feet of coiled tube, which must be navigated by the sperm before they reach the vas deferens. This is the tube which leads from the epididymis to the area of the prostate. It is the tube which is sealed off in a vasectomy. (See p. 87) In the area of the prostate, the sperm are mixed with the fluid of this gland and the other sex organs, and this entire mixture of sperm and fluids is ejaculated through the man's urethra into the vagina. Any blockage in any of these sites, or any lack in quantity of fluid to carry the sperm out during ejaculation, can cause infertility.

Inflammations or infections are most frequent causes of blockage; scar tissue from previous disease can alter the motility of the sperm passages in much the same way that it can alter the motility of the Fallopian tube through which the egg must pass. (See ⋕7 above)

16. Abnormalities in sexual function as a cause of infertility in men

a. A woman does not need to have an orgasm to be fertile.

b. *Impotence,* the inability to have an erection and ejaculation, will, of course, render a man infertile even if sperm production is normal. Other men who suffer from low testosterone (male hormone) production are impotent and sterile as well.

c. *Premature ejaculation* (ejaculation before entering the vagina) may be a cause of infertility if no sperm ever get to the vagina. Other men with neurologic damage suffer from retrograde ejaculation in which the sperm and seminal fluid are ejaculated into the ·bladder rather than into the vagina. This also renders them infertile. (See p. 394)

d. Sperm must be deposited *high* in the vagina for fertilization. Anything which prevents this—for example, injuries that make it hard for a couple to position themselves during intercourse—can cause infertility.

CAUSES OF INFERTILITY IN COUPLES

17. Immunological reaction of woman to man's sperm as a cause of infertility

Some women, for unknown reasons, develop antisperm antibodies to their partner's sperm. These can be detected in the blood stream and are also secreted into the cervical mucus. At the level of the cervix, these antibodies may act to block the passage of the sperm into the uterus. The *postcoital test* screens for this problem. (See ⚮27 below)

18. Problems with capacitation and fertilization as causes of infertility

Once the sperm gets through the cervical mucus, it is altered in some manner not completely understood, by substances in the endometrium and by tubal secretions. This alteration is known as *capacitation* (see p. 40) and must occur if the sperm is to be able to penetrate the coat of the egg and to fertilize it.

Although the exact mechanism of capacitation and fertilization remains mysterious, abnormalities in these functions may cause infertility among couples in which no other cause seems pertinent. Immunologic interactions, for example, may have a role in blocking the processes.

FERTILITY TESTING

19. The fertility work-up

The study of infertility has now progressed to the point where there is a fairly routine procedure for dealing with it, called "the fertility work-up."

This is a series of tests for men and women which can determine the cause of the infertility and lead to measures to overcome it. *It is very important not to expect miracles from a fertility work-up;* as yet, too little is known about some of the causes of infertility—especially the immunological causes—to provide clear answers for all couples.

In addition, there is a psychological aspect to infertility which is very little understood.

One thing that is certain: a fertility work-up is worthwhile. In three fourths of the couples who undergo it, the work-up provides an answer —and even if the answer is that there is no hope for the particular couple to have a child naturally together—it is an answer, an end to worry and conjecture, and the beginning of a new plan of action that can lead to parenthood.

20. When to seek a fertility work-up

When a couple has tried unprotected intercourse, at least two times weekly, for at least a year without a resulting pregnancy, then a fertility work-up should be considered.

21. Whom to consult for a fertility evaluation

The American Board of Obstetrics and Gynecology now certifies superspecialists in fertility and endocrinology. These physicians have knowledge and training beyond the average board-certified obstetrician-gynecologist. Consult them if possible. Unfortunately, there are rather few such specialists and most are associated with medical schools. The American Fertility Society (1608 13th Avenue S., Suite 101, Birmingham, Alabama 35205) will have a listing of fertility centers and physicians in your area with expertise in fertility testing.

If you can't start with a specialist, begin the early tests in a work-up with a local board-certified gynecologist, and if specialized tests such as laparoscopy or tubal surgery are needed, seek referral to an appropriate center.

Make sure that you approach the fertility work-up *as a couple:* some tests are for individual partners, several require the participation of both. The cost may be high if your insurance does not pay for these tests, so check your policy first.

22. Preliminary evaluation for the fertility work-up

a. Complete family and medical histories on both partners should be taken. Questions which must be answered include: Are there others in either of your families with similar infertility problems? Have either of you had children with other people before? Do either of you have any past or present medical problems?

b. The pattern of sexual activity between you must be determined. You will be asked how often you have sexual intercourse, what position you assume most frequently (the woman inferior position is usually suggested to couples having difficulty conceiving). You will get some advice on how to improve chances of conception—for example: that the woman should remain in bed twenty to thirty minutes after intercourse; that she should not use lubricating jelly, and should not douche after intercourse; that the couple should watch the calendar and determine by the woman's menstrual cycle which are her most fertile days (see p. 76), and the couple should attempt to have intercourse at least every other day from days ten to twenty of a twenty-eight-day cycle.

Try to attend these preliminary evaluation interviews *together;* it will save you and your doctor a lot of time. Men are often shy about discussing these matters; they may feel emasculated by the possibility that the infertility is their problem. It may therefore be no easy task to get your man into the evaluation from the beginning. Don't give up; keep after him; if he is the man you want for the father of your children, then it's a worthwhile struggle.

FERTILITY EVALUATION IN WOMEN

23. Basic tests for infertility in women
These include:
a. A pelvic exam with Pap smear and tests for venereal disease
b. Basal body temperature testing
c. Endometrial biopsy
d. Postcoital, PK or Huhner test (a test for couples as well)
e. Hysterosalpingogram
f. Laparoscopy and tubal lavage

24. Pelvic exam with Pap smear and tests for venereal disease
A pelvic exam to begin with may suggest a number of simple physiological reasons for infertility which must be ruled out before further tests are done; the same goes for the Pap smear, to rule out cancer of the cervix, and tests for venereal disease, which may prevent conception. If vaginitis or cervicitis are present these should be treated, for they likewise may decrease fertility. (See p. 300)

25. Basal body temperature testing
The first step in a fertility work-up is to see if the woman is ovulating, best tested for by taking basal body temperature.

Every day before getting up, the woman should take her temperature and record it. If she is ovulating, her temperature will rise in the second half of the cycle. (See p. 78) In addition, if the second half of the cycle is shorter than normal (six to eight days instead of fourteen, for example), then suspect insufficiency of the corpus luteum as a cause of infertility. (See ⚹6 above) Do this test *for several months* before seeing the specialist. It will save time in the work-up.

26. Endometrial biopsy

In this test, a small scraping is taken from the lining of the uterus during the second half of the cycle. The procedure is performed in the doctor's office, takes only a short amount of time and involves some cramping pain, not usually severe. The tissue sample is then sent to the pathologist, who can tell several things upon examining it:

a. Whether the woman has ovulated during that cycle;

b. Whether the endometrium has developed to the point it should have for that day in the cycle. After ovulation, there is a day-by-day change in the endometrium, and if the changes have not occurred in orderly progression, something is probably awry in the development and degeneration of the corpus luteum, indicating a hitch in the hormonal cycle. If the endometrium is out of phase with the cycle, the test will often be repeated during another menstrual cycle—to verify the suspected hormonal imbalance.

c. Whether infection or inflammation is present in the endometrium, preventing successful implantation of the fertilized egg. White blood cells are signs of infection; they will be seen by the pathologist from the biopsy. If infection is detected, the woman can receive antibiotics or other drugs to cure the infection or inflammation and restore the endometrium to a healthy state in which implantation is possible.

27. Postcoital, PK, or Huhner test (a test for couples)

If a woman is ovulating normally, another cause of infertility may be abnormal cervical mucus or incompatibility of the man's sperm with the mucus.

The couple is asked to have intercourse at midcycle; the woman comes to the clinic or office for an examination two to six hours afterward. At this time, some cervical mucus is extracted with a special forceps and examined under the microscope. If the cervical mucus is not thin and stringy—too thick for the sperm to penetrate—that may be causing infertility. (Or it may just be the wrong day of the cycle.) The number of motile (moving) sperm will also show up on the test. Too few indicates a problem in sperm production, or infection or immunologic reaction that has made the cervical mucus hostile to the sperm. *This test may be repeated several times to get an accurate evaluation.* It is painless.

28. Hysterosalpingogram (HISS-ter-o-sal-pin-go-gram)

This is an X ray of the uterus and the tubes: a dye is injected into the cervix which outlines the uterine cavity and the tubes in the X-ray picture. A woman may feel some discomfort in the lower abdomen while the dye is being injected. Sometimes the dye contains iodine, and you will be asked about iodine allergy first.

The hysterosalpingogram can tell several things immediately: Are the tubes open? Are they normal? Is the uterine cavity outline triangular and smooth? A fibroid tumor or anything else distorting the shape or surface of the uterus will show up on the X ray; so will any blockage or scarring of the tubes.

The hysterosalpingogram is usually performed in a hospital X-ray department. Afterward, a pad will have to be worn to keep the dye from staining your clothes. This procedure should be done early in the cycle to avoid the possibility that the woman may already be pregnant.

29. Laparoscopy and tubal lavage

Laparoscopy (lap-ar-OSS-copy) is a surgical procedure by which the tubes and uterus are visualized directly through a scope. (See p. 82) Some physicians believe that they get more information from this procedure and do not do hysterosalpingograms. Others perform laparoscopy if there is an abnormality noted in the tubes on the X-ray study. No matter what the steps in the work-up, the laparoscopy should be done ideally by an infertility expert who will be the one to do the further surgical procedures if abnormalities of the tubes are noted. RECOMMENDATION: Therefore, it is preferable to have this procedure done at a medical center with specialists in infertility.

The procedure has two parts. The laparoscope is inserted into the abdomen and the tubes are observed for any abnormalities. At the same time, another surgeon injects a colored dye through the cervix into the uterus and tubes in the same way as for hysterosalpingogram. The surgeon using the laparoscope can see directly whether the dye is coming out of the tubes in a normal way. The blockage, if there is one, can be identified; endometriosis can be identified; and pelvic scarring or other pelvic pathology can be identified. Surgery may be performed at the same time or at a later date, depending on what condition appears.

30. Not to be depended on: the Rubin test, a non-specific test for tubal potency

Named for Isidor Rubin, an American physician, the Rubin test is a process by which carbon dioxide gas is allowed into the abdomen through the cervix and the pressure needed for passage of the gas recorded on an attached electronic device. For years before the hysterosalpingogram and laparoscopy were available, the Rubin test was used to see if the tubes were blocked.

It still is used by some physicians. If the tubes are blocked, the gas cannot get through; the machine registers a low gas intake and high pressure; the woman feels only mild cramping.

If the tubes are open, she will experience fairly severe shoulder pain due to passage of the gas upward in her body.

This test can be performed simply in a physician's office, but *no woman should depend on it alone because it is very non-specific.* It tells whether the tubes are open, but it does not detect scarring and adhesions which might be interfering with fertility. Today, with the hysterosalpingogram and laparoscopy available as procedures which tell much more about the exact nature of the infertility, the Rubin test is appropriate for very few women. If your doctor suggests that its results will be definitive, take that as a sign he or she is no expert in fertility and seek another opinion.

FERTILITY EVALUATION OF MEN

31. Basic tests for infertility in men
These include:
a. Semen analysis
b. Urological examination
c. Testicular biopsy

32. Semen analysis
Semen analysis is an absolutely essential test to determine if low sperm production or other abnormality is responsible for the infertility of the couple.

Usually, the man is asked to masturbate and ejaculate into a clean jar which has been kept at room temperature. For couples whose religion prohibits masturbation, *coitus interruptus* may be the only way. Under no circumstances should the man submit for testing semen ejaculated into a regular condom, for these contain material which immobilizes sperm and will render the test inaccurate. The man is asked to avoid ejaculation three to seven days before the test; he brings the semen to the lab immediately, no more than one to two hours after ejaculation.

The test can tell several things:
a. the total sperm count per cc. of semen (it should be above 20,000,000 per cc.)

b. Whether enough of the sperm are motile (at least half should be moving in straight lines. If they are moving around in circles, that is a sign of abnormal motility);

c. Whether the sperm are the right size and shape. If the test shows any abnormality in sperm production, motion, or character, the man will probably take the test again to verify a diagnosis.

d. Whether the volume is normal (both too much and too little fluid may cause infertility) and whether the viscosity (stickiness) is normal.

33. Urological examination

A complete urological examination, to determine if any disease or abnormality is causing infertility, is routine in the fertility work-up. It is comparable to the pelvic exam of the woman—*and every bit as important.*

34. Testicular biopsy

This is a simple procedure, done under local anesthetic in the urologist's office, and is indicated if semen analysis has revealed that the sperm count is low or nil or if the sperm are abnormal.

35. Other tests for infertility in couples

If tests on the individual man and woman show no clear reason for infertility, then other tests should be done. These include blood tests for diabetes and thyroid problems, and X ray of the pituitary gland if there is a hormonal imbalance. If hormonal abnormalities are suspected in either partner, more specific tests on blood and urine can be done for estrogen, androgen, and progesterone.

Look ahead for breakthroughs in immunology research. Blood tests for antisperm antibodies are being done routinely on both partners at some centers, usually in medical schools conducting research into male infertility. If the methods of treatment of partners with immunologic incompatibility become successful, these tests may become standard parts of the infertility work-up.

36. The psychological aspects of infertility

If your doctor, having tested you and your partner completely, says your problem is psychological, react with healthy disbelief. Few doctors would dare to give this as the only diagnosis today; too much is suspected, and too little actually known, about the interchange of endocrine function and mental state. It is far wiser to believe that the source of your infertility as a couple is still beyond the ken of medical understanding and hope that, as with so many conditions, your kind of infertility will be soluble for couples in the not too distant future.

The most pressing psychological aspect of infertility is not as cause but rather as effect. Testing, surgery, drugs, endless visits to doctors who have no answers, endless bills for tests that show no results, all this can wear a person down emotionally (and financially) so that the search for fertility actually becomes counterproductive.

Men are particularly sensitive to fertility testing; often, they confuse fertility with sexual health; and the testing is so distressing to them that it just isn't worth the hassle.

If you find yourself and/or your partner growing hysterical, over childlessness, if the tests are beginning to make you anxious and depressed, seek counseling. Or consider taking the pressure off yourself by adoption or (if you can carry a child) artificial insemination.

INFERTILITY TREATMENT

37. Treatments for infertility

A number of treatments are now available that may help certain infertile couples. These include:

a. Fertility drugs—clomid and the gonadotropins

b. Progesterone treatment for luteal insufficiency

c. Surgery to correct endometriosis or tubal scarring in women or blockage in the male genital tract

d. Artificial insemination

e. Psychological counseling may make an infertile marriage happier and, in a few cases, may aid in establishing pregnancy.

38. Fertility drugs

WARNING: *These medications are only for women who are not ovulating and are therefore infertile.* Most women to whom the drugs are recommended have infrequent periods spaced far apart. A few may be menstruating regularly but have found, through the basal body temperature testing method or endometrial biopsy, that they are not ovulating. The Stein-Leventhal syndrome—polycystic ovaries—is also treatable with the infertility drugs. The drugs fall into two basic categories:

a. *Clomiphene citrate (Clomid)*: Most women who are not ovulating regularly still have some FSH and estrogen. What they are missing is the midcycle spurt of luteinizing hormone (LH) which triggers ovulation. Clomid is an anti-estrogen; that is, it tricks the hypothalamus into thinking that the body's estrogen levels are too low. This causes an increased production of FSH-RF and FSH and therefore increases body estrogen. When the estrogen gets to a certain level, the hypothalamus releases LH-RF which in turn stimulates LH release and ovulation occurs.

Generally, a woman will take Clomid once a day for five days following a period (which may have to be induced with progesterone). She takes her basal body temperature daily to see if ovulation has occurred. If ovulation does not occur after three months of treatment, the dose is doubled. When used for the appropriate cases, the results for fertility have been excellent. There is a 5–10 per cent incidence of twins from this therapy, but not the multiple gestations as with Pergonol (see below).

  b. *The gonadotropins—HCG, HMG, Pergonal:* Some women are infertile because of damage to the hypothalamus or the pituitary that cuts down or eliminates gonadotropin production. Follicle Stimulating Hormone and Luteinizing Hormone are two gonadotropins vital for fertility. A woman suffering from the lack of these can take HMG—human menopausal gonadotropin—which is a mixture of FSH and LH extracted from the urine of menopausal women. HCG—human chorionic gonadotropin—is very similar to LH and an additional dose may be given at midcycle to simulate the spurt of LH.

A woman undergoing gonadotropin treatment for infertility needs to be closely followed with daily tests for estrogen levels in blood or urine. At a certain level of estrogen in the blood, the gonadotropins should be stopped. RECOMMENDATION: For this reason, *this type of therapy should always be done at a fertility center.* In addition, the treatment is very expensive, so don't waste any money with non-specialists. These drugs have been associated with multiple births. However, methods for determining the right dosages of gonadotropins are much improved, so that the risk of multiple births is now much lower—*if an expert is administering the drugs.*

39. Progesterone as a treatment of corpus luteum insufficiency

If the endometrial biopsy and the basal body temperature charts suggest that luteal insufficiency (see ✗6 above) is causing infertility or habitual abortion (see ✗10 above), progesterone treatments may be tried. Vaginal suppositories containing progesterone can be administered through the second half of the cycle and during the first three months of pregnancy to correct the deficiency. WARNING: *synthetic progestogens such as medroxyprogesterone or norethindrone should not be used in early pregnancy because of the possibility of fetal damage.*

An auxiliary treatment used by some physicians is a low dose of HCG or Clomid to maintain the corpus luteum.

40. Ovarian wedge resection: a surgical treatment for polycystic ovaries

Many women who do not ovulate and are infertile because of polycystic ovaries have this corrected by the surgical procedure of removing a wedge of tissue from each ovary. This is treatment of last resort; it should be done only if the woman does not respond to Clomid. (See ⚹38a above)

41. Surgery to correct tubal scarring or endometriosis

If a hysterosalpingogram shows that tubal scarring or endometriosis is causing infertility, a laparoscopy is essential to get at the *exact* nature of the problem. It should be done by the same physician who will do any further corrective surgery if this proves necessary. *Be very careful which doctor you choose to perform these procedures. They are complex and difficult and no doctor should do them who is not a specialist, recommended to you by many sources—former patients, your local medical center, family counseling agency, etc.*

Occasionally, a small amount of tubal scarring can be corrected during laparoscopy. Sometimes a laparotomy for infertility is necessary thereafter. An infertility laparotomy has myriad varieties, depending on what the problem is. If adhesions are found, then these are removed and the uterus is often suspended from the front wall of the pelvis so that the adhesions will not reform. If endometriosis is the problem, then it can be scraped off the walls of the uterus, tubes, and pelvis.

If the tubes are blocked at the fimbriated end, then a two-stage operation called a tuboplasty may be suggested. In stage one, the blockage at the fimbriated end of the tubes is cleared away and small plastic hoods are placed over the tubes. They stay there for three to six months. Then in stage two an operation is called for during which the hoods are removed. Essentially, the tubes are being forcibly kept open in the hope that they will reconstruct themselves over time and *stay* open. It doesn't always work. Only about 20–30 per cent of the women who undergo tuboplasty conceive and bear a living child: these are pretty bad odds, considering the strain and risk of two major operations. However, if the tubes are closed, this is the only option unless in vitro fertilization becomes widely available. (See ⚹50 below)

42. Surgery to correct tubal ligation

If the tubes have been tied, there are two surgical procedures to reconstruct them. In one procedure, the two ends of the tube are sewn back together; the physician must employ microsurgery for this procedure, for the tubes are so thin that they can only be seen to be sewn using a microscope. A plastic "splint" is usually inserted into the tube and the uterus to keep channels open until healing is complete. This can be removed at a later date through the cervix. Obviously, this is a very difficult and expensive procedure, the province of specialists only, and the chances of failure are high.

In another procedure, the distal end of the tube is pulled through into the uterus and fastened there, with the fimbria still outside. The success rates vary from 20 to 75 per cent, depending on the procedure and the surgeon. Make sure you know what the success rate of your surgeon is when considering this surgery.

Microsurgery to reverse vasectomy has a higher success rate.

43. Tubal pregnancy is one danger of tubal surgery.

A woman who has had tubal surgery is more likely to experience a tubal pregnancy. (See p. 167) This is the only major adverse effect of the surgery, except of course possible failure.

44. Treatments for infertility due to failure of implantation

Any uterine infection that is preventing implantation of the fertilized egg can be treated and very often cured with antibiotics. If large fibroid tumors are preventing implantation, these can be removed surgically by myomectomy. (See pp. 338–39) If there is a septum in the uterus, this can be removed surgically by an infertility specialist.

45. Treatment of infertility due to abnormal cervical mucus

Some women do not develop the normal stringy mucus (spinnbarkeit) at midcycle. Estrogen treatments at midcycle may help to make the mucus thinner. If the cause of mucus abnormality is infection of the cervix, cyrosurgery (surgery by freezing, see p. 309) and antibiotic creams are often effective.

46. Treatments for immunological reactions causing infertility among couples

a. RECOMMENDATION: The few couples in which a woman is having an immunological reaction against her husband's sperm—that is, if she has antisperm antibodies in her blood—can try a relatively simple treatment. The couple should use condoms during intercourse so that no sperm passes into the woman's body. Blood tests may show that the number of antibodies in the woman's blood will gradually decrease. Antibodies form expressly in response to the challenge of the presence of their specific enemy, in this case, the sperm. Take away the sperm, and the antibodies will have no reason to form.

Once the antibody count in the woman's blood stream is down, the sperm may be able to enter without adverse reaction. Therefore, the use of the condom should be continued except at midcycle, on the days most likely for ovulation. *This is a way of sneaking the sperm past the antibodies before they have a chance to array themselves against it.* If the day is right, and the immune reaction is mild enough to respond to this treatment, pregnancy may result. Other treatments may be forthcoming.

b. Autoimmunity in the man (when he reacts against his own sperm) is a more difficult problem. One treatment that has been tried is testosterone, a male hormone which is taken by the man until the sperm count goes way down and the antibodies in the man's blood that form against the sperm have no reason to form. In some men, the suppression of sperm production leads to the complete elimination of the immune reaction will have stopped as well. In some centers, short-term testosterone treatment is then stopped, and, it is hoped, the autoimmune reaction will have stopped as well. In some centers, short-term high doses of corticosteroids are being used as well. Keep your eyes open for many discoveries in this area of the immunology of conception in the next few years.

47. Treatments for infertility due to low sperm count in the man

a. Abstinence during the first half of the cycle, up to the woman's most fertile days (days ten to twenty), may help to build up the man's sperm count so that he can make the woman pregnant. Clomid (see above ✳38a) may help some men with low sperm counts.

b. If the man has no sperm at all, or very low sperm count, then *artificial insemination* is a possibility. The basic procedure is that for five days at midcycle a woman comes to the doctor's office daily or every other day and semen is placed either directly in the cervix or in a cap which fits over the cervix. There are several sources of semen for the procedure:

1. A man with some sperm but not enough to father children may have his semen mixed with that of a sperm donor, so that the resulting pregnancy has *some* chance of being his;

2. A man who chronically ejaculates prematurely can collect samples of semen to be used in artificial insemination so the baby will be his;

3. Women whose partners have no sperm at all may have to be inseminated entirely with donor semen. One can never know who the physical father of the child is but can take much comfort in the certain knowledge that the father of the child is the man who loves

and nurtures it. And the mother is the natural mother, emotionally and genealogically a very great plus.

48. Artificial insemination is an important option for couples carrying traits for genetic disease

If both the man and the woman carry the trait for Tay-Sachs, for example, or sickle-cell disease, then artificial insemination with the sperm of a non-carrier would insure a normal baby without the need for amniocentesis and possible abortion. (See pp. 218–19)

This is also possible for a woman with Rh sensitization. (See p. 179) If inseminated by an Rh negative donor she will have no problems with the pregnancy.

49. Sperm banks and sperm donors

Men who serve as donors for artificial insemination procedures must be very carefully screened for illness, infection, blood type and Rh, and genetic problems. *Make sure this is done.* Reliable centers keep detailed records on their donors and attempt to match physical characteristics with the woman's partner. Ideally the semen is donated on the day of the insemination, but this is not always possible. If not, the semen is fast-frozen and kept for short periods of time.

There has been much talk lately of sperm banks where semen is stored forever so that if a man wants to father a child ten or twenty years hence, he can do so. In reality, semen does not keep that well and the sperm count in the stored samples decreases with age. Also, there have been several instances of the freezer breaking down and all the semen being destroyed. At this time, no man should undergo vasectomy with the belief that his stored sperm will always be ready.

50. Test-tube babies

In 1978, Dr. Patrick Steptoe and Dr. Robert Edwards achieved what they and many other physicians had been trying to achieve for years: the birth of a living, healthy "test-tube baby." The child's mother had been unable to conceive naturally because of blocked tubes. The doctors extracted an egg from the mother which was fertilized by sperm from the father *in vitro*—in the laboratory—grown to the eight-to-sixteen-cell stage and then reimplanted into the uterus of the mother, where it grew into a little English girl. Couples seeking to solve their infertility problem by resort to this procedure should be aware that it is very, very difficult, not yet widely available and that the failure rate is high. However, the success with Lesley Brown's daughter in England is reason to rejoice. It is important to note that these doctors did *not* create life. They simply replicated in the laboratory a process which could not, for a wide variety of reasons, occur in the mother's body, thereby giving a childless couple the baby whom they so desired.

51. Cloning

Cloning is asexual, single-parent reproduction. It is a way of making cells reproduce themselves on their own, so that the child cell is an exact reproduction of the parent. American and British scientists in the fifties and sixties managed to make it work with frogs—but despite the hold that such a process has on the imagination of novelists (*The Boys from Brazil*) and philosophers, physicians and scientists have not yet seen fit to go to the great trouble necessary to make the process work on humans. Let us hope that their restraint continues unabated.

52. Adoption

Adoption is a legal, not a medical matter, and should be considered by infertile couples who simply have no further medical recourse. Unfortunately, it is not as easy as it once was. The worldwide availability of birth control and the legalization of abortion have drastically reduced the number of children who are actually given up for adoption. Adoptable children are now more often victims of circumstances that have left them orphaned and alone—war, accident, natural disaster.

However, there are a number of miraculous things about adoption, far beyond the realm of medical understanding. One is the uncanny but quite real resemblance that adopted children have to their adoptive parents. If you adopt a baby at a young age, sooner or later, some perfect stranger is likely to say that your son or daughter looks exactly like you.

If your infertility problem is at the point where the only remaining alternatives are risky operations that are more than likely to fail (see ✳41, ✳42 above), or where one partner is absolutely sterile, consider adoption. Millions of people can testify that it is an excellent way to be a parent, and an excellent way to be a child.

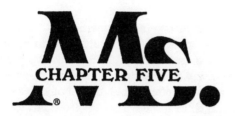

CHAPTER FIVE

HAVING CHILDREN

Pregnancy is one of nature's greatest challenges to a woman, and if this were a different time or society, she would have no choice but to accept it. Today, we are separated by only a few decades from the countless generations of women who had little choice but to bear children as often as their bodies allowed; often, until their bodies gave out. However, just because birth control has allowed freedom to plan and limit families, we're not free of the natural processes that cause women to become pregnant; nor are we free of the political and social forces that conspire to make pregnancy seem a preferred state. Much of the world, and many of us (if we examine our feelings truthfully), still measure a woman's worldly success and status by whether anyone calls her "Mother."

Although it is unlikely that American women would ever want to return to the "natural" state in which they could not help but be pregnant, there is a lot to be said for sustaining "natural" *emotional* reasons for becoming pregnant. In the politically charged atmosphere that surrounds family planning today, a woman may become pregnant (or not) for political reasons; financial reasons; religious reasons; she may begin to feel that having a baby, or not having one, is equivalent to making a *social* statement.

All this has bearing on the decision about pregnancy—but it is not enough to *support* the decision. There is still only one good, basic reason for a woman to become pregnant—and that is because she wishes to have a child by a specific man whose continuation she wishes to link to her own. Denaturalization of the child-creation process is a blessing to women—but dehumanization of the *conception* process could cancel out all our gains.

Pregnancy, with all its hassle, may feel like something a woman does alone, for herself. In fact, some of the great mistakes in mothering are made by women who somehow forget that the end product of the travail is a *separate* human being, who will probably not care about being a "social statement" but will concentrate rather on living his or her own life, and who will remind the mother of the father until the end of time. Take care whose eyes gaze back at you from the cradle.

Pregnancy is a complex process physiologically, and although the process works well for the majority of cases, there are some natural dangers at various stages. Initially, for a woman to become pregnant, an enormous number of processes and circumstances must be perfectly synchronized. (See Chapter 4, Infertility) Many problems can arise between conception and delivery. For a woman to deliver a child safely, without injury to herself or her baby, is a difficult and miraculous occurrence; physicians and midwives and electronic devices can watch over the pregnancy, labor, and delivery, but they cannot guarantee the results. For a baby to be born alive and well requires good personal health care, good medical care, and good luck.

Once a woman makes a decision to be pregnant (ideally, a mutual decision with the father), she must take her pregnancy seriously, and seek help for the rigorous challenge her body is about to accept. Medical advice is essential at this time; self-esteem, self-care, and a loving partner are *crucial*.

CONCEPTION AND DEVELOPMENT OF PREGNANCY

---

1. The moment of conception

Conception occurs when the particular sperm that has outraced all the others in the ejaculate meets and fertilizes the egg in the ampulla (a slightly dilated portion of the Fallopian tube).

For fertilization to occur, capacitation (see p. 40) must have taken place first, as the sperm passed through the uterus. In the tube, the sperm must then penetrate the thick, clear coating that covers the egg— the *zona pellucida* (pell-OO-sidda). The zona is made up of some protein substances, and in order to get through it the sperm releases a protein-digesting enzyme from its head.

Once it has penetrated the zona pellucida, the sperm drops its tail, rather like a rocket separating from its propulsion gear after lift-off. The head of the sperm combines with the egg; the fertilized egg then begins to divide and multiply into a many-celled structure.

2. The fertilized egg reaches the uterus: implantation

It takes about three days for the fertilized egg to move through the tube into the uterus. All the while, it is dividing and multiplying; it has about sixteen cells by the time it reaches the uterus. Once there, it floats through the uterus for another three days, seeking a suitable place for implantation. Having found the right spot, it burrows into the endometrium—the rich, nutrient-filled lining of the uterus, where it will grow through pregnancy.

At the time of implantation it has been about seven days since ovulation and six days since fertilization.

3. The egg differentiates into fetus and placenta

By the time the fertilized egg burrows into the endometrium, it has two distinct sections—the section that will grow into the infant, and the section that will form the *placenta.* The placenta (pla-SEN-ta; derived from the Latin word for cake) is the flat, cake-shaped mass of vascular tissue that filters the substances passing between the metabolism of the mother and the metabolism of the child. *There is no direct contact between the blood stream of the mother and the blood stream of the child* —nutrients and oxygen from the mother's blood reach the fetus through the medium of the placenta; the fetal blood is cleaned of carbon dioxide, nitrogens, and other wastes through the placenta. (See below) The placenta has, in microcosm, the functions of the air and the environment, allowing separate organisms to live together without poisoning each other.

4. Corpus luteum functions are vital in initial stages of pregnancy

Six to seven days past ovulation is the time of peak strength of the corpus luteum in the ovary during the normal cycle. (See p. 17) The corpus luteum assures that the endometrium is thick and rich enough to house the conceptus (kon-SEP-tuss)—early pregnancy. If implantation occurs, the corpus luteum in the ovary continues to grow (it would degenerate if there were no pregnancy) and produce high levels of hormones to support the life of the pregnancy in the first few weeks. The corpus luteum is working so hard to fulfill this support function that the ovary may become enlarged and cystic during the first three months of pregnancy. A routine pelvic exam may detect the ovarian enlargement, which generally reverses by the fourth month. Unless other symptoms arise, it is nothing to worry about.

5. Differentiation: the formation of the fetus' vital organs

When the conceptus burrows into the endometrium, the endometrium actually covers it up. Then the placenta starts to spread out; the conceptus starts to grow an *amniotic sac* (am-nee-OTT-ik) around it, a thin-skinned bag full of fluid that will provide the growth medium for the embryo.

From the moment of fertilization until the twelfth to fourteenth weeks of gestation, the cells of the embryo are undergoing *differentiation*—that is, the cells are differentiating themselves into those that will form the heart, those that will form the brain, the eyes, ears, etc. *These first twelve to fourteen weeks of pregnancy, during which differentiation of organs is taking place, is the time when the embryo is most sensitive to damage by drugs, environmental chemicals, infections, and radiation. A woman should be very careful to avoid such dangers at this time.* (See pp. 212–13 for fuller discussion.)

6. When are the basic organs of the embryo formed?

During the first twelve weeks of pregnancy, a woman is likely not to *look* pregnant to herself or to the world—but the most crucial developments are occurring within her: she is more *delicately* pregnant, her child is in greater danger relatively, than at any other time during the pregnancy.

The following organs form at these times after ovulation:

Brain: 2–5 weeks
Heart: 3–6 weeks
Legs and arms: 4–8 weeks
Eyes: 4–8 weeks
Ears: 6–12 weeks
Mouth, teeth, and palate: 7–12 weeks
Genitals and urinary system: 7–16 weeks

Formation does not automatically lead directly to proper *function.* After the cells differentiate and the organs are formed, they get bigger and stronger continually during the last six months of pregnancy. With all the advanced current technology of neonatology (nee-oh-na-TOL-ogy)—medical specialty dealing with the fetus and newborn—it is still not possible to evaluate how a new human being's body will function after it is born.

7. How a pregnant woman feels is not necessarily an indication of how her baby feels

Pregnancy is the union of two people at absolutely varying stages of growth. What is good for a fully grown woman may be destructive for an embryo which is composed of a few hundred cells. Remember, you are pregnant from the minute of conception.

Thus, during the first twelve to fourteen weeks of pregnancy, when a woman still has not lost her shape and may feel quite unburdened with the weight and pressure of the child, the embryo itself is going through its most difficult stages. Miscarriage is most frequent during this early period, when a woman may feel at her strongest and the embryo is at its weakest.

8. How the fetus is nourished in the uterus

The placenta grows toward the blood vessels of the mother which are lodged in the endometrium. The blood of the fetus flows to the placenta through the umbilical cord. A thin membrane separates the two blood systems. This membrane (the *placental barrier*) allows the waste materials of the baby to flow into the mother's system so that she may eliminate them, and the nutritional donations of the mother to flow into the baby's body, so that the baby can grow.

The amniotic sac around the fetus enlarges constantly through the first three months, and does not fill the entire uterine cavity until three months is over. This may be one reason that miscarriage is so much easier during the first three months—the amniotic sac is floating in the uterine cavity; there is free space around it; it is not firmly held until it expands enough to fill the space.

9. Oxygen from the mother's blood is the vital nutrient for the growing fetus

The growing fetus depends *totally* on oxygen from the mother's blood supply. This is a major nutrient drawn from the blood vessels of the endometrium through the placental barrier to be picked up by the umbilical cord. The mother's blood count must be high enough to carry a good oxygen supply to the infant. Iron is very important in the formation of *hemoglobin* (HEEM-oh-glo-bin), the blood substance that carries oxygen, and most pregnant women will need an iron supplement. (See p. 150)

10. Complications in the flow of oxygen from mother to child

Anything decreasing the oxygen supply in the mother's blood endangers the child, as does anything that decreases the blood flow to the uterus. Usually these conditions only accompany severe diseases—heart disease, high blood pressure, and severe anemia, however, smoking decreases the oxygen supply as well. Good prenatal care is important to detect these medical problems early, and women should cut back or stop smoking during pregnancy.

In late pregnancy, when the uterus is very big, it may press on the *vena cava* (veena CAVE-a), the large vein that carries blood back to the heart from the lower extremities, and this may decrease the flow of blood to the uterus. RECOMMENDATION: One way to alleviate the loss of oxygen flow from pressure on the vena cava is to avoid sleeping flat on your back in late pregnancy; sleep on your side instead, preferably the left side.

Other nutrients besides oxygen that are carried by the mother's blood to the placenta are sugar, amino acids, and all the other substances needed for human growth. (See ✕19–21 below)

11. The corpus luteum and then the placenta produce hormones needed to sustain pregnancy

When a woman does not become pregnant, the hormone buildup that triggers the enrichment of the endometrium stops and menstruation occurs. But when a woman becomes pregnant, the hormones must stay at a high level, to keep the endometrium rich, to sustain the flow of nutrients to the growing fetus.

The maintenance of this hormone supply is crucial to the continuation of the pregnancy; if there are not enough hormones, miscarriage may result. (See p. 95)

Early in pregnancy, the corpus luteum supplies the estrogen and progesterone in large quantities. Later, the placenta produces the majority of the required hormones—estrogen, progesterone, and the *human chorionic gonadotropin* (HCG) a close relative of luteinizing hormone. Production of HCG begins right after implantation, increases steadily for the next fifty to seventy days, then decreases steadily toward the end of pregnancy.

HCG is believed to maintain the corpus luteum during the early weeks of pregnancy until the placenta takes over the production of estrogen and progesterone.

12. Detection of HCG is the basis of current pregnancy tests

Most pregnancy tests now in use depend on the detection of an immunologic (antigen-antibody) reaction to the presence of HCG in the urine. This includes the pregnancy test kits which are now available for home use. The instructions in these kits should be followed exactly. *No test is 100 per cent accurate!* Any woman with symptoms of pregnancy should see a physician, even if her home test is negative.

WARNING: Tubal pregnancy, which is a serious development (see p. 111), may produce a negative urine test, so always double-check with a physician.

Older pregnancy tests involved injecting samples of the woman's urine into the abdomens of lab animals, particularly rabbits. If HCG were present, the animal ovaries would swell and begin to hemorrhage. When they were examined, a day or two after the injection when the animals were killed, the woman's pregnancy could be verified.

Look ahead to more sensitive blood tests that will determine HCG's presence in the blood stream even before the first period is missed. These will be widely available soon.

13. Normal signs of early pregnancy

a. Breasts may enlarge with frequent accompanying burning or tingling sensations.

b. Fatigue is natural during the first few months—and so is the exact opposite, a surge of energy, feelings of great good health and well-being.

c. Frequently the vagina and cervix will have a bluish look during early pregnancy (these are called "Chadwick's Sign," named for James Chadwick, the American gynecologist who first detected them). The blueness is caused by general congestion of blood in the pelvic region.

d. Nausea and vomiting are very frequent. "Morning sickness" is a misnomer, because the nausea can occur at any hour of the day or night.

e. Urinary frequency, common in early pregnancy, is caused by pressure of the growing uterus on the bladder.

PRENATAL CARE

14. Recommended Care

One "unnatural" thing about having children in our era is that most American women can expect, and must demand, regular medical care during pregnancy. For healthy women, prenatal care is preventive medicine—routine weight and blood pressure checks, and blood testing, all of which verify that the correct nutritional exchange is being made and the fetus is growing normally while the woman maintains good health.

15. Select a physician or nurse-midwife early in pregnancy

If you don't hit it off with your doctor, it's best to change to another early in the process. Pregnancy involves a year of care, and it should be with someone you like.

If you are going to a private physician, check out the cost of the *total* pregnancy at the first visit. Try to make sure that you are covered by your insurance *before* you become pregnant; many insurance companies will not cover a pregnancy which has already begun.

The actual medical care involved in a pregnancy may be routine, but the emotional care is not. Make sure the doctor or the clinic you are going to is interested *in you*. Are they pleasant? Do they ask how you are feeling? Do they answer your questions readily, or do you feel intimidated, too intimidated even to ask the questions you want to ask? If so, get yourself to another doctor or clinic. Accessibility is a vital barometer of prenatal care. Can you reach your doctor quickly? Is your doctor responsive, even when you call between visits? Are office or clinic hours convenient for you?

16. Nurse midwives are often excellent prenatal advisers for healthy women

A *nurse midwife* certified by the American College of Midwifery is very well trained to care for a normal pregnancy and delivery, and knows when to call in the doctor who supervises her when there is a problem. For healthy women, such a midwife is an excellent substitute for a physician. In many ways, she may be preferable—for she will frequently answer your questions about the minor discomforts of pregnancy more readily than the physician who may be much more interested in the abnormal than in the normal, run-of-the-mill event. *A nurse midwife must have physician backup;* you should make sure that she does and that the physician is available. In many communities nurse midwives and physicians practice together—an ideal situation.

17. If you plan natural childbirth and breast-feeding, choose your medical adviser accordingly

In the past, obstetricians have not received much training in dealing with women who wish to have their babies naturally and breast-feed. *So a nurse midwife may be a better adviser for you in this instance.*

However, since more and more women wish to have their babies this way, the medical schools, doctors and hospitals are bound to become more responsive in time.

18. Routine medical care during pregnancy

The first visit to the doctor or clinic should be made before the fourth month. The initial visit should include:

a. A complete medical history of the patient (and her family and forebears) and a complete physical examination

b. Pelvic exam

c. Blood pressure

d. Various blood tests: a test to determine blood count and detect anemia; a serologic test for syphilis; blood typing to determine whether the mother is RH-negative; a Pap test; a smear for gonorrhea; and an optional test for rubella (German measles). Jewish women should be tested for Tay-Sachs disease; black women for sickle-cell anemia. (See pp. 218–20)

Visits for a healthy woman without special problems are usually monthly thereafter, through the seventh month; every two weeks during the eighth month; every week during the ninth month.

Blood pressure is checked at each visit to detect any sign of pre-eclampsia (pre-eck-CLAMP-see-a—high blood pressure of pregnancy, see ✳155 below) which may also cause protein in the urine and swelling of the ankles. Urine will be checked at each visit for the presence of protein or sugar. Sugar may be a sign of diabetes (see ✳163 below). Weight will be checked. After about the twentieth week (sometimes earlier), the fetal heartbeat is audible; the new ultrasound devices now make for easy, exciting listening for mother as well as physician. The uterus will be measured with a tape measure or calipers to make sure that the growth is at a steady normal rate.

There should be time at every visit for the woman to ask questions and receive advice, especially on diet and nutrition. *Write down your questions beforehand so you don't forget to ask them.*

19. How much weight should you gain during pregnancy?

The consensus on this question seems to change every generation. Ten to twenty years ago, strict weight control was encouraged and smaller babies were delivered. Today, however, the general opinion holds that bigger babies are healthier and smarter, so optimal maternal weight gain is believed to be twenty-four to thirty pounds.

Essentially, a woman should watch her weight gain if she is fat to begin with, and worry less about it if she is thin to begin with. Excess weight gain may complicate the pregnancy, because it gives a woman a tendency toward hypertension, diabetes and general fatigue; it may complicate the delivery, by putting excess strain on her body in addition to the strain of the swollen uterus; and it may leave her with a weight problem postpartum. Too little weight gain may result in an overly small infant, more susceptible to ill health.

20. Diet during pregnancy

a. It is logical and normal for a woman to experience increased appetite during pregnancy (it is also normal for her not to).

b. A pregnancy diet should be exceedingly well balanced and nutritious; lots of vegetables are a must for vitamins. To satisfy the enormous protein needs of the growing fetus, eat milk, meat, fish, eggs, or dried beans in increased amounts. Milk and milk products like cheese and yogurt supply protein, carbohydrate, and calcium. (See p. 268)

Often, a woman's body will instruct her which foods to choose; a confirmed coffee drinker may find coffee intolerable during pregnancy; a woman who hardly ever touches cooked vegetables may find they are exactly what she wants above everything; a woman who has always loved citrus will find that oranges give her heartburn. Follow your instincts; *eat what makes you feel good; but keep your dietary choices within the realm of the nutritious.*

c. *Junk food is no good for you when you are not pregnant; when you are pregnant, it is no good for you and your baby.*

d. Vitamin supplements in moderation are helpful for pregnant women; excess supplies do you no good, and in the case of the fat-soluble vitamins (see p. 253) may actually prove dangerous.

e. In pregnancy folic acid supplementation is advisable.

f. Calcium supplements may be needed by women who are not getting the equivalent of a quart of milk per day.

g. The need for protein escalates greatly; about 70–80 g per day is suggested.

21. Women need extra iron during pregnancy

As the fetus produces blood cells and the woman's blood volume increases, the diet requires extra iron. An average diet contains 5–15 mg of iron and a pregnant woman must have 18 mg or more. Most obstetricians recommend iron supplements for all pregnant women; usually in the form of 300–600 mg of ferrous sulfate or ferrous gluconate per day. If a woman is anemic to begin with or if she has had a pregnancy within the last two years, more iron may be required. (See Anemia, p. 369) Even if a woman is not anemic, her bone-marrow stores of iron will become very low if extra iron is not given.

22. Don't go on a weight-reduction diet while you are pregnant

Whatever problems you may be having with your weight, don't try to solve them during pregnancy. Every nutritious thing you don't eat is being denied to the fetus as well, and the fetus is *not* overweight. A woman cannot in good conscience make her unborn child pay for her own dietary excesses before she becomes pregnant. So gain at least twenty to twenty-five pounds, and if that leaves you fat, diet after delivery.

23. Pica: outlandish food cravings during pregnancy

Some women develop fairly outlandish cravings for various foods during pregnancy—this is probably related to the signals transmitted from the gastrointestinal tract to the "appestat" (the appetite control center in the brain) and the sense of taste. When the foods you crave are healthy (pickles, ice cream), then you can indulge yourself. But some "unnatural" foods, frequently craved by pregnant women, are very dangerous to them and their unborn children: laundry starch, clay from the soil, ice scraped off the walls of the freezer compartment in the refrigerator, even kitchen cleansers. These substances irritate the stomach and can cause severe anemia. Avoid them at all costs.

24. What to wear during pregnancy

During pregnancy, women frequently perspire more heavily; therefore, choose comfortable, absorbent clothing and try to avoid synthetics. Wear comfortable shoes that give you support; high heels or clogs which distort the alignment of your spine or throw your body forward generally only contribute to any back discomfort you may have from the forward-pull of the baby. *For breast tenderness in early pregnancy* a slightly padded brassiere may help. *If you feel pressure in your lower back,* a girdle may help. Maternity shops carry special girdles that make room for the bulging baby but give extra support in the back. *If you feel excess pressure or experience swelling in your legs in late pregnancy,* take the pressure off by every device available—wear a pregnancy girdle; wear sturdy, low-heeled shoes; wear stockings or support hose and elevate your legs frequently. *Your breasts will enlarge gradually during the pregnancy.* Even if you don't normally wear a brassiere, you may find that you want one now. Make sure it isn't too tight *or* too flimsy; the breasts are filling up with milk in late pregnancy and need support. *If you plan to breast-feed your baby,* start wearing a nursing brassiere in your last month.

25. Loss of balance is common in late pregnancy

By the seventh month, a woman may be carrying around twenty pounds of extra weight, much of which is the body and environment of another human being. It is common under these circumstances to experience a loss of balance that is akin to but is not actually dizziness. A woman may, for example, take a step and find that the floor is not exactly where she expected it to be; she may sit down and find that the chair is actually higher, or lower, than she expected it to be. *This is normal.* Wear low shoes at this time, to minimize the chance of twisting an ankle and actually falling. Stick to a pattern of exercise in which loss of balance cannot result in injury. Make sure someone helps you in and out of the tub or shower in late pregnancy.

When riding in a car, do not place the seat belt across the fetus. The lap strap should be pulled across your pelvis *below* the fetus. Use the shoulder strap. This helps avoid injury to the fetus in case of an accident or sudden stop or sharp collision from the car behind you.

26. Exercise during pregnancy

Exercise is important during pregnancy for all women (unless specifically restricted for medical reasons): it improves circulation, and minimizes many ordinary discomforts, such as swelling of the legs and back pain due to pressure on weakened muscles. Sports which were standard before pregnancy should be continued as long as there is no danger of losing balance and falling in the later months.

Every pregnant woman should begin a program of exercise early in pregnancy, especially if she wasn't in good shape when she started. Try walking or swimming every day for thirty minutes, at least. Exercises given in natural childbirth classes are helpful, especially sit-ups and straight-leg raising with one knee bent to strengthen the abdominal muscles. Remember that the pull you feel when doing leg lowering exercises, for example, is *not* a pull on the fetus: it is a pull on the abdominal muscles, which will need to be strong for delivery.

27. Recommendation: Avoid douching during pregnancy

Unless your physician suggests that you douche for a specific reason, don't do it. The cervix is soft during pregnancy and sometimes a little bit open: douching could allow some water to pass through the cervix up into the uterus, if the nozzle were improperly placed, causing the bag of waters (the amniotic sac) to break prematurely, or causing infection. If douching is suggested, keep the bag low so that water pressure is not too great, do not insert the nozzle more than an inch or two into the vagina and do not hold the labia closed. (See p. 229)

28. Sexual intercourse is perfectly all right all through pregnancy

The old-fashioned practice of limiting intercourse after the seventh month is senselessly punitive to both man and woman, and in fact, drives them away from each other at a time when they need to be especially close.

For both partners, there are frequently many changes in sexual drive during pregnancy—on a psychologic and physiologic basis. During early pregnancy a woman may feel less interested in sex, especially if she is suffering from fatigue and other minor discomforts. (See ✷30 below) Interest in sex frequently increases during the middle three months, sometimes more than before the pregnancy. In late pregnancy, because of increasing discomfort, interest in coitus may decrease.

The pain of the episiotomy (see ✷96 below) may interfere with sex for several weeks postpartum. If a woman is breast-feeding, her vagina may be dry, with some resultant burning or pain during intercourse. Lubricating jelly can be used. In addition, the great emotional involvement which the mother has in the child after delivery may decrease her interest in sex temporarily. This should normally return after a few weeks.

A man may experience a wide range of sexual feelings during the pregnancy. He may unjustifiably fear injuring mother or baby during intercourse. He may not find the woman sexually attractive in late pregnancy, but this feeling should pass. Most men take great pride in their potency; and this makes them feel sexually even closer to the mother of the child.

Postpartum, both partners must make adjustments. A new human being is around, demanding a huge amount of attention, usually disturbing the parents' sleep. Both partners may feel quite exhausted for the first few weeks; therefore, sexual activity may decrease.

Certain adjustments in sexual technique will be necessary as the pregnancy advances. The male-superior position may become more uncomfortable than other positions. The man may find that he cannot thrust so deeply in later months, no matter what the position is. Many couples use alternate forms of sexual expression such as oral sex and mutual masturbation if intercourse isn't feasible.

If a woman is experiencing a leakage of fluid or bleeding during late pregnancy, she should avoid intercourse until she is examined by a physician.

29. Orgasm and premature labor

Some physicians believe that orgasm experienced by a woman in late pregnancy may initiate labor. This has not been proven conclusively and is not really a problem unless labor begins prematurely. A woman may wish to avoid orgasm in the last six to eight weeks of pregnancy if she has had premature deliveries in the past.

DISCOMFORTS OF PREGNANCY

30. Minor discomforts of pregnancy

These include:

a. Nausea and vomiting
b. Constipation
c. Increased salivation
d. Heartburn and belching
e. Increased heart rate
f. Nosebleeds
g. Light-headedness and dizziness
h. Varicose veins and hemorrhoids
i. Shortness of breath
j. Urinary frequency
k. Skin changes
l. Breast changes

m. Vaginal discharge

n. Mild abdominal pains and spotting

o. Orthopedic problems

p. Leg cramps and pains

q. Edema (swelling of ankles)

r. Insomnia

s. Eye problems

t. Psychological changes

All of the above are usually normal; easily anticipated; nothing at all to worry about. They can almost invariably be lived through without special medication.

Most pregnant women experience a couple of these discomforts. Some experience none at all. Even if you experience every single one, and feel absolutely miserable, *you can still assume that you and your baby are healthy.*

Medical treatment will do little to help the woman suffering the normal discomforts of pregnancy. The advice of other women will serve just as well. However, *if a symptom persists or worsens, seek a medical opinion to assure yourself that nothing serious is happening.*

31. Nausea and vomiting

Nausea and vomiting in pregnancy is probably a gastrointestinal reaction to hormonal changes. Although many women feel sick in the morning, many will feel sick at any time of day. Usually, the condition starts about the fifth week of gestation and ends by the twelfth week; but some women experience it (and are still healthy) throughout the pregnancy.

Treatments to try include:

a. Sipping carbonated soda

b. Nibbling a dry cracker or a piece of dry toast

c. Eating frequent small meals

Nausea occurs most often with an empty stomach (that's why it occurs so frequently in the morning). So keep crackers in your purse for munching on during the business day, or in other circumstances where you're far from a pantry. The cracker works often because it absorbs the saliva and thereby rids the palate of the nauseating taste. Avoid dreadful odors that make you feel sick.

Nausea may be related to the taste in your mouth. Some women find that it is relieved by a morsel of sharp taste-changing food: a strong peppermint or a stick of cinnamon.

Some physicians believe that nausea and vomiting come from vitamin B-6 deficiency. If you are vomiting all the time and losing weight, medications must be used if natural remedies have failed. (Also see Pernicious Vomiting, ⚹149 below)

32. Constipation

Constipation is very common, especially in later pregnancy, when the swelling uterus presses on the descending colon. It may also be related to decreased muscle tone in the intestinal tract due to high hormone levels. It is also a major side effect of the iron pills often prescribed.

Try adding fresh fruits, bulky vegetables, and bran to the diet; drink more fluids. If all this doesn't work, try bulk stool softeners such as psyllium seed or cellulose. Do not expect a bowel movement every day, even when you are not pregnant. Constipation occurs when stools are hard and when you have been unable to move your bowels for *several* days. Once a woman has moved her bowels and broken the cycle of constipation, she should attempt to defecate without additional aid as always, while adjusting diet appropriately.

If the iron pills you are taking cause constipation, switch to another type which contain stool softeners.

Avoid laxatives. Stool softeners are much better. If you *must* have a laxative, use milk of magnesia. Mineral oil may inhibit absorption of vitamins from the intestinal tract, and other laxatives contain substances which have not been proven safe for use in pregnancy. (See p. 242)

33. Increase in salivation

Women who are severely affected find they must carry tissue and spit frequently. Increased salivation often accompanies other digestive problems of pregnancy. No treatment is effective; delivery ends the problem.

34. Heartburn and belching

Heartburn and belching, extremely common effects of pregnancy, are caused by the lessening capacity of the cramped stomach to hold down food. Increased pressure on the abdomen as the fetus grows leads to a kind of backup of the stomach juices into the lower part of the esophagus (e-SOFF-a-gus), the muscular tube leading from the throat to the stomach, with concurrent irritation from the acid. The causes of heartburn are related to those that cause nausea: the food you eat does not pass smoothly into the lower stomach; you taste it long after you have eaten it; you may experience a rising bitterness in your throat, a feeling that you have incompletely digested what you have just eaten. Certain foods may increase heartburn: coffee, citrus fruits, vegetables like cabbage and squash. Avoid the particular foods that seem related to the problem; try the same treatments recommended for nausea (see ※31 above); try over-the-counter antacids; don't lie down after eating because this will further hamper digestion. Some women find it possible to "walk off" heartburn.

35. Dental problems

Pregnancy in itself does not trigger increased tooth decay, but it is important that routine dental care continue during pregnancy. The old taboo against dental care and extractions during pregnancy is no longer medically valid. If X rays are absolutely needed, the abdomen can be shielded to protect the fetus. However, (*warning!*) *do not have major dental work requiring general anesthesia during pregnancy.* The work should be done under local anesthesia, because the risks of general anesthesia involve decreasing the oxygen supply to the fetus.

Two conditions of the gums seem to be peculiar to pregnancy.

a. *Gingivitis* (jin-ji-VY-tis), an inflammation of the gums, is common in non-pregnant women as well, but one particular type gets much worse during pregnancy and then dramatically subsides after delivery.

b. Small *"pregnancy tumors"* may grow on the gums during pregnancy; they are benign, but should be removed by the dentist (novacaine is sufficient anesthesia) because they will probably grow again during the next pregnancy. The "pregnancy tumor" looks like a small red polyp on the gum, and is related to gingivitis.

36. The volume of blood in a woman's cardiovascular system grows steadily throughout pregnancy, causing several minor side effects

By the time a woman is nine months pregnant, the volume of blood in her body is about 1½ times that of her normal non-pregnant state. This occurs in response to the nutritional requirements of the fetus. The increased blood volume may cause accelerated heart rate and/or nose bleeds. These are *minor* side effects—uncomfortable, but no danger to general health.

37. Increased heart rate

To pump the greater volume of blood, the heart must beat faster, and occasionally, this will cause palpitations—a feeling that the heart is racing. Anemia, a deficiency of red blood cells, aggravates palpitations. Iron is an important dietary supplement to avoid this side effect. (See ※150 below)

38. Nosebleeds

Nosebleeds are common during pregnancy because the increased volume of blood makes the little blood vessels in the nose break more easily. The high hormone levels in pregnancy may also have this effect. The nose bleeds are nothing to worry about and will usually stop of their own accord, in a few minutes.

39. Light-headedness and dizziness

"Postural hypotension" is the name given to the dizziness that pregnant women sometimes experience when they change their position suddenly—get up quickly; sit down quickly. It is probably related to a momentary lag in circulation, when the large uterus presses on the vena cava (the major abdominal vein) and the larger volume of blood is trapped below the waist, unable for a second or two to get to the brain. As a result, a woman may feel dizzy—or experience a stabbing headache that disappears almost immediately. *This is nothing to worry about.* Lie down on your left side, so the blood supply can even out through your body; then get up again, slowly. Postural hypotension is one major reason that many ordinarily athletic women find it hard to continue active sports later in pregnancy. If this happens to you, substitute slower, more controlled exercise like calisthenics or yoga. If a woman actually faints, she should be examined by a doctor. But this may also be due just to changes in circulation.

40. Varicose veins and hemorrhoids

As pregnancy progresses, women may notice that the veins of their hands and arms as well as the legs become more prominent. This is caused in general by increased blood volume. Because there is greater pressure on the body's lower area, varicose veins of the legs are a very common complaint at this time, as are hemorrhoids—varicose veins of the anus. "Varicose" implies that the veins have stretched and expanded abnormally. Take care to wear supportive clothing and hose for varicose veins, and avoid constipation which will aggravate hemorrhoids. (See p. 384)

Varicose veins may also appear on the vulva or the labia majora, the large outer lips of the vagina. These can be very uncomfortable. Alleviate the pressure that causes them by wearing special elastic panties, available from maternity shops and hospital-supply stores.

41. Shortness of breath

In late pregnancy, the growing fetus may push the diaphragm (the major breathing muscle) upward, causing pressure on the lungs and shortness of breath. There is little to be done about this except to coddle it—lie down on your side with your head elevated so that the weight of the baby falls away from the diaphragm. The symptom will disappear in very late pregnancy, when the baby drops in preparation for birth.

Women who report shortness of breath in *early* pregnancy are probably responding to the increased fetal need for oxygen. Sit down; breathe deeply. WARNING: If shortness of breath occurs at night or is persistent or severe, consult your physician.

42. Urinary frequency

In the first three months, urinary frequency is so common a complaint that it can be taken as a *sign* of pregnancy. It is caused by pressure of the uterus on the bladder. *It requires no treatment. Do not limit intake of liquids—these keep the bowel functioning well:* just stay within range of a bathroom. The symptom may be alleviated in the middle months and may reappear in late pregnancy, when the baby's head —in preparation for birth—sinks down and puts new pressure on the bladder. WARNING: If frequency is accompanied by pain or fever, this may be a sign of kidney or bladder infection. (See p. 316) See a doctor.

43. Increased skin pigmentation and chloasma

It is quite common for a dark pigment to be deposited around the nipples, in the genital region and/or in a straight line down the middle of the abdomen during pregnancy. Some women will be annoyed by a brownish discoloration over the face, called chloasma (klo-AZ-ma) or the mask of pregnancy. These changes occur because the pituitary is producing higher levels of melanocyte stimulating hormone, which spurs the growth of cells containing *melanin* (MEL-a-nin), a skin pigment. Exposure to sun aggravates these changes. There is nothing to be done about them; they are almost never very serious; and usually, when the pregnancy is over, they remain, although they may fade a good deal. Oral contraceptives cause the same problem in some women. (See pp. 46–47)

44. Stretch marks

Overweight people, or people who have been overweight and have reduced, sometimes acquire stretch marks, watery-looking striations. Very often, in men, they appear on the upper arm; in women, on arms, hips and breasts. During pregnancy, a woman may experience stretch marks on her breasts and abdomen.

There are two theories of causation. First, the enlargement of the breasts and abdomen may cause the skin tissues to tear, the marks may indicate where the tissue separated. Second, high levels of adrenal hormones during pregnancy may cause these skin changes. (They also appear in people with adrenal disease.)

Often the marks are bright pink in color: they may appear in the fifth and sixth months of pregnancy, when the general weight gain begins to wear on the body and will often fade to white after delivery. Home remedies, such as application of cocoa butter and olive oil, generally are not harmful but not effective either. *It may help more to keep body weight under control before and after delivery, and to exercise to firm up the fleshy areas.*

45. Increased perspiration and body odor

This is perfectly natural for the pregnant woman. Use normal hygiene—frequent bathing, deodorants if you feel the need; absorbent, cotton clothes.

46. Changes in hair distribution and quality

Hormonal changes may cause some increase in facial and abdominal hair, some hair loss around the temples and throughout the head. Hair that held a curl well before pregnancy may straighten out and become limp and resistant to any amount of dressing. After delivery, hair will return to normal. WARNING: *Avoid coloring your hair during pregnancy.* Although it is unlikely, you may be allergic to chemicals in the hair color that never affected you at all before. (See p. 234)

47. Itching and dryness of the skin

During pregnancy, the skin of the abdomen is severely stretched and may become dry and itchy as a result, especially over the hip bones and belly. Frequent bathing, to control increased perspiration, may aggravate the dryness. Most women find that oil or a dry-skin cream (*not a hormone cream!*) applied to affected areas controls the problem.

Very severe itching and dryness may indicate that liver functions are changing in reaction to the increased estrogen levels of pregnancy; it will end with delivery, but should be reported to your physician so that liver problems can be ruled out.

48. Breast changes

Early in pregnancy, the nipples may be very sore and the breasts very tender. This usually stops by the third or fourth month, as the body adjusts to the new hormone levels. Expect your breasts to enlarge continually through to term. Small amounts of watery fluid leak from time to time. The little bumps around the areole (dark area), called Montgomery Tubercles, will also tend to enlarge and occasionally drain. All this is normal and nothing to worry about.

49. Vaginal discharge

As hormone levels increase during pregnancy, a woman normally experiences increased vaginal discharge, generally watery, whitish in color, not foul-smelling and not irritating to the vulva. (If these latter signs occur, suspect vaginal infection, and have yourself checked.) Don't be alarmed if your underwear seems rather wet all the time; cotton underpants are recommended for their absorbency. Vaginal infections, with the exception of moniliasis (see p. 302) do not increase unduly during pregnancy.

50. Abdominal pains, cramps, and spotting

Throughout her pregnancy, a woman may experience a multitude of various aches and pains which suggest nothing except the reaction of her body to the demands of housing a different body within her. Sometimes, in early pregnancy, a woman may feel cramps that would normally make her think she was about to get her period. When the uterus grows out of the pelvis, this usually stops. If bleeding accompanies the cramps, that may be a sign of something more serious.

Bleeding is very common in early pregnancy. A day or two of spotting with a small amount of cramping may occur at the time of implantation of the conceptus into the endometrium (about a week earlier than the normal menstrual period). Between 20 and 25 per cent of the women who carry to term report bleeding during the first three months. Only rarely is the bleeding as heavy as that of a normal period, although if a woman has lost track of her menstrual schedule, the bleeding can confuse her sufficiently so that she actually doesn't realize she is pregnant. Off and on bleeding or spotting during the first three months is usually nothing to worry about; if it is continuing or heavy, or accompanied by severe pain, it probably constitutes the beginnings of a spontaneous abortion (or miscarriage) and should take a woman to her physician immediately. (See ⚹121 below)

Later in pregnancy, gas pains are frequent and often severe. They can usually be relieved by a diet heavy on fruit, bran, and other whole grain cereals; to prevent constipation, avoid gas-producing foods.

Between four and six months, a woman may experience sharp, distinct pains in the lower abdomen or on either side of the uterus, especially when she changes position and the uterus moves. These are *round ligament* pains: the round ligaments attach the uterus on each side to the pelvis, and when they are stretched and the uterus moves, there is a corresponding pain on the pulled side. This is to be considered a normal abdominal pain.

In the second half of pregnancy, the baby itself is moving. If the baby kicks and hits a woman's liver, she will feel a very sharp pain. It will not persist, but it may recur, and nothing can relieve it except possibly a change of position and ultimately the delivery of the baby.

Abnormal abdominal pain during pregnancy has these features:

a. it persists for hours;

b. it is unrelieved by a change in position that allows the uterus to move;

c. it is unrelieved by a bowel movement.

d. If the uterus is tender *to the touch,* that is abnormal. The organ itself should not be hurting.

e. If fever or bleeding accompanies the pain, that is not normal and medical attention should be sought.

51. How a moving baby feels

Nothing can be told about a fetus from the way it moves. Some seem to be slumbering in the womb, and occasionally stir a little; some seem to be wrestling with the womb—a woman's stomach can actually be seen moving suddenly and violently this way and that way—it bulges and bumps and has, again literally, a life of its own.

WARNING: *Do not take anything to calm the baby down;* and do not be offended if people seem to be staring at your stomach. Old Wives' Tales (OWTs) that predict the sex and/or personality of the child from the way it moves in the womb are all nonsense; movements in the womb are quite involuntary, and sex and personality were meant to be surprises.

In late pregnancy the baby gradually moves less because the space becomes more cramped. A sudden cessation of movement should send you to your doctor, who can listen to the baby's heart, or perform a stress test (see ✗180 below) to see if the fetus and placenta are well.

52. Backache

This can be a nagging problem, especially in late pregnancy, and is due to the change in posture created by the pull of the growing child. Many women tend to arch their backs and lean backward to counter the forward pull of the abdomen. *Backache can be largely prevented* by a program of exercise begun in early pregnancy—sit-ups and leg-raising exercises strengthen the abdominal muscles so that they are better equipped to carry the weight of the baby and take the pressure off the back. A pregnancy girdle can help. (See References for information on exercises.)

53. Relaxation of the pelvic joints

In some women, the sacroiliac and the pubic joints relax excessively during pregnancy, causing backache and a nagging ache in the pubic area that can become very aggravating if you stand on your feet too long. The problem, if it occurs, usually starts in the seventh month. A pregnancy girdle is helpful, but sometimes nothing will help except resting and putting your feet up.

If these symptoms are so severe as to be crippling, ask your doctor for referral to an orthopedic specialist.

54. Problems with the joints of the legs and hips

In late pregnancy, when the weight buildup is relatively great and loss of balance (see ⚹25 above) can distort a woman's sense of just how and where her legs are carrying her, there may be pain in the hips or knees. Occasionally, the knee joints may give out—the leg will just collapse. This is not a problem unless a woman is injured herself in the fall. Try to walk with someone when you get really big; make sure you've got something, or someone, to hold onto when you get in and out of the bathtub.

55. Women with pre-existing orthopedic problems should take special care when they are pregnant

Some orthopedic problems, such as *scoliosis*—a congenital twisting of the spine—are aggravated by pregnancy. If a woman has a weak back, weak hips or legs, she should consult with her orthopedist before she becomes pregnant, and allot a great deal of time during the pregnancy to lying and sitting down, or to physical therapy if indicated.

In the case of arthritis, pregnancy can be a blessing as well as a danger: the increased weight that must be borne by the inflamed joint may make the condition more painful; on the other hand, the higher hormone levels of pregnancy may relieve the pain considerably. *No woman with a chronic disease should become pregnant without fully understanding the conditions and complications that might surround the pregnancy and delivery.* (See High-risk Pregnancy ⚹162 below)

56. Leg cramps

In the second half of pregnancy, severe muscle spasms (cramps) in the calf muscles of the legs are very common. Some say this is caused by too much calcium; others say too little. Diuretics—substances which some pregnant women take to prevent water buildup and edema —may cause potassium loss and resulting cramps. If you must take diuretics, make sure potassium loss is not a side effect; adjust your diet and vitamin supplements; drink lots of orange juice and eat bananas— both are rich in potassium.

Frequently, leg cramps occur at night. Try these treatments: pull the toes up forcefully with the leg extended straight; this will stretch the muscle that is in spasm and help relax it. Or have someone massage the muscle very briskly. Or place a pillow at the foot of the bed at night to prevent the legs from straightening out completely during sleep.

57. Pinched nerves and numbness in the legs

Toward the end of pregnancy, as the uterus enlarges, and the head of the baby settles into the pelvis, the nerves of the upper legs may be pinched by the pressure. In some women this causes numbness in the legs; in other women, the simple act of walking may complicate the pressure and cause pinching of the nerves in the thigh. Shake your leg; change position; get off your feet. The pinching will probably stop after delivery.

58. Edema (swelling) of the feet and ankles is extremely common in late pregnancy

It is a rare woman who gets through a pregnancy without experiencing (ed-EE-ma) of the feet and ankles, usually most pronounced at the end of the day. It is primarily due to increased pressure on the veins of the legs because of slowed circulation as the blood must flow around the enlarged uterus: some fluid that is normally cleared just stays in the lower extremities.

Varicose veins aggravate the problem. Tight garters, excessive salt intake (salt causes water retention), and a lot of standing during the day, will also aggravate the edema.

Try elevating your feet often. Whenever you sit down, put your feet up, on a stool, another chair, whatever is handy. Do not cut down on salt intake too much, because this will lead to sodium deficiency, which is not good for the pregnancy. Cut down a little but *do not use salt substitutes routinely*. If you have varicose veins or must be on your feet continually, wear elastic stockings, and *always* avoid garters. WARNING: If edema spreads to the hands and face and is as bad in the morning as it is at night, this may be a sign of toxemia. (See ⚹155 below) Have your blood pressure and urine protein checked.

Diuretics should not be prescribed for uncomplicated edema of pregnancy. They may be dangerous to the fetus.

59. Headache and fatigue

These two complaints are almost universal among pregnant women, especially in the first and last trimesters. Fatigue is due to the extra metabolic needs of the baby and the sheer weight of the pregnancy. Rest when you need to.

Headaches are generally mild.

WARNING: *Do not take anything for them if possible until the fourth month, and then, take only acetaminophen or mild pain-killers.*

Avoid aspirin in the last three months because excess aspirin intake has been associated with bleeding tendencies in babies.

60. Insomnia

In late pregnancy, it is sometimes very difficult to find any comfortable position in which to sleep. A woman may have to be satisfied with napping for short periods during the day; if she has been sleepless the night before, her household will just have to adjust to her irritation and fatigue the day after. WARNING: *Do not take any sedatives in early pregnancy. This includes over-the-counter drugs.* Avoid any but the mildest sedatives recommended only by your physician in late pregnancy, and use them only if you are wild from sleeplessness, and have tried every sleeping position, including sitting up in a chair, with your feet elevated, and lying on your *left* side (this position allows for maximized blood flow to the fetus by avoiding pressure on the vena cava by the uterus).

61. Eye problems

Some women experience relatively great changes in their eyes during pregnancy; it is not clear why. If at all possible, do not invest in new glasses while you are pregnant, because you will probably need your old ones back again right after you deliver the baby.

62. Psychologic changes

Hormones have enormous influence on the mood of the individual, and a pregnant woman is undergoing an *upheaval* in hormone levels.

Anticipate mood changes; don't attach too much importance to them; make sure those around you are likewise prepared. Remember: you are just as likely to feel elated as you are to feel depressed.

a. *The emotional circumstances under which a woman becomes pregnant in the first place have as much to do with her mood as hormone levels.* If she wants the baby and cares about the father, she is likely to have a happier time being pregnant than if she is having her fourth or fifth child, accidently conceived by a man she no longer likes.

b. *Depression is frequent during pregnancy. Never medicate it without medical advice.* It is absolutely normal when you have been throwing up and running to the bathroom every half hour, to feel furious with the man who got you into this predicament, and also very down about life in general. If your depression is severe and unceasing, seek reliable professional help.

c. *If this is your first child, it is natural to fear the pain of labor.* Don't talk to older women about this, talk to your contemporaries, to women at your clinic, discuss pain relievers with your obstetrician, and attend childbirth classes. (See ✂69 below)

d. *If you are worried about genetic defects in the child, try to think things through carefully. Unless there is a specific genetic disease in your family, you have a greater than 95 per cent chance of bearing a perfectly normal child once past the third month of pregnancy.* Many familial diseases can now be detected by amniocentesis. (See p. 216) If you are over thirty-five, you should ask for genetic counseling and amniocentesis.

e. *The last thing a pregnant women needs is an internal crisis about the loss of her looks. So before you become pregnant, make peace with the fact that you will soon lose your shape.* Aside from your waistline, there is no reason to believe that you will lose any feature that makes you attractive. In fact, most pregnant women look better in many ways. Your skin may have more tone, your mood may be *better,* and the father of your child may think you are more wonderful than ever before. Few women bulging with child can get through their pregnancy without feeling their vanity assaulted. But now is not the time to be vain. Now is the time to be healthy.

f. *Dependency on the obstetrician* is a common phenomenon among pregnant women and certainly is encouraged to varying degrees by doctors who, like most people, love to be loved. It happens mainly to women who mistakenly discount their own ability to control their situation.

Remember, in the majority of cases, the presence or absence of your particular doctor is not critical to the outcome of the delivery. *You* are having the baby and the most important determinant of successful delivery is generally your health and preparedness—not a particular physician's skills. Of course, in case of emergency, the doctor's skill is important, but most deliveries do not end in emergencies.

g. *Changes in libido*—sexual responsiveness and desire—often occur during pregnancy. (See ✂28 above)

NORMAL LABOR AND DELIVERY

63. Labor and delivery

Most women can expect normal labor and delivery. Don't expect emergencies or complications, but provide for them in the back of your mind and in your plans for where you are having your baby.

64. Preliminary contractions and "false labor"

Small uterine contractions occur from time to time throughout pregnancy; they are not usually painful or even noticeable. In the last month or two, many women begin to *feel* preliminary contractions which are sometimes so strong that they are hard to differentiate from true labor. These Braxton Hicks contractions (named for John Braxton Hicks, the English gynecologist who discovered them) are more prominent in women who have had children already. Probably they help to soften the cervix and stretch it for labor. Try not to feel too disappointed if the labor you thought you were having turns out to be false. The real thing will start soon enough.

65. Lightening: engagement of the baby's head in the lower pelvis

Lightening occurs typically about two weeks before labor, *in women having their first child.* Suddenly, the baby seems to drop; a woman will feel less pressure under her heart; she will be able to breathe better; she will feel "lighter," and will also experience urinary urgency, for the baby has now pushed its head between the bones of the pelvis and is probably pressing on the bladder too.

Lightening is a good sign. First, it signals that the pregnancy (which may feel by now as though it has lasted ten years) is soon to be over. Second, it signals that the pelvis is probably wide enough for the baby to get through. Observers may notice that the baby is pushing the stomach outward in more pronounced fashion.

If lightening doesn't happen, there is nothing to worry about; it will usually occur closer to actual labor. *Women who have previously borne children should not expect it.*

66. Bloody show and loss of the mucus plug

For some weeks prior to labor, the cervix is effacing (thinning) and dilating (stretching). A few days before labor, there may be a little bleeding and/or loss of the plug of mucus that has served as a cervical barrier throughout the pregnancy. This may happen naturally, or it may be brought on by a pelvic examination close to term, or it may not happen at all. Bleeding, if it does occur, may be only a tiny spot or as much as can be trapped on one sanitary napkin. If there is more, notify your doctor right away.

67. Rupture of the membranes

The rupture of the membranes and escape of the amniotic fluid may occur as an immediate prelude to labor, which will begin right away or in a few hours. Most women do not experience it until labor is in progress.

But some women who haven't had a labor pain yet will suddenly experience the gushing release of the fluid. This may feel like a constant slow leak or it will come pouring down your legs in a relatively heavy stream. Call your medical advisers and go to the hospital.

Labor should start within twelve hours after the rupture of the amniotic sac. If it does not, labor should be induced, because once the membranes have broken, there is some danger of infection. Do not wait at home alone for labor to start; by doing so, you are running unnecessary risks. Temperature and heart tones must be monitored. If the fetus is not term size when the membranes burst, then the birth may be more complicated. (See ✗138 below)

68. Labor

There are two points of view in the labor and delivery rooms: that of the woman giving birth, and that of the medical people attending her. They *see* the labor; she *feels* it.

a. Medical people observe a birth by palpating the cervix and measuring the stages of labor by its *dilation*—the widening of the opening of the cervix—and its *effacement*—the thinning of the cervical wall as it stretches. As labor continues, the cervix becomes progressively wider, until it is wide enough to allow the infant through.

To a doctor, or midwife, the stages of labor look like this:

Stage 1-A: Called *the latent phase,* this is the first half of the first stage of labor. The cervix is dilating rather slowly, and the woman says that her contractions are rather far apart. When the cervix is 5–6 centimeters dilated, the first half of the first stage is ending.

Stage 1-B: The second part of the first stage usually starts when the cervix has opened to about five to six centimeters width. This is actually the shorter part of the first stage, and is called *the dilation (or accelerated) phase.*

The first stage in its entirety can last a variable length of time: sometimes more than twenty-four hours, sometimes only an hour.

Stage 2: The second stage starts when the cervix has dilated completely, and lasts until the baby is delivered. It should not last more than two to three hours (see below).

b. Many medical people will say that "true" labor only starts when the cervix begins to dilate at a steady rate. Women, however, tend to measure labor from the first pain to the last; thus, the process may seem much longer to a woman than it does to those attending her.

To the woman, the stages of labor feel like this:

Stage 1: She feels distinct, separate cramps which at first feel the same as the occasional Braxton Hicks contractions she may have had before. (See ⚥64). They may start in the back and pass around to the front of the abdomen. (The difference from the Braxton Hicks contractions is that contractions of labor gradually become more regular and last longer. They may start at thirty minutes apart, but then a pattern develops and they get closer and closer together.)

By the time the contractions are five to seven minutes apart, you should be on your way to the place where you are having your baby. (Start out earlier, or later, depending on how many children you've had and how far you live from the hospital. Discuss this with your doctor ahead of time.)

A labor pain is caused by the movement of the uterus, as it contracts to help push the baby toward the birth canal. In the latent phase of labor (Phase 1-A, above) these contractions are relatively weak, and the pain should be relatively easy to take. Depending on a woman's personal pain threshold and the particular circumstances of her labor, the pain may be bad or not—but there is time between the contractions to recover from one and prepare for the next.

Stage 2 has three parts: dilation, transition, expulsion.

During dilation, the contractions are three to five minutes apart and becoming more forceful. Most of the work in dilating the cervix is done at this time.

During transition, the cervix reaches 8–9 cm of dilation, the contractions begin to come very close together and the woman may feel severe pressure on her rectum and an urge to push, although it is too early to do so. (See ⚥70). This is the most difficult part of labor because the contractions are so close together that it is almost impossible to recover from one before another starts. Luckily, it doesn't last too long.

During expulsion, observers report that the cervix is completely dilated, and the woman can push with her contractions; this is a great relief; it means the end is near; the pain is about to be over; many women report a kind of euphoric feeling.

Don't every imagine that you should have your baby alone!

Both points of view are needed if a birth is to be handled properly. A woman who is trying to deal with the labor needs another voice besides the voice of her own nervous system to reassure her; the physician, midwife, or husband trying to assist her delivery needs to be told by the woman how she feels, how bad the pain is, how frequently it is coming. There should be a lot of communication in the labor room and the delivery room.

Pain, of course, is relative. Some women will swear they had an easy time in labor; some will say afterward that it was absolutely dreadful. No woman can really know what her labor will be like, even if she has had children already. Assume then that labor will be hard (it may surprise you and be easy); prepare for it by exercising regularly during pregnancy; seek instruction from groups that will teach you breathing exercises, which are *extremely helpful* in ameliorating labor pains. And when you are in labor, keep your mind firmly fixed on one idea—that the stronger the pain is, the closer you probably are to giving birth to your baby.

69. Where to seek training for labor

Both the Lamaze* method group and the Childbirth Education Association in your locality will provide information and training for both mother and father to prepare for childbirth. Many hospital prenatal clinics and departments of obstetrics and gynecology provide their maternity patients with exercise and training classes too. You will probably be able to avail yourself of these services at little or no cost. Even if you are not planning to go through labor without anesthesia, these classes will improve your muscle tone, help eradicate anxiety about labor and teach you invaluable aids for dealing with the pain of labor.

70. When to "push" during labor

By the time the cervix is dilated 8–9 cm, the emerging baby will be pressing, quite often, on the rectum, and the woman will feel a strong urge to push as though she were defecating. This is what makes transition, the stage immediately before expulsion and birth, so difficult. Resist the urge and listen to the advice of your medical attendants. If you start pushing too soon, before the cervix is completely dilated, you may cause it to tear and complicate the delivery. Wait until the people with you say the cervix is completely dilated. *Then* push or bear down along with the contractions. Since there is usually extreme rectal pressure at this point, you probably wouldn't be able to resist pushing even if you wanted to. For a lot of women, the signal that the cervix is sufficiently dilated for them to bear down is a joyous moment. When you can push with the contractions, a lot of the pain may be relieved. Some women experience a feeling at this juncture akin to orgasm. Whatever your physical reaction, you know now, the labor is about to end—and that's enough to make anybody happy. Childbirth classes and books on natural childbirth (see References) will give a woman a good idea of efficient methods of pushing.

* The Lamaze method is named for a French obstetrician who developed it for use among working-class people who could not expect to have anesthesia during childbirth.

71. Try not to lie flat on your back during labor

Blood flow to the uterus is best if you lie on your left side, and this strengthens contractions. Many women find that if they sit up, the pains are easier. If your pains are far apart, try walking around between them. Good circulation is vital to the labor process.

72. Yelling does not strengthen contractions

Some women believe that if you yell during a labor pain, the contraction is stronger and labor progresses more quickly. This is an Old Wives' Tale (OWT). If you need to cry out during labor, go ahead; but don't make a philosophy of it. It may waste your strength, diverts the people around you from their job, which is to watch over the delivery, and won't do anything at all for your contraction.

73. Episiotomy

An episiotomy (eh-PEEZ-ee-otomy) is an incision in the bottom of the vagina, made at the time of the delivery of the head of the baby, to give it more room to get through. At best, it prevents *random* tearing of the vagina and the rectum by the emerging baby; at worst, it is unnecessary. If your physician thinks it is necessary, he or she should *tell* you on the spot; it is no fun to be surprised by a surgical incision, with stitches, that may hurt a lot after you've given birth. The stitches will absorb. (See #96 below) Episiotomies *may* be overused in this country. *Make sure* that your physician does not expect to do one on you as a matter of routine, but only if the birth requires it. Women who have had children before are much less likely to need an episotomy than those who are delivering for the first time.

74. Delivery of the placenta, or "after-birth"—Stage 3

About three to five minutes after the baby is delivered, the placenta will follow, usually painlessly. The woman feels her uterus contract, and she can push the placenta out. The physician will inspect the placenta to make sure that no pieces have been left behind in the uterus to cause excess bleeding.

75. Contraction of the uterus after delivery

The uterus will begin to contract naturally after delivery, shrinking back to a size it has not been for many months. This causes minor "after-birth" pains for a few days. To help the uterus shrink, many women may receive a shot of Pitocin or ergonovine. If the infant nurses immediately at the breast, this will help contract the uterus as well. The uterus is back to normal size by six weeks after delivery.

ANESTHESIA FOR DELIVERY

76. Many women prefer to have some anesthetic during labor

Natural childbirth is much praised in our time, and for many women, it is manageable. However, if you happen to feel the need during your labor, remember that there are a number of analgesics and anesthetics which can ease your pain and still not interfere with the baby's well-being or your own enjoyment of the birth. *If you find you cannot go through childbirth totally unsedated, don't feel ashamed or guilty.* Your pain threshold is yours alone, and only you know what you are going through. Don't stand for your partner (who feels expert since he came along to all your natural childbirth classes) saying, "Your friend Millicent had natural childbirth; what's the matter with *you?*" There's nothing the matter with you. There is something the matter with people who think all women are alike.

77. Pain relief during labor

a. *Recommendation: General anesthetics should not be used during a normal delivery.* First, when a woman is asleep, she cannot push when she needs to and otherwise help her labor along. Second, general anesthesia puts the baby to sleep too, may depress her breathing after birth, or slow down her heart rate, decreasing the oxygen supply to the brain during birth. Third, a sleeping baby and a sleeping woman can prolong labor unnecessarily, increasing the risk of unnecessary complications, requiring the use of unnecessary outside aids, such as forceps. Finally, if you are asleep when the baby is born, you are cutting yourself off from one of life's more indescribable joys. (General anesthesia should be reserved for emergencies.)

b. *Analgesics:* Early in the first phase of labor, a woman who needs pain relief can receive a narcotic and/or tranquilizer by injection or intravenously. This makes it possible to relax or even doze off between contractions without actually going to sleep. Too much sedation can lengthen the latent phase, so bear with the early labor if possible. If given too close to the time of delivery, narcotics may cause a baby to have a low Apgar score. (See ✂91 below)

c. *Epidural anesthesia* (eh-pee-DUR-ril) is an option for a woman entering the active (dilation) phase of labor. (Stage 1-B, ✂68 above) A needle is inserted into her back, *near the spinal canal but not into it.* Then a small plastic catheter is inserted into the epidural space, and the anesthetic is injected through it. It will make a woman feel numb from the waist down and should almost completely relieve the pain of labor and delivery. Epidural anesthesia should not be confused with a spinal block, in which anesthetic is injected into the fluid of the spine, causing a temporary paralysis. With epidural anesthetic, a woman can usually still move.

Epidural anesthesia is a technique which requires a lot of training. Some obstetricians can handle it, but in most places, an anesthesiologist will be needed. When the anesthetic is being given, great care must be taken that the catheter is not inserted in the spinal fluid; for this reason, a test dose is inserted first, to make sure the right area has been located.

WARNING: *The anesthetics injected through the catheter are in the Novocain family, so if you know from your experience with the dentist that you are allergic to Novocain, tell your doctor first; a substitute anesthetic material can be found.*

As the lower extremities become numb, blood pressure may decrease. To guard against this possibility, a woman will have fluid running intravenously into her arm throughout the procedure, maintaining volume in her blood vessels.

One relatively frequent problem with epidural anesthesia is a definite increase in the number of patients who require forceps delivery; lacking feeling below the waist, they can't bear down and push the baby out as well. Episiotomy is also more frequently needed with epidural anesthetic. A woman should remember that even though she will feel no pain, she will feel a pulling sensation when the baby is delivered.

(A non-medical problem of epidural and other anesthesia is that many insurance policies do not fully cover anesthesiologists' fees. Check this out beforehand.)

d. *Caudal anesthesia* is essentially the same as epidural anesthesia, except that it is administered lower in the back, in the region of the tailbone.

e. *Nitrous oxide gas* can be given to a woman in light doses in the second stage of labor, to lessen the pain without putting her out. This is given by an anesthesiologist who places a mask periodically over the woman's mouth and nose.

f. *Saddle block* is an injection of anesthetic into the spinal canal which numbs only those areas of the pelvis that would touch the saddle if you were riding a horse. It is usually given when a woman goes out of the labor room into the delivery room. Low blood pressure is a risk here as well, and intravenous fluid must be used to prevent it.

g. *Paracervical block, a questionable technique.* As delivery approaches and the pain worsens, the cervix can be injected with local anesthetic. (This technique is also often used during abortion or D & C.

(See p. 196) Relief is almost instantaneous and lasts for about an hour. The overall safety of this method for use in labor is currently being debated. There have been reports of excess anesthetic being absorbed by the fetus, causing changes in fetal heart rate and other problems. Therefore, paracervical block should only be considered if other methods are not available. (There does not seem to be any similar safety issue when it is used for abortion.)

h. *Pudendal block* (poo-DEN-dal): The pudendal nerve supplies sensation to the perineum (per-ee-NEE-um), the area around the vagina and the vulva. A pudendal block is a series of two injections given just prior to delivery, just inside the vagina into the pudendal nerve on each side. This numbs the lower third of the vagina and the external genitals. For forceps deliveries and for episiotomy, it provides excellent relief.

78. The environment of the labor room

If you are going to have your baby in the hospital, take a look at the labor room while you are pregnant. Most of the time unfortunately, it will be a bare and spiritless place—blank walls, nothing to divert the eye; a large clock, ticking loudly, which guarantees that time is your primary companion. Some hospitals have begun to realize that this is the worst environment for labor—silent, lonely, and starkly oppressive —and have actually built new wings for family-centered maternity care, with all the comforts of home. All the family can be present in a very congenial and relaxing atmosphere, with the added advantage that if anything goes wrong with the delivery, the hospital is right there.

If your hospital has not already made an effort to warm up the labor room, bring your own diversions. Bring magazines to look through between contractions; bring a radio with earpiece and set it on the all-music (not the all-news) station; bring your partner and make sure he knows when he should talk to you. Bring some small hard candies to suck on: the sugar in them may add to your strength. Bring a crossword puzzle or a deck of cards. Diversions make the time go faster. If you just lie there, timing your contractions, listening to the clock ticking, the time—and the pain—will be unnecessarily heavy burdens.

Talk to the nurses and physicians who come to check you periodically so that you know what your progress is. If they are cold or uncommunicative or pleasant and helpful, inform the hospital administrators when you go home with your newborn baby. Like other institutions that serve the public, hospitals are sensitive to what they hear. It will certainly improve the environment of labor rooms if you take the trouble to criticize a bad performance by hospital staff and heap praise on a good one.

79. Back labor

Some women feel the pain of labor most acutely in the lower back; this may mean that the baby's head is coming into the pelvis in a posterior position. This is nothing to worry about. The position of the head will rotate usually by the latter part of the first stage.

80. Recommendation: It is a good idea to involve men in labor and in delivery

At one time, husbands were virtually never invited into the labor room or the delivery room. Now they are generally included in the birth process at the request of the mother. If your hospital refuses to allow men to attend the birth of their children, find this out early in pregnancy, when there is time to choose another hospital. Likewise, if your doctor refuses to allow your man to be with you, and you disagree, thrash out the issue early in pregnancy so, if you must, you have time to find another doctor.

A man needs some preparation for labor. Almost all natural childbirth classes encourage the presence of the man as well. If you expect your man to be with you, make sure he knows generally what to expect; it will be something of a surprise to him anyway. Try to be understanding if he cannot stand to see you in pain and runs away when the going gets rough. And don't let your man, high on a little bit of knowledge, become the "expert" on your labor. He is part of the supporting cast. *You* are the star.

81. Fetal monitoring with ultrasound is a must for high-risk pregnancies; but its use for all pregnancies is highly debatable

A fetal monitor is a relatively new electronic device which monitors the strength and frequency of contractions as well as the fetal heart beat. Two "receivers" are strapped around the mother's abdomen and attached to a small screen which registers, in patterns of light, what is going on inside the belly. One measures the contractions and the other the fetal heart rate. It gives hospital personnel added information about the baby's heartbeat and general progress during labor. For the woman, it is a rather cumbersome device and can be annoying during labor. Later on in labor, part of the device can be replaced by a small clip that can be attached to the baby's scalp, and this is more comfortable for the woman. At other times a pressure transducer is placed inside the uterus to measure the intensity of the contractions. The fetal monitor shows two patterns:

a. the fetal heart rate and
b. the frequency and strength of the contractions of the uterus.

Certain patterns in the baby's heart rate may suggest that not enough blood and oxygen are getting to the brain. In these cases, if oxygen administration and change of the mother's position do not work, a Caesarean section would be advisable.

Fetal monitoring is necessary for women who have high-risk pregnancies—such as diabetics, or women with hypertension. (See ⚹162 below) Women who are having induction of labor with Pitocin should be monitored to make sure the contractions are not too strong or too close together. *Some maternity centers require routine fetal monitoring because of malpractice problems. Of course, you can refuse this, but you will be asked to assume the risk, however slight.* If you have any complications of pregnancy, it would be best to have monitoring in labor.

As far as the safety of ultrasound which is used to monitor the heart rate, most experts say that it is very safe; others question whether routine use is really acceptable. There are rare reports of minor scalp infections from the clips. *Watch for reports* on the pros and cons of routine fetal monitoring.

82. Fetal blood sampling

If mild irregularities in heart rate are noted on the monitor, a tiny sample of blood may be taken from the scalp of the baby and tested for acidity and oxygen content. If the baby's blood is too acid or too low in oxygen, the diagnosis is fetal distress—and a Caesarean section should be performed to avert the possibility of brain damage, which might occur if the decreased oxygen flow were allowed to continue.

83. Artificial rupture of the membranes (bag of waters)

Sometimes during labor, a quantity of amniotic fluid collects in front of the baby's head and actually prevents the head from descending into the pelvis. In these cases the obstetrician or midwife may rupture the membranes with a sterile instrument. This procedure does not have to be done routinely, for in most cases the membranes will break naturally. Some physicians even believe that the routine practice is dangerous and may increase the chances of fetal distress. (Ref.1)

84. Labor should not be induced for the sake of convenience

Labor can be induced by the administration, intravenously (through a vein in the arm) of oxytocin, which stimulates contractions. This is the same preparation used to stimulate stronger contractions when a woman has been in labor a long time with irregular contractions.

This procedure should be saved for special circumstances, and avoided otherwise.

Elective induction is when the mother wants to have her baby on a specific day (so that she can be assured of being up and around in time for her brother's wedding, for example) or when the doctor wants her to have the baby on a specific day (so that he can be assured of being able to make his plane to the Caribbean the day after). This kind of reordering of the priorities of life is not recommended, since induction may involve a certain amount of extra risk to the fetus, and it should not be electively run. One of the major risks of elective induction is prematurity: if someone has miscalculated the dates, labor may be induced too early.

Medically indicated inductions may occur when the risk for continuing the pregnancy to term is too great either for mother or child. Induction might also be indicated for a woman with a history of very fast deliveries who suspects she might not make it to the hospital in time, or when a woman is two or more weeks late.

WARNING: *Induction of labor by rupturing the membranes and then sending the woman home to await labor is not acceptable medical practice. Do not allow it!*

85. Forceps are for special cases only

Every effort should be made to allow the mother to deliver the child naturally, without any outside assistance. However, in some cases, forceps—various instruments which help pull the baby's head farther into the birth canal—are helpful and necessary.

If a woman has epidural or general anesthesia, her body may be too relaxed to bear down in the final stage of labor and push the baby out. A physician may have to assist the baby by pulling its head an inch or two lower with forceps. This should only be resorted to when the baby's head is very low in the pelvis.

When the baby's head is still up in the mid-pelvic area, the forceps should only be used in special or emergency cases—for example, if the fetal heart rate becomes suddenly irregular, indicating that the baby is in distress and the birth process must be speeded up right away. Another situation requiring forceps would be a prolonged second stage of labor. Generally, it is considered dangerous to the infant if labor continues for more than two to three hours after the cervix is completely dilated.

Forceps may leave red marks or swellings on the cheeks of the baby which should disappear in a few days.

86. Anxiety may complicate labor

Studies have shown that the higher the woman's level of anxiety during labor, the more likely she is to have an abnormal labor. Adrenalin (a-DRENN-a-lin), the hormone that is secreted when a person becomes very agitated, may actually cause uterine contractions to become erratic and ineffectual. It is a relatively simple matter to avoid extreme anxiety during labor: use the nine months you are given to prepare for it by reading and learning relaxation exercises for labor.

87. The baby's environment immediately after delivery

Doctors should not slap a baby's bottom when it is born; they can upon occasion dislocate a baby's hips that way. If the mother is awake, she can hold the baby immediately. If the baby wishes to breast feed immediately, that is fine; it will help contract the uterus. The baby may make a loud outcry after it is born, or a small noise, or no noise; medical people will check the baby's vital signs in all cases, and make sure that it is all right. If a woman has had general anesthesia, the baby may be asleep when delivered—and in that case, medical people may go to some lengths to wake the baby up, to make sure that it does not "forget" to breathe.

RECOMMENDATION: *Heed LeBoyer and discuss his theories with your obstetrician.* (Ref. 2) The French obstetrician LeBoyer has recently brought forth a whole set of theories on how to calm the environment in which the baby is born; to create a pleasant, tensionless atmosphere in which there is no loud noise, no extreme of temperature, no machinery, no forceps. *As long as neither baby nor mother has a problem, this or a modification of it is the recommended method of delivery.* (It remains to be proved, however that this type of delivery makes the child grow stronger and healthier, as LeBoyer contends.)

On the other hand, if there is a problem, the machinery—such as fetal monitoring and forceps—may be critical to the baby's well-being, and should be available just in case.

88. Home delivery is usually safe but not always so

If a woman wants to have her baby at home, she should make sure there is hospital backup within minutes of her house. Some of the major risks in pregnancy occur just at the time of delivery—for example, postpartum hemorrhage or fetal distress—and *they cannot be adequately handled outside of a hospital.* Obviously, there are excellent financial and emotional reasons for wanting to have a baby at home, where everybody loves you and the environment is warm and welcoming. And for most women most of the time, it would probably work fine. But for the occasional woman and the occasional baby who gets into trouble, home delivery can be terribly dangerous. Discuss this with your obstetrician. Family-centered childbirth units *in hospitals* are to be preferred.

89. Midwives, an excellent alternative

For a thousand generations, the people who helped women deliver their babies were midwives—other women, skilled and experienced in the childbirth event. In many countries, they are still the normal attendants at a birth. In America, however, childbirth has increasingly become a medical occasion with a marked decrease in fetal and maternal deaths over the past eighty years. It is now possible to screen out the low-risk pregnant women who do not necessarily need a physician in attendance. For these women, nurse midwives are gaining in popularity.

90. Emergency delivery

Sometimes a woman goes into labor very quickly, and the labor is so rapid, she simply has no time to get to the hospital and the physician or midwife who was supposed to help her with the delivery is unable to get to her quickly enough. In these cases, call the police or the fire department; they will come immediately. Almost any police officer and most firemen have emergency training sufficient to assist at the delivery of a baby.

If no one can get to you fast enough, and you are alone when your baby is born, *don't panic*. The swiftness of the labor and delivery probably indicates that things are going *well*.

If you can, find a clean sheet and put it under you, so that the baby is born onto a clean surface. You can reach over and catch the child as it comes out.

Make sure the baby is breathing. Rub its back and/or throat and try to keep the baby's head down. This will help free the mucus secretions from nose and mouth so the baby can breathe easily.

If the child is not breathing, put your mouth over his nose and mouth and suck inward. This will help clear mucus. Then give the baby artificial respiration, about twenty to thirty puffs per minute.

Wrap the baby in something warm.

If you have time, tie the cord in the middle with any material available. This is not absolutely necessary, for the vessels in the cord will close off themselves after a few minutes. Usually the placenta will deliver itself within five to ten minutes. This can be assisted if the baby nurses at your breast. If the placenta seems slow in coming out, try bearing down, it may be in the vagina.

Also, it is important to rub your uterus through the abdomen so that it will contract and make the bleeding minimal. Don't pull on the cord, you may break it and cause more difficulty delivering the placenta.

By this time, help should have arrived. Even if everything went well and your baby is fine, make sure you and the baby see a doctor afterwards.

Lightning-fast emergency births of this kind are frightening, but they can be handled if you keep your cool and remember throughout that *a fast delivery is usually a sign of good health* in both mother and child.

91. The Apgar score

Named for Virginia Apgar, the noted anesthesiologist, this score is a way of evaluating the general health of infants immediately after birth. It scores an infant on heart rate, color, cry,† muscle tone, and reflexes. The test is made one minute after birth and again five minutes after birth. A perfect score is 10; a fine healthy baby usually scores between 7 and 10. Babies born under general anesthesia often score lower, and in fact, it was the application of this test which placed general anesthesia into such discredit for routine deliveries. If a baby scores lower than 7 on the Apgar score, it may need some added treatment (oxygen)— but this only means that the baby is not in peak health at the time this is made; it does not necessarily forebode future ill health and should not be used for prognosis, unless there is later evidence that the baby is not well. The baby will be watched more closely by pediatric staff if the Apgar score was low.

NORMAL POSTPARTUM COURSE

92. Normal postpartum care

The postpartum period begins after delivery of the placenta and lasts six to eight weeks. The care that a woman gives herself at this time, when her body is gradually returning to its non-pregnant state, is vital for her general health in the future.

93. Three to four days in the hospital is the normal stay; a few hours is the normal minimum

Most American women who have had normal deliveries remain in hospital for three to four days afterward. If a woman wants to take her baby home right away, that is fine too—as long as the baby is in good health and the woman assumes responsibility.

Walk as soon as you feel well enough, to improve circulation and speed healing.

† Even a baby born under optimal LeBoyer conditions will make some sound when it is born.

Urinate and move your bowels as soon as possible. It is *normal* to need a laxative in the first few days, for the pressure of the baby's head on the rectum during delivery may have left rectal muscles sore and stretched. If you have had an episiotomy, you may be afraid to defecate, for fear of tearing the stitches. Usually, this fear is groundless, for the incision does not extend into the rectum except in rare instances. (If it does, your doctor should tell you.)

Follow your own preference when deciding how long to stay in the hospital. Keep two considerations in mind:

a. Is the baby strong enough to go home, away from the surveillance of the pediatric staff?

b. Can you get the baby back to the hospital at forty-eight to seventy-two hours? The baby must have a blood test on the second or third day of life, and must be brought back to the hospital for it if discharged earlier. (This test is to check for the disease phenylketonuria, which causes mental retardation.)

c. Will you have assistance at home if you leave earlier than three days?

d. Are there other children at home who are unlikely to understand that their mother needs extra rest at this point? Many women find that they need the three- or four-day breather away from the busy family life.

94. Recommendation: "Rooming in" is the best postpartum arrangment

"Rooming in" means that the baby stays with the mother after delivery, and usually that the father can visit at any time. The alternative— preferred by many hospitals—is to keep the babies separate from the mothers, to bring them to the mothers only at "feeding time," every four hours, and requires that fathers observe strict visiting hours. While you are pregnant, check which method is used in your hospital—*and try to place yourself and your family in the "rooming in" situation.* A woman who has had a baby is not sick; she should not be separated from her baby as though she were sick; a well father should not be separated from his baby. "Rooming in" satisfies family emotional needs and dissipates the feeling that the postpartum days are somehow postoperative days. If your hospital does not allow rooming in, and you would prefer it, seek out another hospital.

95. Lochia: postpartum bleeding

Lochia (LOW-key-a) is a normal postpartum bleeding. For the first two to three days after delivery it is quite red: small clots are normal; large clots are not. The amount of flow may increase when a woman nurses her baby, for the uterus usually contracts during nursing. (See

✕101 below) From one to two weeks, the bleeding becomes thin and pinkish; this then changes to a whitish-tan discharge (still a form of lochia) which generally lasts no more than another two weeks. The first menstrual period should occur six to eight weeks postpartum, unless a woman is breast-feeding. (Breast-feeding may delay the renewal of menstruation. (See ✕104 below) Lochia should not smell foul; it has a distinct odor, like that of menstrual blood. But if it smells really bad, this may signify infection. See a doctor.

96. Care of the episiotomy

The pain of an episiotomy depends on the size and location of the incision and the number of stitches that were taken. The stitches will either absorb themselves or may fall out fifteen to twenty-one days after delivery. The pain will let up in two or three days, and the best way to relieve it is with hot water; try sitz baths, or stand in the shower, spread your buttocks and let the water run on the stitches. Perineal tightening exercises help the healing. (See ✕99 below)

It is also a good idea to take a look at your episiotomy with a hand mirror. First of all, this reassures you that it is healing. Secondly, it reassures you that the incision is not right in the anus (it sometimes *feels* as though it is there) so that the psychological trauma of moving your bowels will be relieved.

If pain is especially severe, your physician can suggest a topical anesthetic ointment to relieve it.

97. Sexual activity after delivery

Obviously, sexual activity other than intercourse can resume immediately after delivery. Normal intercourse should feel comfortable two to three weeks after: if episiotomy pain interferes, wait for further healing. Birth control should be started as soon as sexual intercourse is—your partner should *use a condom* if you are still bleeding. As long as lochia is present, the cervix is still open, and only a condom or abstinence will protect against infection. WARNING: *Never imagine that you are not fertile after delivery.* Some women (and they can never be sure who they are) start to ovulate again very quickly. Even breast-feeding is not a reliable protection for everyone. *Don't take any chances: use birth control.*

98. Postpartum "blues"

A lot of women feel depressed after delivery, probably aggravated by hormonal changes. It may seem odd that a blessed event should make you miserable, but if it is any comfort, you should remember that writers often feel that way after they finish their great novels and swimmers often feel that way after they have won their great races. You will probably snap out of it in two to three days. If the depression lasts for weeks, or interferes with sleep, then something else may be wrong; seek counseling.

99. Postpartum exercises

Many exercises taught at childbirth classes before delivery can help retone your abdominal muscles after delivery.

a. Wear a girdle to support the abdomen in the postpartum period before starting exercises.

b. If you have had an episiotomy, put off strenuous exercising until three to four weeks after delivery.

c. *Exercises for the abdominal muscles:* Sometimes after delivery the abdominal muscles will separate, leaving a woman with what seems like a hernia at the midline of her stomach. The following exercises, done daily, will pull the muscles back together again. Lie on your back, lift your legs and lower them slowly to a count of ten of fifteen, one leg at a time with the other knee bent. Do sit-ups—lie on your back, lift head and shoulders off the floor.

d. *Exercises for the muscles of the perineum* (Kegel's exercises): These can begin almost immediately after delivery and include—stopping and starting the urinary stream each time you urinate, and (after lochia has stopped) placing two fingers inside the vagina and contracting the muscles in around the fingers. These exercises should be done regularly *for many weeks* to restore full muscle tone. (These exercises can also be helpful in treating urinary incontinence. (See pp. 321–22)

100. Breast-feeding

The very best nutrition for most newborns is mother's milk, and more and more women are breast-feeding today. Breast-feeding is also convenient; no bottles, no mixing, no boiling, no cost. Although some babies are allergic to cow's milk, virtually none are allergic to mother's milk. Breast milk is better absorbed than other milk, and some studies show that breast-fed babies are less obese throughout life since they control their own food intake. Important antibodies to fight infections are passed from mother to baby in the milk. Breast-feeding provides contraception (not 100 per cent safe) for as long as it is continued as the only form of feeding for the baby (an advantage for women whose religious beliefs prohibit contraceptives). Finally, psychological studies have shown positive effects from early and prolonged contact between mother and baby.

Any woman who is interested in breast-feeding should do it; and if she isn't interested, she should try to be. True, other children, even a husband, may feel jealous; mothers from the generation that gave up breast-feeding entirely, may object; a certain amount of outdated social convention may suggest that breast-feeding is somehow "primitive." However, it is possible to breast-feed, even in public places, without exposing the breast and offending anybody.

If you work outside the home you may be unable to get home and feed: but even in this case, breasts may be pumped and milk stored to be administered by bottle. If you decide that the whole scene is not for you, don't feel bad; there are several very good premixed formulas on the market.

RECOMMENDATION: There are scattered reports of environmental pollutants appearing in breast milk. *Don't let that deter you from breast-feeding.* Prepared milk undoubtedly has its own pollutants.

RECOMMENDATION: If you are not breast-feeding, keep your breasts tightly bound in a bra or breast binder to prevent the collection of milk in the breasts. OPINION: Some physicians and hospitals regularly give high doses of estrogens to prevent the production of milk in the postpartum days. Don't accept this treatment. The binders work just as well and do not have the side effects of the hormones. (See p. 160)

101. How breast milk is produced: prolactin, oxytocin, and colostrum

Prolactin is a hormone produced by the pituitary which triggers production of milk in the breasts. Normally, it is inhibited by substances secreted by the hypothalamus. But after delivery, there is an effect on the hypothalamus which stops the prolactin-inhibiting process and allows prolactin to be released, producing milk.

As the baby sucks, more prolactin is released—and more milk produced.

The milk is formed in the glands of the breasts; it is transported to the nipples through many ducts. This process is called the "let-down" of milk to the nipples. The hormone that triggers let-down is *oxytocin,* also produced by the pituitary gland. Suckling causes further release of oxytocin, and increased let-down of milk. (Oxytocin also causes the contractions of the uterus felt during nursing.)

Colostrum, a very nutritious, watery substance, is the advance signal of milk production: During the last few weeks of pregnancy, it usually drips from the nipples. It is important that the infant nurse early when colostrum is still present because it contains antibodies from the mother that protect the infant against infectious illness.

102. Problems with "let-down" of milk

The most common problems with breast-feeding are with "let-down." If a baby doesn't suck hard enough, there may be insufficient oxytocin to stimulate adequate milk flow to the nipples. A woman who is very nervous or anxious may secrete other hormones which inhibit oxytocin production. Mild sedatives, or a drink of wine or liquor before feeding, have been known to help in this case. In addition, nasal sprays of oxytocin may give the needed extra push. Once the baby is breast-feeding regularly, and suckling energetically, then "let-down" is continuous and sure. The first day or two of nursing are usually the toughest, if there is any problem at all.

103. Do not smoke or take drugs while breast-feeding, and watch what you eat

a. The nicotine in cigarettes passes through the milk. Don't pass these poisons to your baby or assail her sensibilities with this relatively strong and stimulating substance. (See p. 260)

b. Do not take medication while breast-feeding. If you must, check with your pediatrician to make sure it will not have an adverse effect on your baby. Do not take oral contraceptives while breast-feeding.

c. Diet during lactation should be similar to that in pregnancy:

1. high in all the nutritious foods,

2. especially high in calcium and the B vitamins (except Vitamin B-6 which, in high doses, may inhibit lactation). Drink lots of fluid because you are losing so much in the milk.

d. If your baby is suffering from gas pains or colic, suspect your diet. Some foods, eaten by the mother, can aggravate the child's stomach or cause gas—chocolate, cabbage, Brussels sprouts, broccoli, and garlic are frequently distressful to nursing infants.

104. Breast-feeding as contraception

Breast-feeding provides contraception, but not 100 per cent protection—so use a *mechanical* backup method, a condom or diaphragm. Although women in many parts of the world breast-feed their babies for a year or several years, without supplementary food, American women often start their babies on solid food earlier. As soon as you start adding other items to the baby's diet, the contraceptive effect of breast-feeding begins to diminish.

105. How to prepare breasts and nipples during pregnancy

During the last few months of pregnancy, a woman can prepare her nipples for the challenge of a nursing baby by rubbing them firmly with a towel, rolling the nipples between her fingers, then applying lanolin or cocoa butter. These mild abrasions toughen the nipples so they will not be susceptible to fissures and cracks later on. This preparation is not necessary for all women but helpful for many.

106. How to start breast-feeding

Start immediately after delivery or in the recovery room.

Breasts should not be tender unless they are engorged. It may hurt if the baby grabs only the nipple and not the whole areolar area (the dark area around the nipple). Break the suction with your finger and get her to start again with more of the areola in her mouth.

In the beginning, feed the baby frequently, every one and a half to three hours, as she demands. This stimulates milk production and let-down. Feed from both breasts each time.

Plan ahead: Rooming in is best when breast-feeding. If you don't plan for a rooming-in situation, the baby will be brought to you every four hours, just like children who are being bottle-fed. This means that milk comes into the breast less easily and out of sync with the baby's needs. Women who breast-feed in this situation therefore tend to have more problems than those who are rooming in and can feed their babies any time it is necessary.

Try not to feed the baby supplemental bottles during the first few weeks. Until her sucking is strong, she will find the bottle easier to get milk from and thus may learn immediately to prefer it.

107. Premature infants can be fed with breast milk

A premature baby is usually small and relatively weak and needs the best nutrition possible. *Breast milk is preferable to anything else.* The milk can be expressed out of the breasts by hand or with a pump and fed to the baby through a bottle or stomach tube. If you have your child prematurely, be sure to discuss this method of feeding with the pediatrician.

108. Breast-feeding has little effect on cancer

Some researchers claim that the virus which causes breast cancer and which is dormant in women is passed on to a baby through breast milk. Other researchers say that the incidence of all types of cancer is lower in people who were breast-fed as babies. Recent large studies have shown no significant difference between the two groups. It is currently believed that the effect of breast-feeding on breast cancer is probably not significant. (Ref. 3) (See p. 346)

109. Weaning from breast to bottle

Start with one feeding a day from the bottle; continue this way for a week or more. Then gradually add more bottle feedings. The slow method is easier on the baby, and it helps avoid the problem of breast engorgement as less breast milk is used. Again, the breasts should be bound tightly if engorgement is a problem.

110. There are groups of nursing mothers in most areas of the country

If a woman plans to breast-feed she should find out about organizations of nursing mothers. Childbirth Education Association and LaLeche Leagues throughout the country are available to assist women during breast-feeding. Keep close contact with your pediatrician, midwife, or obstetrician if any problems arise. (See References)

ABNORMAL PREGNANCY AND CHILDBIRTH

111. Problems and abnormalities of pregnancy and birth

A number of things can go wrong for mother and child during pregnancy and delivery. Fortunately, they happen in a small minority of cases; most can be anticipated with good prenatal care and handled successfully in a well-equipped hospital. But the possibility of complications should motivate any woman to have her children in or very near to a good hospital, with the direct or indirect supervision of a skilled obstetrician.

112. Breech birth

In 3 per cent of all pregnancies, a baby moves into the birth canal feet first or behind first, instead of head first. This is called a *breech birth*. Its major problem is that the largest part of the baby—the head —comes *last*. When the head comes first, during labor, the baby's bones can mold themselves to fit the pelvis. When the head comes last, the thin parts of the baby's body come out easily, and then it is critical that the head comes out quickly, lest the baby be hurt. (In a breech birth, only about three minutes remain for the baby's head to come out before the child is in real danger of brain damage from decreased oxygen flow.)

Even if the pelvis is wide enough for the baby to pass through in breech position, there is still danger to the child in this type of delivery. Damage to the nerves of the neck and arms is common, and so is *cerebral palsy*—various defects (ranging from small speech defects to total crippling) in motor power and coordination caused by damage to the brain during delivery.

To avoid these dangers in a breech birth, many physicians will deliver the baby surgically. (See Caesarean section ✕141 below) Some breech babies can deliver safely in carefully selected cases. (Ref. 4) Discuss this with your obstetrician.

113. Breech birth and other abnormal presentations can usually be detected at regular prenatal examinations or in early labor

Before twenty-eight weeks of pregnancy, the fetus is frequently in the breech position but usually will rotate around before delivery. If it does not, a woman can discuss with her obstetrician beforehand the possibility of Caesarean section. Sometimes, ultrasound will be used to determine the size of the baby's head, and X rays will be taken to determine the size of the bones of the pelvis to see if the baby will have trouble fitting through. Even if there is room for the head to pass through, many medical experts now recommend Caesarean section for almost all breech deliveries because of other risks.

114. Other malpresentations which may require Caesarean section

A "presentation" in obstetrical language is the way in which the baby presents itself over the cervix as it opens during labor. A "malpresentation" is any way that the baby has of entering the birth canal which is not the simple, head-first way. Many of the malpresentations require Caesarean section because it would be impossible to deliver a live, normal baby in that position. For example a transverse presentation means that the baby is lying horizontally across the mouth of the cervix. A compound presentation means that two parts are presenting together, for instance a hand and a foot.

115. Warning: external version—a dangerous way to handle malpresentation

External version is an outdated and dangerous obstetrical practice by which the doctor, faced with a breech or other malpresentation, pushes and pulls the abdomen and the baby to get the child into a head-first position. (The doctor is turning—*version*—the baby from the outside —*external*.) *Don't let this happen to you or your baby.* While you are pregnant, discuss the possibility of breech or other malpresentation with your doctor and discuss the possible options including Caesarean section.

116. Twins

Twins occur in one out of eighty-five American births; the rate is slightly higher for black families.

a. *Identical twins:* One egg is fertilized by one sperm and early in its development splits into two identical halves and becomes two identical people. In the uterus, the placentas are usually joined.

b. *Fraternal twins:* Two eggs are produced during ovulation and fertilized by two different sperm, producing two people who may look alike to any or no degree. Fraternal twins don't have to be brothers;

they can be sisters; they can be brother and sister. In the uterus, the placentas are sometimes joined, sometimes not.

c. *"Siamese twins"* originally referred to twins from Thailand (then Siam) who were both joined at the rib cage. Today, the term refers to any twins who are joined at any point. This is a rare phenomenon and occurs because the split of the egg for identical twins has been incomplete.

Fraternal twinning is by far the most common type and is hereditary. Usually, the parents have family histories of twins on either or both sides. In addition, it is more common in older women.

About 25 per cent of all twins are identical twins. This type of twinning is not hereditary and is not influenced by fertility drugs (see ⚹117 below).

Most twins are fraternal and born healthy and normally through the vagina if both are presenting head first. A physician, hearing two heartbeats, feeling two heads, may be able anticipate twins prenatally. Sometimes, one baby is concealed by the other and comes as a surprise at delivery. The uterus of a woman carrying twins will generally be bigger than that of a woman carrying one child. Breast milk should be sufficient to feed both babies.

117. Fertility drugs increase the chance of multiple births

Gonadotropins (see p. 109) seems to increase the incidence of twins and multiple births by causing greater egg production and therefore multiple ovulation. This does not always happen, but if you are taking these drugs for fertility, be on the lookout for a multiple pregnancy.

118. Problems with twins and multiple births

a. *Prematurity* is the biggest problem with twins. Perhaps because the sheer size of the babies distends the uterus and creates excess pressure that triggers labor, most twins do *not* go to term.

b. *Smallness:* Even if a woman carries twins to term, they are likely to be smaller than other babies, simply because they have had to share the same uterine space and the same inflow of nutrition.

c. *Toxemia* (see ⚹155 below) is a greater danger to women carrying twins because of the greater metabolic demands on their bodies, as is

d. *Anemia* (see ⚹150 below), red blood cell deficiency, caused by the increased nutritional drain on the mother.

e. *Complications in delivery* occur sometimes with the second-born of the twins, which usually comes within fifteen minutes after the first. Most twins enter the world head first; the one lying farthest down in the womb exits, and the second follows. The second most common presentation among twins is that the first baby comes out head first, and the second baby is a breech birth. The diagnosis of twins can be made by ultrasound and usually the presentation of the two babies can be determined too. However, in some cases, an X ray of the abdomen is needed to which way the second baby is coming. RECOMMENDATION: Caesarean section is increasingly considered the best type of delivery if either baby is not presenting head first.

f. *Postpartum hemorrhage* is a greater danger in having multiple births because the uterus stretches and may have more difficulty contracting.

g. *Emotional problems* seem to be more worrisome to identical twins as they grow older because it is hard, in a world where everyone else is at the very least unique, to be *the same* as someone. If a woman has had identical twins, she should be on the lookout for emotional crises and have the advice of psychological counselors familiar with this syndrome when her children are still very young.

119. A woman who knows she is having twins should be sure to have them in a hospital

Because the risks in multiple births are greater in general, home delivery will only compound an already risky situation.

120. Pseudocyesis: false pregnancy

This is one of those physiological phenomena whose roots seem to be totally psychological—at least, at our current stage of medical diagnosis. A woman is convinced that she is pregnant. Her periods cease. Her belly grows large. She has many of the discomforts of pregnancy. But she is not pregnant. Every other cause of the signs and symptoms of pregnancy must be ruled out, but then the woman and her doctor must consider the psychological factors. Usually, women who experience false pregnancy have conflicts about childbearing: they want to be pregnant but they are afraid of pregnancy. Or they don't want to be pregnant but they wish they could satisfy the desire of husband or lover for a child. Many cases occur among teen-agers who for some deep-rooted reason wish to punish or frighten their parents or please their boy friends. Whatever the reasons, pseudocyesis is a serious emotional disorder and even if it ends of its own accord, it should be treated with psychological counseling. (For a good description of a pseudocyetic woman, read Edward Albee's play *Who's Afraid of Virginia Woolf.*)

121. Miscarriage—spontaneous abortion

Miscarriage is the death of the fetus and the passage of tissue and blood from the uterus before the twelfth week of gestation. It is estimated to occur in about twenty per cent of pregnancies, and the percentage may even be much higher (including very early pregnancies which were undetected). The signs of miscarriage are bad cramps and bleeding; if the miscarriage is occurring early, there may be very little bleeding—a woman may go to the bathroom and pass what seems to be a clot: this is the miscarriage. Sometimes, early abortions are caused by genetic abnormalities in the embryo.

For many women who are having problems with fertility, the conceptus simply isn't strong enough to hold to the uterus, and miscarriages will occur repeatedly. (See p. 94) Heavy smokers have a higher incidence of miscarriage.

Sometimes what looks like the beginning of a miscarriage is just a little cramping and bleeding during the first few months, and the baby grows to term and is delivered safely. WARNING: *Do not take drugs to prevent miscarriage unless you have a specific infertility problem.* (See p. 109) Most have not been proven effective and *may be dangerous to the fetus.*

If you are bleeding significantly, more than during menstruation, get to a hospital immediately. If it is a smaller amount, ask your doctor for advice. Most miscarriages occur without complication, but a woman should be examined to make sure no fetal tissue remains inside the uterus thereby increasing the risk of bleeding and infection.

a. *Incomplete abortion* occurs when a woman is passing clots of tissue and her uterus is open but the total conceptus does not pass out. She will probably need a D & C (see p. 328) to remove all fragments of tissue so that the womb will close and the bleeding will stop.

b. *Complete abortion* occurs when the whole conceptus is passed and the bleeding stops on its own. If an examining physician finds no damage, then the woman can go home—no D & C is needed. Very early abortions are usually complete.

c. *Missed abortion* occurs when the fetus dies but does not pass out of the uterus. The uterus does not grow any more; the pregnancy test becomes negative, but the periods do not return as they would in a complete abortion. A D & C must be done to remove the conceptus.

122. Immature delivery: loss of the baby during the middle three months of pregnancy

Once a baby is past three months in the womb, its loss becomes more complicated. There are three major reasons that women lose babies up to six and a half months of pregnancy:

a. Maternal illness

b. Incompetent cervix, a condition whereby the cervix opens prematurely

c. Severe genetic disorders in the fetus

123. Maternal illness (See High-risk pregnancies ⚹162 below)

If a woman becomes very sick during her pregnancy, this can upset the flow of nutrients to the fetus, causing it to die. Severe heart, kidney or liver disease can cause fetal death. However, other serious diseases (arthritis) may not affect the child. Sometimes, if the baby has been in the womb long enough, it can be delivered surgically or by induction, and kept well in an incubator until it is big enough to go home with its mother. This may be necessary (for example with certain diseases) to protect both mother and child. Congenital anomalies of the uterus, or large fibroid tumors, may prevent the uterus from stretching enough to house the baby. In these cases, a woman will usually go into labor and deliver a child prematurely. Pediatric intensive care units can do much to save and restore to health a baby born alive under these circumstances. *Plan ahead:* if you have an illness that may complicate pregnancy, plan to deliver in a hospital equipped with intensive care units for you and your child.

124. Incompetent cervix

The cause is unclear, but in some women the cervix loses its strength and begins to open up in the middle of the pregnancy, typically, at four to six months. There is no labor. Suddenly, a woman has the feeling that everything is "dropping out"—and it is. Sometimes the membranes break early and then labor begins.

The cervix should not open before twenty-eight to thirty weeks, even in women who have had many children. A woman who has a history of second-trimester losses should be examined *weekly* starting at twelve weeks to see if the cervix is opening prematurely. If it does begin to open, she can go to the hospital and under anesthesia the obstetrician can take *a stitch* in the cervix, to hold it closed so that the baby can grow to term. This is called *cerclage*. It is not foolproof, but it has allowed many women who would otherwise lose all their children to bear several normally. When labor begins, the stitch is cut, allowing the woman to deliver the baby. Sometimes, the stitch pulls out and has to be replaced later in the pregnancy.

Once incompetent cervix has been diagnosed, a woman should have the stitch placed at about fourteen weeks of each pregnancy. She should not wait to see if the cervix will open again—the likelihood is that it will. Early prenatal care is, therefore, essential. Some physicians place the stitch while the woman is not pregnant, but this procedure is still being debated. DES-daughters have a higher chance of this complication. (See pp. 365–66)

125. Genetic disorders (See Chapter Seven for complete discussion)

Fetuses with severe chromosomal or developmental disorders have a higher frequency of aborting in the second three months of pregnancy. (See p. 217) Any fetus thus aborted should be studied in the lab to determine whether there was any gross disorder, for this will be pertinent to the way the mother and her physician treat future pregnancies.

126. Ectopic pregnancy

Ectopic (eck-TOP-ic) pregnancy occurs when the fertilized egg implants elsewhere than in the uterus and begins to grow there. It is almost impossible for such a pregnancy to succeed. Ectopic pregnancies usually occur in the Fallopian tube (tubal pregnancy)—98 per cent—but they can also occur in the ovary, cervix, and in very rare instances, in the abdominal cavity itself.

Tubal pregnancy is more common among women with damaged Fallopian tubes, either because of infection, venereal disease, endometriosis, corrective or exploratory tubal surgery, or an IUD. The incidence today is about one tubal pregnancy per 200 live births—but because of the widespread use of IUDs and the gonorrhea epidemic, the incidence is increasing. Of the pregnancies that occur in women who have an IUD in place, about five per cent are ectopic. (See pp. 63, 64)

127. Symptoms and treatment of ectopic pregnancy

Frequently, the first sign of tubal pregnancy occurs when the fetus grows so large that it splits the tube and blood escapes into the abdominal cavity. This generally happens about six to eight weeks from the time of the last period and causes abdominal pain. Usually some vaginal bleeding has occurred prior. *Seek immediate medical attention* for severe abdominal pain at any stage of pregnancy; ectopic pregnancy is one of the causes in early pregnancy.

Sometimes the ectopic pregnancy can be detected before it bursts. In these cases the woman may be having lower abdominal pains, and the physician detects a mass on one side of the pelvis. An ectopic pregnancy must be differentiated from a corpus luteum which may also be swollen in early pregnancy, so a laparoscopic examination may be performed to look directly at the tube. (See p. 105)

Another method of detecting a ruptured (or leaking) tubal pregnancy is to perform a culdocentesis (cull-duh-sen-TEE-sis) (from the French word *cul-de-sac,* literally "the bottom of a bag," in this case referring to the space between the rectum and uterus, and from the Greek word *kentesis*—to puncture). A needle is inserted into the top of the vagina, through the wall into this space behind the uterus where blood collects if the tube has ruptured. If blood is found, surgery is indicated.

The surgical procedure usually is the removal of the Fallopian tube on the affected side. This may be achieved by

a. an abdominal incision;

b. Some physicians prefer to operate through the top of the vagina in specially selected cases.

Sometimes the conceptus (early pregnancy) can be squeezed out the end of the tube and the tube repaired. This procedure may leave a damaged tube, which may lead to another ectopic pregnancy in the future. *However, if one tube has already been removed, this is the treatment of choice.*

WARNING: *The ovary does not usually have to be removed in case of tubal pregnancy. Many surgeons do this routinely. Make sure yours does not, unless the ovary has been damaged.* The loss of the Fallopian tube is necessary in most cases but the removal of the ovary with its supply of eggs and hormones is needless.

128. Emotional aspects of losing a baby

The loss of a baby through miscarriage or fetal death almost has to affect a woman emotionally; the psychologic results may range from simple regret to morbid depression. Very often, the effect is delayed. In the rush and emergency of miscarriage, a woman has no time to think about what might have been. Weeks or months later, she may find herself terribly blue and anxious. This is a kind of grieving; it may stem from the natural fear that, since once pregnancy aborted, others may not be successful. *It is normal to feel very bad after losing a baby.* Try and take other emotional pressures off yourself at this time. And if you cannot shake the depression, seek professional help.

129. Prematurity: the greatest single danger to newborn babies

Every baby needs a full nine months in the womb to grow strong and big enough to withstand the onslaught of life in the outside world. Therefore, premature babies—born before full term—tend to be smaller and weaker and at a serious health disadvantage.

In a recent study, the death rate among premature babies who weighed less than 2,500 grams (5 pounds, 8 ounces) was 109.8 per 1000. Among larger, full-term babies, the death rate was only 4.48 per 1000. (Ref. 5) The over-all neonatal death rate in this country has stabilized between 13 and 16 per 1000 live births.

130. Causes of prematurity

Most common among these is a serious illness of the mother. Placental dysfunction, in which the placenta is unable to provide adequate nutrition to the baby, is also often a cause. And very frequently, there will be no reason at all that is obvious.

131. Dangers of prematurity

a. *Low birth weight* in itself predisposes a newborn to many illnesses and injuries; growing awareness of this has led physicians to revise upward their old estimates of how much weight a woman should gain in pregnancy. (See ⚡19 above) Premature babies are almost always smaller than healthy babies need to be. The exception to this general rule is the baby of a diabetic mother, in whom excess weight may signify ill health. (See ⚡163 below)

b. *Respiratory-distress syndrome* is the biggest problem among premature infants. When the baby is born, the lungs are not yet fully developed and oxygen cannot penetrate the lung membranes to get into the blood stream. This creates a serious danger of *brain damage and cerebral palsy.*

c. *Jaundice* is common among premature babies, for their livers are often underdeveloped.

132. Respiratory distress syndrome, brain damage, and cerebral palsy

Brain damage is a general term for injury to the baby's brain during pregnancy and birth; cerebral palsy is a disease which results from brain damage during pregnancy or at birth; usually it is due to a loss of oxygen to some part of the brain. *The kind of injury that occurs in cerebral palsy is usually not an injury to mental process. It is a loss of motor coordination elsewhere in the body. A child with cerebral palsy may be handicapped, but unless there has been other injury as well, he is frequently not retarded.* This distinction is vital—for too often, people with cerebral palsy who can think as well as anyone else are treated as though they are retarded, because their speech may be slurred or their movements impaired. Cerebral palsy and brain damage can cause a vast variety of damage, ranging from the slightest limp to total crippling.

It is very rare in America that brain damage at birth is caused by the trauma of a rough delivery; usually it is caused by respiratory distress syndrome associated with prematurity or loss of oxygen to the brain sometime during pregnancy. Therefore a woman who is going into premature labor should make every effort to place herself in a hospital with the equipment and the skilled personnel necessary to meet the emergency. *Plan ahead. Check out the nursery facilities of the hospitals near you while you are pregnant and have your baby in the best one or near it, if you have a high-risk pregnancy.*

133. Treatment of respiratory-distress syndrome in newborns

A premature infant with immature lungs must receive higher than normal levels of oxygen from people who are well trained in this procedure. If too much oxygen is given, there is a risk that the retina of the eye will be affected and blindness will result. In high-risk centers, special respirators are now available to deliver oxygen directly to the infant's lungs, assisting with breathing and the movement of the chest muscles. Blood transfusion techniques, similar to those used in treating jaundice (see ✕134) help in some cases.

134. Treatment of jaundice in babies

If jaundice from immature liver function in premature babies, or from any other cause such as Rh disease (see ✕158 below) becomes severe, the pigment which builds up in the blood stream (bilirubin) can deposit in the brain and cause damage. Frequently premature babies who begin to show signs of jaundice are treated with ultraviolet light several times a day, a treatment which breaks down the pigment and decreases the jaundice. (The safety of this treatment has not been proven by long-term studies.) Some babies will require exchange blood transfusion to remove the bilirubin.

135. Nutrition and environment for premature babies

An incubator is a kind of transparent box or covered crib, in which the environment of a premature infant is controlled to maintain the right levels of oxygen, the right temperature and humidity. It picks up where the womb left off, helping an infant continue to grow and gain strength until he is ready for the outside world. Most hospitals have incubators for premature children or full-term children who need them.

Nutrition for the premature infant must be decided on at the time of the birth. The baby cannot feed at the mother's breast; it must be fed intravenously or through a tube slipped through her throat or nose into the stomach. Sometimes breast milk (if the mother has it available) can be expressed manually by the mother and then tube-fed to the baby. (See ✕100 above)

136. Good prenatal care is the best way to prevent prematurity; good hospital staff and facilities are the best way to prevent prematurity from damaging your baby

Choose your hospital according to its capacity to care for you and your baby *in an emergency* or make sure they can easily transfer your baby. If the delivery is normal, without complications, as it almost certainly will be, then all you did was waste a little time and effort. If there is a complication, such as prematurity, your time and effort will be worth everything to you and your child.

137. Treatment for premature labor

If a woman goes into premature labor, there are several methods of stopping this medically. In one of these a solution of 10 per cent alcohol is given into her blood stream through a vein. This treatment has been very effective in stopping labor and allowing the pregnancy to continue. After the labor is stopped, a woman may be advised to drink a glass of wine each day to keep the contractions from returning. Apparently, alcohol stops the natural production of oxytocin by the pituitary which leads to uterine contractions. This treatment has not been associated with the birth defects of fetal alcohol syndrome. (See ⍟169 below) However, other more widely used drugs—ritodrine, Vasodilan and magnesium sulfate—may be safer, although long-term studies are not available.

138. Premature rupture of amniotic membrane. (See ⍟67 above)

If the bag of waters ruptures *before* the onset of labor, a woman who is near term will probably go into labor very shortly. If she does not, labor should be induced.

If the fetus is very small, however, when the membranes rupture, some physicians will try to forestall further leakage of amniotic fluid by instructing the woman to stay in bed, hoping that the pregnancy will continue for a few more weeks. The risk of this method of treatment is that once the membranes have broken the amniotic sac and the fetus may become infected. This risk must be weighed against the risk of prematurity in each individual case.

Premature rupture of membranes is usually without specific cause; sometimes it can be related to cervical infection, vaginitis, poor nutrition, or incompetent cervix.

139. Steps to take if amniotic membranes rupture

If a woman finds herself leaking fluid without control (enough leakage so that it runs down her leg), she should call her physician or get to a hospital immediately. WARNING: Some doctors will react by telling a woman to get into bed and stay there. *Do not accept this advice.* Insist on being examined immediately, to make sure that it is amniotic fluid which is leaking, and to make appropriate plans for managing the delivery of your child.

140. Warning: Amniotomy to induce labor is an outdated practice to be avoided

Amniotomy is a practice whereby a physician ruptures the membranes artificially as a method of inducing labor and sends the woman home to await its onset. This is bad medicine. If artificial rupture of membranes is absolutely necessary (see ✕83 above), it should be done in the hospital and if labor has not commenced twelve hours afterward, a woman should receive Pitocin (which stimulates contractions) intravenously and should be checked very frequently to see that she does not have a fever.

141. Caesarean section

Named for the delivery of Julius Caesar, who was reportedly cut from his mother's womb, a Caesarean (se-ZAIR-ian) section is the major surgical alternative to normal vaginal birth. If you or your baby get into trouble during delivery, it can be done as an emergency operation. If you have had a previous Caesarean section, the delivery can be planned.

142. Incisions of the Caesarean section

An incision is made in the abdominal wall, either
a. vertically at the stomach midline, or
b. horizontally, at the uppermost edge of the pubic hair.

RECOMMENDATION: *If there is time to plan the Caesarean, ask for the horizontal incision.* It is usually stronger while healing, and later on will be almost invisible, camouflaged by the pubic hair. (For this reason, it is called the "bikini scar.") Ask for it if you are having any abdominal surgery, e.g., a hysterectomy or surgical removal of ovarian cysts.

143. Caesarean-section procedure

The uterus is right in the middle of the abdomen, and easy to see after the incision. The intestines are *behind* the uterus, so they do not obscure the surgeon's view. The bladder must be pushed downward, away from the uterus, so the incision can be made. (A catheter must be placed in the bladder before the operation to drain all the urine.) The incision is usually made horizontally, low in the uterus, in the area of the baby's head; the head is then pulled out and the rest of the body follows as in a vaginal delivery. The placenta is removed. The uterus is sewn back *in two layers.* The bladder is then placed back over the uterus and pinned there; then the abdomen is closed. The whole operation takes about an hour. The reason that the incision in the uterus is made as low as possible is that the uterine wall there is thinner and contains fewer of the major contracting muscles, making the scar stronger, making healing easier. In addition, the lower scar makes it easier for a woman to have another pregnancy and another Caesarean section.

In other emergencies and in breech deliveries, an incision may be made higher in the uterus—but these indications are rare. *Make sure to ask your doctor what type of scar is left in your uterus.*

Postpartum course is essentially like that in normal delivery. However, there is more pain, because there has been an abdominal incision, and postpartum contractions feel worse in an already sore belly. Because of the movement of the bladder during the operation, a catheter will be in place for about twenty-four hours afterward, and even after it is removed, the woman may feel cramping when her bladder is full. Naturally, because of the healing of the abdominal incision, it takes longer to regain full strength.

By the first day a woman who has had a Caesarean section will be able to breast-feed if she desires.

144. When is Caesarean section necessary?

a. *Cephalopelvic (SEFF-al-lo-pelvic) disproportion* is a common cause for Caesarean section. This means that the baby's head is too big for the pelvis. Usually a woman will start off making good progress in labor and then the head fails to come down into the pelvis. A physician who suspects this disproportion may order X rays (pelvimetry) before making a decision for surgery, but these are frequently not required. In this case the operation saves the life of the child and the mother who might have died of this complication otherwise. (In underdeveloped countries, cephalopelvic disproportion is a common cause of infant and maternal mortality. The mother labors and labors; the baby, squeezed between the pelvic bones, dies; the uterus ruptures; the mother dies.)

Breech babies and other malpresentations are often delivered by Caesarean section because of the fear that either the head or any other presenting part will not fit through the pelvis. (See ⚹113–115 above)

b. *Fetal distress:* If fetal monitoring (see ⚹81 above) shows that the baby's heart rate is severely depressed or irregular or if estriol (see ⚹180 below) values are very low and a woman's labor for some reason cannot be induced, then Caesarean section is indicated.

c. *Maternal illness:* If a woman has heart disease, for example, or other serious illness and cannot safely carry her baby to term, Caesarean section may be performed to save the life and health of the mother, and the baby too, again, if induction is not possible.

d. *Previous surgery on the uterus:* Women who have had myomectomy procedures which have entered the center of the uterus (see pp. 338–39) and women who have had hysterotomy procedures for abortion (see pp. 197–98) usually will need Caesarean section if they deliver a term-size baby.

145. Anesthesia for Caesarean section

In an emergency, when the woman does not already have an epidural anesthetic in place, general anesthesia will be used. An epidural or spinal anesthetic can be used if there is no rush about the surgery. (See ⌗77 above)

146. Caesarean section can be performed repeatedly on the same woman

Until only a few years ago, doctors believed a woman could only have three Caesarean section deliveries. Today, advances in surgical technique permit a woman to have several more babies in this manner. Usually, if there was a good reason for the first Caesarean section, the same reason will motivate the next one: for example, cephalopelvic disproportion. However, in some cases—for example, if a section has been done because of fetal distress—a woman may be able to deliver her next child normally, with careful monitoring. Discuss this with your doctor. Make sure you know what type of incision is in your uterus. The low incision makes laboring safer. *Never consider labor and delivery outside of a hospital if you have had a previous Caesarean section.*

147. Delivery by Caesarean section is increasing

The percentage of babies delivered by Caesarean section has been increasing dramatically over the last few years. A major of this increase is the widespread use of fetal monitoring and the detection of abnormalities in the fetal heart rate. It is very difficult to say whether all of these procedures are necessary. One must approach the subject with an open mind at this time. Caesarean sections are done in effort to prevent a decrease in blood flow and oxygen to the brain (as suggested by abnormal heart rates on the monitor). The major problem is that no one really knows how severe damage will be if an abnormal pattern lasts for a prolonged period of time. Most obstetricians and their patients are not content to wait and see, once an abnormal pattern is detected.

The other major factor in the increase is that, today, almost all abnormally presenting infants (e.g., breech) are delivered by Caesarean section. This has substantially reduced the neonatal death rate and other brain damage among such babies. (See ⌗112 above)

148. Postmaturity

There is nothing to the OWT that no pregnancy lasts longer than nine months; occasionally one does. This is nerve-racking for the mother, whose perceptions of the day she conceived are now being challenged by everybody. In most cases, she will go into normal labor and have a normal child without problems. The only time that postmaturity is a danger is when the function of the placenta begins to decline, the baby actually begins to lose weight in the womb and may die. Generally, if a pregnancy lasts two weeks past its expected termination, a physician will check the estriole (an estrogen) in the woman's urine and will do some stress testing to make sure the placenta is still functioning normally. (See ⚭180 below) If placental function is declining and the woman is still not having her baby, labor will be induced.

149. Hyperemesis gravidarum—pernicious vomiting of pregnancy

A great many women experience nausea and vomiting routinely during pregnancy. (See ⚭31 above) However, in a few cases, vomiting is continual; the woman begins to lose weight steadily; she becomes dehydrated (her body loses water). Food and sometimes the mere mention of food make her sick. If the continual retching tears the lower part of the esophagus (the lower throat) she may vomit blood. Sometimes, the woman becomes jaundiced. Any or all of these symptoms differentiate normal vomiting from pernicious vomiting. An additional sign is that the medications usually given to control vomiting do not work at all.

Hyperemesis (hy-per-EM-eh-sis) gravidarum (gra-vi-DAR-um) usually starts in the second month—at the same time that normal nausea and vomiting start. The treatment is hospitalization and intravenous fluids to build up her strength again and sedation so that her stomach muscles relax out of the spasms that accompany vomiting. She gets no food by mouth for several days, then gradually is started on fluids, then solids.

As with many diseases, hyperemesis gravidarum may have both psychological and physiological causes, and the relative importance of the two causes is not known. The disease can be successfully treated medically, however.

150. Anemia—iron deficiency

Anemia—deficiency in red blood cells—is more common in pregnant women, because greater demands are being made on the blood supply for the nutrition of the fetus.

Most anemias of pregnancy are related to deficiency in iron. If, as is often the case, a woman is borderline anemic to begin with, the extra strain of pregnancy may deplete her iron stores completely and push her into anemia. (See p. 369) Therefore, to avoid anemia before it begins, *all* pregnant women should take an iron supplement. (See ⚹21 above) Some women cannot take pills, or liquid supplemental iron, or their bodies cannot absorb iron in this form. In these cases, the iron can be given by injection but this has side effects. Iron deficiency in pregnancy is a possibility in all women. Particularly affected are those women who have had a child during the previous two years, or women who just don't eat well.

151. Folic-acid deficiency anemia in pregnancy

A simple blood smear will frequently tell which kind of anemia you have. In iron deficiency, the red cells are very small; in folic-acid deficiency, they are usually large. Of course, the two causes may exist together and the distinction would be impossible. An additional blood test for folic acid can be done.

Folic acid is found in leafy green vegetables and liver. Most pregnant women show a marked decrease in folic acid by the last trimester, no matter how well they have been eating. Some physicians believe that folic-acid deficiency may cause premature detachment of the placenta (see ⚹157c below, Abruption), pre-eclampsia (see ⚹155 below), and infant anomalies. Folic-acid deficiency severe enough to cause these problems is very rare, and affects mostly badly undernourished women. REMEMBER: *multiple vitamins taken in pregnancy should contain folic acid.*

152. Effects of anemia in pregnancy

It is rare in this country (but common in poorer nations) for anemia to be so pronounced in a pregnant woman that her baby is affected. Mostly the effect is on the American mother. She may suffer from fatigue, get headaches, or palpitations of the heart, for it pumps harder when there is less hemoglobin available to carry oxygen to the baby. If a woman is suffering normal shortness of breath and dizziness, these may be aggravated by anemia.

153. How to prevent anemia in pregnancy: EAT WELL!

To prevent anemia, take vitamin supplements with iron and folic acid; eat plenty of liver and green leafy vegetables. If you become anemic anyway, you may have a different form of anemia and this should be tested. (See p. 369) *Adolescent mothers* (see pp. 29–30) are prime targets for severe anemia because American teen-agers as a group eat rather poorly to begin with. If you know any teen-age girl who is pregnant and have any influence on her at all, make sure she gets excellent prenatal care and eats wisely.

154. Urinary-tract infections

Between 5 and 10 per cent of pregnant women show bacteria in their urine, and 25 per cent of these women will develop symptoms of kidney or bladder infection. (See pp. 315–16) There is a higher incidence in pregnancy because as the uterus grows, it presses on the ureters (the tubes that draw urine out of the kidney to the bladder) which are already sluggish and dilated because of the rise in hormone levels during pregnancy. Infection is more likely in the stagnated urine. The symptoms of these urinary tract complications are burning and pain on urination, and urinary frequency. The additional symptoms of kidney infection are often high fever and pain in the back, under the ribs. Treatment is by antibiotics—and if there are any such symptoms, treatment should be sought immediately.

155. Toxemia

Literally, toxemia (tox-EE-me-a) means blood poisoning. In pregnancy, this is characterized by hypertension (high blood pressure) and some kidney changes.

Pre-eclampsia—a mild form of toxemia—has these symptoms:

a. Excess urinary protein (usually associated with kidney changes)
b. Edema—swelling because of water buildup, and
c. High blood pressure.

In the most severe cases (eclampsia), the woman has seizures or fits.

156. Treatment of toxemia in pregnancy

The best treatment for toxemia is good prenatal care, so that it can be detected quickly and treated before it becomes severe. For this reason, have blood pressure checked at every visit; have urine checked for protein buildup, legs and feet checked for swelling. If toxemia is detected in its early stages, bed rest is the best treatment; sometimes mild sedatives are prescribed. If the blood pressure goes dangerously high, the woman will be hospitalized for treatment. When a woman has severe toxemia, and is a likely candidate for seizures, she may be given injections of magnesium sulfate—a seizure preventive.

Because of widespread good prenatal care, toxemia rarely reaches an aggravated stage. Why some women get it and most women don't is still unknown; statistically, it is more frequent in women having their first child; in younger and adolescent mothers generally; and in women who are predisposed to hypertension, for example, women who are extremely fat or have a family history of high blood pressure. It may be related to an immunologic reaction of the mother to the fetus. Toxemia usually abates very quickly after delivery.

157. Bleeding in the third trimester is not normal

The *only normal* vaginal bleeding at this time is the scanty blood show that precedes labor—anything else is a sign of trouble and always should be reported to a physician.

a. *Cervicitis:* severe inflammation of the cervix may bleed quite a bit, especially after intercourse. It can be treated by vaginal suppositories or creams.

b. *Placenta previa:* rarely, the placenta attaches to the uterus at an abnormally low point, covering the cervix completely or partly. The first symptom is painless bleeding, usually in the seventh or eighth month. A physician may perform an ultrasound test or amniography (see ※180 c and d) to check where the placenta has attached. Placenta previa usually requires a Caesarean section delivery. If the baby is still very small, a physician will admit the mother to hospital and try to get the bleeding under control so the pregnancy can continue for a few weeks. If the bleeding is severe, the operation may have to be done immediately, and the prematurely delivered baby kept in an incubator until it is big and strong enough for the outside world.

Placenta previa is more common in women who have had many children or who have had a Caesarean section or other uterine surgery.

c. *Abruptio placenta:* Sometimes the placenta separates partly or completely from the wall of the uterus. This can occur before or during labor. The symptoms are severe pain in the uterus and bleeding, although sometimes there is no external bleeding because the blood is accumulating in the uterus.

Abruptio placenta may be associated with hypertension, pre-eclampsia or folic-acid deficiency, and heavy smoking, but the exact cause is unknown.

Treatment is emergency Caesarean section unless the woman is well along in labor and the baby's heart rate is stable.

158. Rh disease in pregnancy

The Rh factor (so named for the Rhesus monkeys in which it was first discovered) is found on the outside of the blood cells of 85 per cent of the population. From the other 15 per cent it is missing. Women with Rh-negative blood in the past could expect problems if they were giving birth to a second or later child with Rh-positive blood. The mother's blood can react against the baby's blood (an immune reaction —the normal way the body has for fighting a foreign element). When, during her first pregnancy, a number of fetal cells entered the circulation of the mother by the breakdown in the placental barrier, the mother can develop antibodies—the body's defense against foreign elements—against the baby's cells. The first baby is usually born unscathed. But the second Rh-positive baby can be developing in a maternal body with predeveloped antibodies against its blood. The antibodies from the mother's blood can pass across the placenta, attack the blood cells of the fetus, making it severely anemic and in the worst cases, causing such severe loss of blood cells that the baby has heart failure and dies.

159. Detection and treatment of Rh disease

First, the Rh negative mother's blood can be analyzed for the presence of the antibody. If it is there, then the chance of Rh disease exists and the pregnancy can be managed accordingly.

If the antibody levels in the mother's blood rise during pregnancy, then the threat to the baby is yet more serious. *All mothers* who harbor the antibody should have amniocentesis (see ※180e) at around twenty-eight weeks of pregnancy. A little amniotic fluid can be drawn off. If it contains high levels of bilirubin, the substance that the baby's red-blood cells produce when they are breaking down, then the physician knows that the baby is being affected.

If the amniotic fluid test shows that the fetus is severely affected, a blood transfusion may be given to the fetus in the uterus. Universal donor (O-negative) blood is injected into the abdomen of the fetus, using special X-ray monitors. Depending on how far along the pregnancy is, this procedure may have to be repeated two or three times, up until the thirty-second week of pregnancy. The baby will probably need another transfusion immediately after birth. It is difficult and nerve-racking, but the baby is frequently saved. These procedures must be performed at high risk centers by specialists.

In less severely affected babies, a total blood transfusion may be performed after delivery if the level of bilirubin in the infant's blood stream is dangerously high.

A woman with severe Rh disease can consider artificial insemination with an Rh-negative donor to avoid future problems. (See p. 113)

160. Prevention of Rh disease

Thankfully, today, most Rh disease can be prevented. A shot of gamma globulin (RhoGam), rich in antibodies, can be given to the woman after any incident in which fetal Rh-positive cells may have entered her blood stream. These incidents include

a. delivery of an Rh-positive child,
b. abortion or miscarriage,
c. an ectopic pregnancy,
d. amniocentesis for genetic testing. (See p. 219)

Gamma globulin antibodies attack any Rh-positive cells which may have entered the mother's blood stream and destroy them *before* she develops her own antibodies against them. This means that the next pregnancy has the same chance for success as the first. *The injection must be given in each case listed above. Essentially, it keeps the woman's immune system from going to work against her Rh-positive child, by doing the job the antibodies would have done before they can even get started.*

The shot should be given within seventy-two hours after the incident. A blood test must be done twenty-four to forty-eight hours later to see if the antibodies from the gamma globulin are adequate; if they are not, another shot can be given.

Some physicians recommend additionally giving RhoGam at twenty-eight weeks of pregnancy to prevent the small number of failures (1–1.5%) which occur when RhoGam is given only postpartum. (Ref. 6)

All pregnant women should have routine blood-typing. Even if therapeutic abortions are performed, Rh-negative women should always receive the shot of gamma globulin. (*RhoGam* is the most common product.)

161. Too much or too little amniotic fluid can be a danger

a. Sometimes, a woman develops extraordinary amounts of amniotic fluid. Her uterus swells much more than normal. This is called *polyhydramnios* (polly-high-DRAM-nee-ohs). It frequently accompanies twins and diabetes and fetal abnormalities, but may occur in otherwise normal pregnancies.

b. Since amniotic fluid protects the baby, too little fluid (*oligohydramnios*) (oh-LIG-o-high-DRAM-nee-ohs) can allow injury to the fetus. This latter defect is especially found in postmaturity.

162. Medically high-risk pregnancies

Pregnancy carries its own risks even in the healthiest of women, delivering under the best conditions. Some women, however, are in such bad health that they risk doing great damage to themselves and their children just by becoming pregnant. The maternal mortality rate in the United States is about 14 deaths per 100,000 pregnancies (including abortions, miscarriages, and all types of deliveries). Many of these women died because of severe additional illness or because of criminal abortion. For babies, the risk of death or injury is much greater with a very sick mother.

Despite the dangers, some high-risk women will decide to have children anyway. This should be a well-thought-out *decision*, not an accident. *Be aware of the risks if you are considering running them.* Place yourself within reach of a center that specializes in high-risk obstetrics (usually a medical school hospital); these facilities will have the doctors you need and the intensive care units your baby may need.

Yours is a high-risk pregnancy if you suffer from

a. Diabetes
b. Hypertension
c. Kidney disease
d. Heart disease
e. Sickle-cell anemia or related diseases
f. Cancer
g. Alcoholism
h. Drug addiction

163. The risk of diabetes

It may be easy to control diabetes in a young woman with insulin and diet; it is much harder to control it during pregnancy. Higher doses of insulin are needed as the fetus grows. Frequently, a diabetic woman will have to be hospitalized for periods during pregnancy for regulation of her disease. Her baby will tend to be heavier than other babies unless the disease is well controlled; or, if the placenta is affected, the baby may be smaller than expected.

Gestational diabetes develops only during pregnancy, usually in women who have a family history of diabetes. Other likely candidates are women who have had overweight (more than eight and a half pounds) babies previously and women with sugar in their urine. These women should have their blood sugar tested repeatedly during pregnancy. Screening for blood sugar should be done two hours after a large meal. Diabetes is not inherited by the fetus, but the tendency toward it later in life is inherited. Infants of diabetics have higher risks of congenital abnormalities.

164. The risk of hypertension

This is a common disease, especially among older women, obese women, and among black women. During pregnancy, high blood pressure can complicate the flow of blood to the placenta, resulting in smaller babies. A woman can have both pre-eclampsia and hypertension in pregnancy. (See ╳155 above) Any severe elevation of blood pressure requires aggressive treatment and close monitoring of the baby. Another possible effect of hypertension is kidney damage during pregnancy, which in turn carries a high risk to mother and child.

165. The risk of kidney disease

Women with pre-existing kidney disease have many problems with pregnancy. If kidney function deteriorates greatly during pregnancy, abortion or early delivery may be the only ways to prevent maternal death. *Remember: pregnancy is a nutritional interchange.* The waste-elimination function of the kidney is overloaded during pregnancy and therefore it must be in good working order.

166. The risk of heart disease

The work of the normal heart must increase 50 per cent during pregnancy. For the damaged heart this strain may be too great. No matter what the origin of the heart damage—congenital, rheumatic, or hypertensive—the risk to the mother increases during pregnancy.

167. The risk of sickle-cell anemia and other related diseases

Women with sickle-cell anemia have great difficulties with pregnancy. Some studies show as high as 50 per cent infant mortality and 25 per cent maternal mortality. The great danger is from blood clots which frequently occur in the lungs and are sometimes fatal. In high-risk care centers, such women are able to receive effective therapy in the form of transfusions during the pregnancy, and the risks are lessening. Women with sickle-cell trait may run increased risk of urinary infection in pregnancy. (See pp. 216–17)

168. The risk of cancer

Cancer anywhere in the abdomen is an absolute contraindication for pregnancy. If not the cancer itself, then the radiation and drug therapy required to treat it will almost certainly damage the child. Carcinoma-in-situ of the cervix may be treated conservatively during pregnancy, then more aggressively after delivery. (See p. 364) Breast cancer may be treated during pregnancy, but radiation and mammography constitute some danger to the fetus, if not shielded.

169. The risk of alcohol excess

Children born to alcoholic women are reported to have many congenital defects. And some reports suggest that children of mothers who drink just moderately may be smaller and more jittery than the average. Pregnant women should try not to drink and should never take more than two drinks per day. (Ref. 7, 8) Binges that go beyond that amount are particularly dangerous to the fetus in early pregnancy.

170. The risks of smoking during pregnancy

Recent studies have shown that babies born to women who are heavy smokers are smaller in size, and more likely to be premature. The incidence of early abortion (see ✄121), bleeding during pregnancy, abruptio placenta (see ✄157c), placenta previa (see ✄157b) and premature rupture of the membranes (see ✄138) is higher in heavy smokers. (Ref. 9, 10) Women must cut back to less than one pack per day during pregnancy; and preferably stop the habit altogether, both for their own and their baby's health.

171. Recommendation: Avoid radiation and X rays during pregnancy

Any woman who is sexually active and requires abdominal X rays should only have them in the first half of the menstrual cycle when she is sure she cannot possibly be pregnant. If X rays are absolutely needed in pregnancy, make sure the abdomen is shielded. The risk to the fetus of a diagnostic X-ray series study is very low. The risk of X-ray therapy is very high.

172. Severe environmental pollution is dangerous during pregnancy

In this era when the world is just beginning to recognize the devastating effects of environmental pollution, there are not yet enough laws, there is not enough environmental control technology, to lessen the danger to a pregnant woman and her baby. *Therefore, a woman has to control her own environment as much as she possibly can.* In July 1976, for example, an industrial accident at the Ismesa Chemical plant in Meda, Italy, created a poisonous cloud, containing the toxic chemical dioxin, that spread over several communities. Doctors warned women in their first three months of pregnancy that they might bear deformed children as a result of the exposure to the poison. Although abortion was at that time against the law in Italy, the government consented to it for these women; the Roman Catholic Church did not. Each woman had to make up her own mind about what to do.

There is no way to avoid this terrible sort of calamity except by much stricter government regulation of (particularly industrial) pollution. However, an individual woman who ordinarily works with toxic substances must inform herself of the dangers to her baby and should transfer to another job or get off the job as soon as she decides to become pregnant. This is not easy, but it may save your baby's life.

WARNING: If you work with paint, lead, mercury compounds; if you work under the pall of a big industrial incinerator; in a plant that produces chemical waste; around an operating room or any hospital or industrial area where anesthetics are used or produced. (Women working with anesthetics experience an increase in spontaneous abortion.) *Get out before you become pregnant.* Science cannot yet give definitive answers on industrial pollution; sometimes the poisonous effects are not felt for years. So don't wait around for scientists to tell you yes or no; they may not be able to until it is too late.

173. The risk of drug addiction

If a woman with a drug habit continues to take hard drugs while she is pregnant, the baby will be born addicted—and will suffer the horror of withdrawal symptoms after delivery. (Even Darvon, taken during pregnancy, has been shown to cause withdrawal symptoms in newborns.) In addition, there is a higher rate of complications in the pregnancies of addicted women—mainly prematurity. If a woman is a heroin addict, she should try to get into a methadone program or a withdrawal program during her pregnancy.

Early but as yet unproven reports indicate that women who take LSD or smoke a lot of marijuana during pregnancy may cause chromosomal damage leading to genetic damage in their babies. *Stay off these drugs if you are pregnant or contemplating pregnancy.*

Other medications are dangerous as well. (See p. 212 and Table 4, Chapter Seven)

174. Infectious diseases contracted by the mother may affect the fetus

Particularly in early pregnancy, some infectious diseases of the mother can cross the placenta and damage the child, or infect the child at the time of delivery. These diseases include rubella (German measles), herpes genitalis, and syphilis and gonorrhea.

175. The risk of rubella

If a woman has been exposed to rubella in early pregnancy, she should have blood tests to determine whether she has become infected with the disease (see p. 221) for it will almost invariably hurt the fetus.

176. The risk of herpes

Women who have genital herpes (see p. 309) in the last five to six months of pregnancy may pass this to the infant during delivery and, some physicians believe, while the infant is still in the uterus. If the baby is infected, it develops a disease which looks like smallpox and is frequently fatal. Most physicians advise delivery by Caesarean section if there are any lesions in the vaginal area in the last few months of pregnancy, but even this doesn't completely protect the baby.

177. The risk of syphilis

Syphilis may infect the fetus in the uterus during the last six months of pregnancy and cause severe damage to several organs (brain, bones) if not treated. This is why all women should have blood tests for syphilis during the first and third trimesters of pregnancy. If detected early and adequately treated, the baby *may* come through it all right. (See p. 314)

178. The risk of gonorrhea

Gonorrheal infection may cause blindness in the baby if it is present in the birth canal during delivery. Testing for this infection should be routine in all pregnant women. To prevent gonorrhea eye infections, drops of penicillin or silver nitrate are placed in the baby's eyes at time of delivery. (See p. 312)

179. The risk of other infectious diseases

Several other infectious illnesses are known or strongly suspected to cause fetal defects. (See Table 3, Chapter Seven)

180. Tests used to monitor high-risk pregnancies in late pregnancy

a. *Estriol detection.* During the last eight to ten weeks of pregnancy, large amounts of *estriol,* an estrogen, are excreted in the urine. Estriol excretion should remain at a constant level up to thirty-four weeks, then increase dramatically. This shows whether the baby's adrenal glands are working well (the adrenal glands of the fetus produce the original substances of estriol), whether the placenta is normal (for the placenta metabolizes the fetal adrenal substance and changes it to estriol), and whether the mother's kidneys are normal (the kidneys control the amount excreted in the urine). Estriol is usually measured in a twenty-four-hour urine sample or in a blood sample. If the estriol excretion is abnormally low, further tests will generally be used to evaluate the fetus. WARNING: *Estrogen cannot be given by injection to correct the estriol levels!* This in fact may be dangerous. (See p. 367)

b. *Stress testing.* In women with low estriol levels or who are overdue, a stress test may be given to determine the condition of the fetus or placenta. In the "non-stress" test, the baby's heart rate is monitored as during labor. If the condition of the pregnancy is good, the heart rate of the infant should go up about fifteen or more beats per minute after the infant moves. If this does not occur, the Pitocin stress test may be performed. In this test, Pitocin is given in dilute solutions intravenously to start some contractions. The baby's heart rate is monitored through several contractions. If there are abnormal changes in the heart rate, this signifies that the fetus is in danger and that (generally) Caesarean section delivery should be done.

c. *Amnioscopy.* This is a test whereby a small cone is placed through the already open cervix; through this cone, the physician can see the amniotic fluid. If there are greenish-brown stains on the fluid (known as meconium), that means the fetus is under some strain and has been defecating into the amniotic fluid. This is not necessarily an indication that the fetus is in trouble; but it does suggest that the baby should be monitored carefully, and that other tests (the estriol test; the Pitocin stress test) should be made to check out the situation. This is not widely performed in the United States.

d. *Ultrasound: safer than X ray.* This is a method of bouncing sound waves off various structures in the pelvis to determine their size. Early in pregnancy, an ultrasound scan can determine the size of the sac in which the conceptus is housed. This is useful if a woman who wants an abortion is unsure when she became pregnant and does not know which type of abortion to have. It is usually done before amniocentesis for genetic testing. (See p. 219) Later in pregnancy, ultrasound can be used to measure fetal size—the waves bouncing off the head of the baby indicate the size of the rest of the fetus. They can also determine the location of the placenta. Ultrasound can identify multiple pregnancies. At present it seems a much safer alternative to X ray in many instances. The long-term safety of this diagnostic method, and its use in fetal monitoring as well, remains to be confirmed. OPINION: There is *no excuse* for its routine use at every visit, in all pregnancies as is the practice in some places.

e. *Amniocentesis.* This is a test done at various stages of pregnancy, in which a needle is inserted through the abdomen into the uterus to remove a little amniotic fluid for testing. It can tell several things:

—How mature the baby is: in late pregnancy it is especially important information when early delivery may be necessary.

—If the baby's kidneys are working. Creatinine can be measured in the amniotic fluid. This substance, produced by the fetal kidneys, begins to rise after thirty-four weeks of gestation.

—If the baby's lungs are working. By measuring the lecithin-sphingomyelin (L-S) ration in the amniotic fluid, the maturity of the fetal lung can be determined. Lecithin and sphingomyelin are lipids, fatty substances, found in the fetal lungs; they increase normally after thirty-five weeks of gestation. If the ratio is high, then the risk of respiratory distress syndrome is less.

—If there are significant numbers of fetal fat cells in the fluid. This suggests that the fetus is mature.

—If there are genetic problems. (See Chapter Seven)

—If there is serious Rh disease; bilirubin in the fluid is analyzed.

f. *Amniogram: a less desirable alternative to ultrasound.* Some hospitals do not have ultrasound equipment, and will try to gain information about the placenta by amniogram—injection of dye into the amniotic fluid which then outlines the placenta on an X ray.

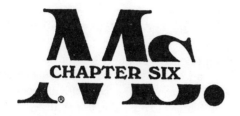

CHAPTER SIX

ABORTION

No woman can claim that she has control over her own body unless she is able to secure a legal, safe, and reasonably priced abortion, when and if she wishes.

Proper usage of birth-control methods cannot absolutely prevent unwanted pregnancies; and today, the most effective methods are being seriously re-evaluated because of the possible dangers to a woman's health. (See Chapter Three) Thus, the possibility that she may one day have to make a decision about abortion faces every sexually active woman—and she should try her best to know what she thinks before that day arrives.

Any state control over a woman's decision to have or not to have an abortion is an intolerable infringement of her civil rights, and must be guarded against by all. If the power to grant abortion resides in anyone but the woman herself, she is simply not a free person. Nor should this freedom be abused. The woman who thinks that the law should force her convictions about abortion upon others must remember that by the same process, she herself could be forced to accept ideologies that are abhorrent to her. This century has already seen this dramatically demonstrated in Nazi Germany, where women of the "Master Race" were prohibited from having abortions, and women of races considered "inferior" were forced to have them.

An abortion is the removal of the tissue of pregnancy from the womb before the time of "viability"—the time that a fetus might be able to live outside the womb (presently thought to be about twenty-six weeks).

The word "abortion" comes from the Latin word *aborto*, to miscarry. And in fact, when an abortion results from natural causes, it is called a miscarriage. (See pp. 164–65)

Until a few years ago, abortion was illegal in this country, except when occasionally sanctioned as treatment vital to save health or life. Many otherwise law-abiding people felt compelled to violate the abortion laws. Often, they found themselves in the hands of quacks and criminals, or well-meaning physicians forced to work under conditions they would never have tolerated were secrecy unnecessary.

While abortion was illegal, healthy women were regularly crippled and killed. Good doctors were ruined. Evil ones made illicit fortunes.

Wealthy women could flee to foreign countries where abortion was legal, performed under sanitary conditions. Poorer women had to put their lives in the hands of strangers in motel rooms, in locked offices and empty buildings. Some of the methods used were reminiscent of medieval torture; red rubber catheters, knitting needles, coat hangers, corrosive douches, and packings soaked with Lysol and phenol and placed in the uterus, methods that often caused massive infection, perforation and hemorrhage, ultimate sterility, terrible pain, death.

The sheer carnage was agonizing testimony to the fact that large segments of the public had already withdrawn consent from the ideas that had prompted the laws against abortion in the first place—and this, essentially, is why the laws were changed.

On January 22, 1973, the United States Supreme Court ruled that the performance of an abortion before three months of gestation was strictly the decision of a woman and her doctor. After three months, the same holds true—except that the states are allowed to more stringently regulate the medical practices of facilities where abortions are performed.

Since that original decision, this freedom has progressively eroded. In 1977, the Supreme Court declared that states had the right to prohibit payment for abortion for poor women on medical assistance. More recently, regulations written for federally funded medical programs have prohibited abortion payments except in cases of rape and incest and the chance that the mother may die. Military dependents no longer have insurance coverage for abortion.

Women who are not actively fighting this trend should reconsider their silence, for it could eventually return our daughters to the sad situation of our grandmothers.

Under current American law, every woman makes the decision about abortion *for herself.*

For many women, abortion involves ethical issues which must be resolved by the individual conscience, not by the law.

For all women, abortion involves health issues of vital importance: abortion is an operation involving the risks of blood loss and infection. Like other surgery it should be avoided if possible—in this case by careful attention to birth control. *Abortion should never be thought of as a birth-control method.* However, as stated before, even properly used methods have a predictable failure rate, and the choice for abortion must therefore be available.

Abortion should be used as the method of last resort—by women who are *absolutely convinced* that it is the proper course for them. It must always be a personal decision, not the decision of friends, parents, or boy friends and husbands; *advice* is helpful, but women should see to it that the *consent* of others is not a legal requisite.

1. Abortion is legal—but not equally available in all states

Federal law does not automatically override state antiabortion laws, and in some states, this means that legal battles over abortion reform are still being fought. A woman may have an easier time obtaining a late abortion in New York, for example, than in some areas of neighboring New Jersey, where the status of the law is somewhat different. Women on medical assistance will have increasing difficulty obtaining payment, and all women should fight to secure new equal treatment.

2. No physician is obligated to perform an abortion

If the physician you normally see is unwilling to perform the operation, he or she should refer you to another doctor or clinic. *It is just as important that a doctor have the right to refuse to perform an abortion as it is for the woman to have the right to have one;* however, neither patient nor doctor may restrict the other's rights. If the doctor refuses a referral, Planned Parenthood can usually provide free information on clinics and physicians in your area who are ready and qualified to perform abortions.

3. Check your insurance plan for abortion coverage

Blue Cross/Blue Shield covers abortion in many states, but some other insurance plans do not. If abortion would be your option for an unwanted pregnancy, check your current plan and plans you are considering to see whether it is covered.

4. Medical reasons for abortion

Although the vast majority of abortions are requested by the woman with no overriding medical problem, some medical reasons may compel a woman to abort when she would have preferred to deliver the child. These include:

    a. Risks to the woman's own health, from diseases such as:

        1. Severe heart disease

        2. Severe kidney disease

        3. Severe hypertension

        4. Severe diabetes with kidney disease

        5. Sickle-cell anemia or other related disease (see p. 370)

        6. Cancer of the genital tract

        7. Some cases of myasthenia gravis, a neurologic disease, that does not respond to drugs

    b. Risks of severe genetic defects or illness in the child:

1. Development of rubella (German measles) or other viral illnesses in early pregnancy (see p. 222)

2. Exposure (during early pregnancy) to drugs known to cause deformities or disease (see pp. 223–24)

3. Excessive X-ray exposure

4. Serious or fatal genetic disorders in the child which can be detected by amniocentesis (see Chapter Seven) (Ref. 1)

Seek another opinion if abortion is recommended for any other "medical reasons," and you do not want it.

5. Legalization has vastly improved the safety of abortion

In 1976, approximately 1,000,000 legal abortions were performed in the United States. The death rate for legal abortions in 1976 was 1 per 100,000 (Ref. 2): a *low* estimate of the death rate from criminal abortions is 40 per 100,000. Some experts estimate that 70 per cent of the women who had legal abortions would have had illegal ones if the law had provided them no other recourse. (Ref. 3) Thus, it can be said that the availability of legal abortions probably saved the lives of at least 250 women in 1976. The complication rate, for example from infections that lead to infertility, is likewise much lower now that abortions are legal.

Other beneficial effects on public health arise from the availability of abortion when major genetic abnormalities are detected. And there are immeasurable benefits to the woman who suffers from chronic disease and who can now abort before her pregnancy further taxes her already weakened health.

METHODS OF ABORTION

6. Recommended techniques of abortion

Only these techniques should be considered.

a. *Menstrual extraction* can be used in very early pregnancy or suspected pregnancy up to the second week past the missed menstrual period.

b. *Suction abortion* is the preferred method of abortion for pregnancies between six weeks and fifteen weeks after the last menstrual period. (Some centers perform suction abortion and D & E up to twenty weeks.)

c. *Saline instillation* will be used between fourteen and twenty-six weeks of pregnancy.

d. *Prostaglandin administration* is an alternative to saline instillation in later pregnancies and is increasingly being used in early pregnancy on an experimental basis.

e. *Urea instillation* is being widely tested as an alternative to saline instillation in later abortions.

WARNING: There is no safe way to induce abortion with medications taken by mouth or by injection.

7. Routine pre-abortion procedures

a. *The physician who will perform the abortion must know the woman's medical history in detail.* This includes history of previous pregnancies as well as all past and present medical problems and allergies. *Be honest. Conceal nothing.* If you do, you are preventing yourself from receiving the best possible care.

If a physician or clinic does not ask for a *complete* medical history, pick an alternative site for the procedure.

b. Certain laboratory tests are essential before an abortion: *a good clinic will do them all.*

1. A *pregnancy test* and *pelvic exam* must be done to verify that you are pregnant, and how far along you are.

2. A *blood count* must be done to rule out anemia.

3. *Blood type* and Rh type must be determined. (See p. 179)

4. *Blood pressure* must be taken.

5. *Urine* must be checked for sugar and protein.

6. A *Pap smear* for cervical cancer should be taken if a woman has not had one in the last six months. (This is an optional test but performed by most good clinics.)

7. *Tests for VD,* especially gonorrhea, should be taken. If a woman has undetected gonorrhea in her cervix, she risks infection of the uterus, tubes, and ovaries after the procedure. (See p. 311) The abortion procedure should be postponed until the disease is treated—usually only a matter of a few days.

c. Be prepared to make two visits to the clinic or doctor's office—one for tests, one for the abortion.

8. Menstrual extraction

For women who recognize that they are pregnant within two weeks after their first missed period, menstrual extraction is the ideal method of abortion.

It can be done with or without local anesthetic and involves only minor discomfort.

First, a speculum (SPECK-you-lum) is inserted into the vagina as in an ordinary pelvic examination. The vagina and the cervix are grasped with a tenaculum (ten-ACK-you-lum), a small surgical clasp. If local anesthesia is used, it is injected at this point into the cervix—causing a little pain. A flexible plastic cannula (CAN-you-la) attached to a syringe is then inserted into the cervix. (*Cannula* comes from the Latin word for cane or reed, and that's what a cannula looks like—a reed, thin as a drinking straw.) Suction is applied with the syringe and the lining of the uterus—including the pregnancy, is removed.

9. Routine procedures after menstrual extraction

After menstrual extraction, the woman should wait at least thirty minutes for a blood-pressure test. Bleeding should be checked. A follow-up examination should be scheduled for no more than three weeks later, to make sure there are no complications or side effects, including the possibility that the procedure has failed and the pregnancy has not been ended. (See ⚮35 below)

10. When should menstrual extraction be performed?

Menstrual extraction should be performed no later than two weeks after a missed menstrual period, and no earlier than the date the period was expected.

11. Who should perform menstrual extraction?

Only a physician trained in sterile technique and with experience doing pelvic examinations and abortion should perform menstrual extraction. The procedure should not be done by the woman herself, because of the greater risk of infection.

12. Where should menstrual extraction be performed?

Menstrual extraction may be performed in a doctor's office or an outpatient clinic; hospitalization is not usually necessary.

13. Advantages of menstrual extraction

a. *Menstrual extraction can be performed before the routine urine test for pregnancy is positive.* Since the safest abortion is the earliest possible abortion, the procedure is the safest of all abortion techniques.

b. *Menstrual extraction involves very few side effects.*

The immediate complications of the procedure appear to be very few —a 1 per cent incidence of infection, excess bleeding, cramps, and spotting. In about 2–5 per cent of cases, the procedure does not work and the pregnancy has to be ended at a later date by another procedure. This is why the examination at two to three weeks is very important.

The biggest advantage of menstrual extraction is that the cervix does not need to be dilated. This is important because some practitioners believe that dilation of the cervix during abortion leads to future incidence of premature delivery. (See ⚹37 below)

14. Is menstrual extraction really an abortion?

Because menstrual extraction can be used to treat the *possibility* of pregnancy, some states believe it is not really an abortion at all. This difference of opinion affects the matter of regulation. In New York, for example, menstrual extraction is considered an abortion procedure, is regulated for medical safety in the same manner as other abortions, and must be reported to state and federal statisticians. In some other states, the status of menstrual extraction is not clear, and the procedure is not regulated so closely.

Whether or not a state considers menstrual extraction an abortion, the woman herself should do enough checking to make sure she is having it done under excellent medical conditions—to guarantee her own safety even when the state does not. (See ⚹39 below, How to Choose a Safe Abortion Clinic)

15. Suction abortion

Suction abortion is the preferable procedure for terminating pregnancies of six to fifteen weeks' duration.

Anesthesia is always used—either general or local (paracervical block, an injection of local anesthetic into the cervix). If local anesthesia is used, a woman will sometimes receive a sedative before the procedure begins.

A speculum is placed in the vagina. The cervix is grasped with a tenaculum and the anesthesia is injected into the cervix. Both of these steps may involve a short-lived pain until the anesthetic takes hold. There should be very little pain during the procedure after that.

The cervix is gradually widened with a set of successively larger dilators until it is just wide enough to receive the cannula, the plastic tubing that is connected to a suction pump. The pump sucks the tissue of pregnancy into the tubing and thence into a container in which it is collected and sent for pathological examination. After the suction, some physicians scrape the inside of the uterus with a metal curette, to make sure all the tissue is removed from the uterine wall. ("Curette" comes from the French word *curer*, which means "to clean.")

16. Routine procedures after suction abortion

The woman should rest several hours in a recovery room after the operation, where her blood pressure and pulse will be monitored frequently, and she will be observed for amount of bleeding. She should be prepared to stay until the sedative wears off and she feels well enough to go home. Some centers routinely give prescriptions for medications to take to contract the uterus, and for infection if it develops later. While the woman is still in the recovery room she will usually receive the first dose of Ergotrate (URG-oh-trate), the drug to contract the uterus and to lessen the bleeding. Do not expect to take any other drug at this time.

Before leaving the clinic, schedule a follow-up examination for within the next two to four weeks.

17. When should suction abortion be performed?

Suction abortion may be performed up to fifteen weeks of pregnancy —*but it is much preferable to do the procedure before twelve weeks,* for the complication rates rise sharply thereafter.

18. Who should perform suction abortion?

Try to use an obstetrician-gynecologist who has performed the operation frequently before. The more procedures any physician performs, the lower the rates of complication.

19. Where should suction abortion be performed?

Suction abortion can be done very safely in outpatient clinics up to twelve weeks of pregnancy. However, women who are further along than this, or who have any medical problems, should use a hospital, not a free-standing clinic.

20. Dilatation and evacuation: (D & E) a supplementary procedure for suction abortions at thirteen to fifteen weeks

WARNING: Do not allow D and E *alone* for abortion performed prior to twelve weeks. The suction procedure is preferable, with lower blood loss and fewer complications.

However, between twelve and fifteen weeks, dilatation and evacuation is frequently used *in addition* to suction. In this procedure, the uterus is scraped with a curette after the suction.

Some physicians use the procedure up to twenty weeks with great safety—but this is still debatable practice for later pregnancies (Ref. 4, 5). Watch for news about this matter.

21. Saline instillation

Saline instillation is a procedure frequently used between fifteen and twenty-six weeks of pregnancy. In this procedure a concentrated solution of salt is introduced into the uterus in exchange for the amniotic fluid around the fetus.

The woman empties her bladder, lies on her back, and the lower part of her abdomen is washed with antiseptic solution. A small amount of local anesthetic is injected into the skin over the uterus. Then a long needle is inserted through the abdomen into the sac around the fetus. The fluid is removed through the needle and replaced by the saline solution. Some physicians will use a small plastic catheter rather than leave the needle in place.

A general anesthetic will not be given, for the woman must be awake during this procedure. The reason for this is that occasionally the saline solution is injected into a blood vessel causing dizziness and headaches which the woman must be able to report immediately to her physician.

Within two to twenty-four hours, the uterus begins cramping. This will last for several hours until the fetus is delivered. Frequently, as the cramps begin, some fluid will leak from the vagina. To strengthen contractions and shorten the time of the procedure, the woman may have an intravenous bottle containing a dilute solution of Pitocin (pi-TOE-sin), a drug that causes the uterus to contract, attached to her arm. The placenta will be delivered after or with the fetus. The whole procedure takes between twelve and thirty-six hours. Sometimes the placenta does not deliver itself, and a curettage (a scraping of the uterine lining) must be performed. The cervix is already open, so dilatation is not needed. During the contractions with a saline abortion, a woman will need analgesic drugs.

Sometimes, in pregnancies earlier than sixteen weeks, the saline solution will be introduced through a needle or catheter that is passed through the lower part of the uterus via vagina. This route, however, has a somewhat increased rate of infections. The obvious advantage is that the woman does not have to wait until sixteen weeks.

RECOMMENDATION: At present, the suction abortion—D & E combination is safer for thirteen to fifteen-week pregnancies. (See ⊁20 above)

22. Routine procedures after saline abortion

Remain in the hospital until the abortion is complete. If you find that your hospital or doctor suggests that women go home to await cramps, choose another site for your abortion. Blood pressure, bleeding, pulse should be monitored for at least six to twelve hours afterward. Allot several days for recuperation at home and schedule a follow-up appointment for no longer than four weeks later.

23. When should saline instillation be performed?

Saline abortion should be performed preferably *after* the fifteenth week of pregnancy—the complication rate is lower then.

24. Who should perform saline instillation?
Only a qualified obstetrician-gynecologist.

25. Where should saline instillation be performed?
Only in a fully equipped hospital.

26. Concentrated urea solutions as an alternative to saline
Urea is found normally in the body: in concentrated solutions it has the same effect as saline solution in starting uterine contractions. It is currently being widely tested throughout the country. Early studies suggest that it *may* have fewer side effects than saline, and *may* be the treatment of choice for women with medical problems. The procedures are the same as for saline abortions.

27. Prostaglandin adminstration: alternative methods of early and late abortions
Prostaglandins are fatty acids which function as hormones in the body and can cause strong contractions of the uterus. (See p. 325) They have been found effective in inducing abortion when given:
a. Into the amniotic sac
b. Into the space between the membrane and the uterus
c. Into the vagina and
d. Into a vein by injection.

A major problem with the use of prostaglandins is the occurrence of severe, although not life-threatening, side effects such as nausea, vomiting, and diarrhea. Usually these symptoms can be controlled with appropriate medications, and in many centers prostaglandins are being used routinely in place of the saline for late abortions. A vaginal suppository of prostaglandin is now commercially available.

The role of prostaglandins in early abortions is less clear. If a simple method of administration can be found, then it may well replace suction procedures in years to come. At present, the gastrointestinal side effects as well as the problem of a significant number of incomplete abortions, make prostaglandin administration inappropriate for routine abortions in the first twelve weeks.

Look ahead! The methods of second-trimester abortion may change greatly over the next few years, so watch the media for reports.

28. Hysterotomy and hysterectomy are not proper methods of abortion
a. *Hysterotomy,* a kind of mini-Caesarean section, was used widely for abortion in the fourth to sixth month of pregnancy before saline instillation became available. It is a major operation with a high mortality rate as well as other complications. Hysterotomy should only be used

as an abortion technique in the rare eventuality that saline instillation fails several times or if infection or hemorrhage occur.

b. *Hysterectomy,* the removal of the uterus, is sometimes recommended to women who want an abortion and no further pregnancies.

WARNING: *If either of these procedures are recommended to you, refuse, unless you have a very serious gynecologic disorder as well*—such as cancer.

Suction curettage or saline abortion are safer forms of abortion; tubal ligation (see p. 80) is a vastly safer form of sterilization (in terms of medical complications). *Hysterectomy should only be used to treat a serious illness, and neither pregnancy nor fertility is an illness!* Never accept hysterectomy as an abortion procedure on any other basis, for it is major surgery with much higher risks than other abortion procedures. (See p. 333)

29. Laminaria, a seaweed product that helps dilate the cervix

To assist in dilating the cervix before an abortion, some physicians and clinics recommend the use of laminaria (la-min-AIR-ee-a). The laminaria is inserted into the cervix twelve to twenty-four hours before the abortion. It swells and gently starts to dilate the cervix, making mechanical dilation easier later on. This is especially useful for a woman who has never had children, whose cervix may be difficult to dilate, for it decreases the risk of laceration. (See ✕35d below)

NORMAL POSTABORTION COURSE

---

30. Routine care and normal after effects of abortion

a. Do not leave the clinic or hospital without a twenty-four-hour-a-day phone number to call in case of emergencies.

b. Even if you feel fine, have an examination 3–4 weeks after the abortion, which you should schedule before you go home from the abortion procedure.

c. Bleeding from an abortion usually lasts one to two weeks—it may last only a few days or up to four weeks. The bleeding is usually very light (less than a menstrual period) after the first two days. A series of a few small clots in the days immediately following the procedure is normal. Large clots and constant heavy bleeding are not normal. If the amount seems too great, contact your physician or clinic *immediately.*

d. Mild cramps are normal for the first few days after the abortion. Frequently medications are prescribed to help the uterus contract back to normal size and these may cause more severe cramping in the first two to three days. Also, the later the abortion, the more frequent and severe the cramping, for the uterus has to shrink back to normal from a much larger size. After early abortions it is also normal to experience no cramping at all. If constant, severe pain is experienced, especially if accompanied by heavy bleeding or fever, a woman should contact her physician or clinic *immediately*.

e. Infection sometimes occurs after abortion, so a woman should check her temperature several times daily for the first few days after the procedure and notify her physician if it is over 100. A foul-smelling vaginal discharge is another sign of possible infection.

f. The first period after an abortion should occur within fifty days. If it does not, see a physician.

g. Breast tenderness may occur, especially after late abortions. Medications are sometimes given to counteract this at the time of the procedure, *but a tight bra or binder is the best and safest treatment*. (See p. 158)

h. Resume showering, bathing, washing hair, and eating immediately after abortion.

i. Douching should be avoided for at least two weeks after the procedure, or else fluid may get past the still-open cervix and cause infection.

j. Intercourse should be avoided for the first few days. If resumed within the first two weeks, the man should use a condom for the same reason as stated above.

k. Fatigue is normal after an abortion, even an early one—because of blood loss and the release of tension. Plan for at least two days' recuperation to get your strength back completely.

31. Resume contraception soon after abortion

Many women ovulate very shortly after abortion, so plans should be made before the procedure for the use of contraception. Birth-control pills may be started immediately after the procedure. They may also be started after the first period; have your partner use condoms until that time.

The IUD is usually inserted during the first menstrual period but not before six weeks after the procedure (to decrease the chance of perforation, see p. 58). Use condoms until this time. Some physicians insert IUDs immediately after an *early* abortion procedure and this is safe. However, IUDs should not be inserted immediately after a *late* procedure because the uterus is still too large and expulsion rate very high.

If a woman uses a diaphragm, this should be fitted at least three to four weeks *after* an abortion so that all the relaxation effects of the pregnancy on the vagina will be gone.

32. RhoGam administration is routine postabortion treatment for women with Rh-negative blood

Even in the termination of early pregnancies, a woman may become sensitized to Rh-positive red cells and therefore have problems with future pregnancies. (See pp. 178–79) For this reason, all women having abortions should be tested for blood type and, if Rh negative, should receive RhoGam after the procedure. Check with the clinic or doctor ahead of time about RhoGam if you know you are Rh negative—at some places the shot is included in the fee, in others it is not.

33. Warning: Do not accept hormone treatment to bring on your period until you are sure you are not pregnant

Sometimes women who are late with their periods are given progesterone shots or tablets to bring it on. *Recent warnings suggest that synthetic progestogens given during pregnancy may cause fetal malformations.* So don't accept this medication until you have had a pregnancy test and are absolutely sure you are not pregnant. These medications do not induce abortion, they only bring on a period if you are *not* pregnant.

34. The earliest abortion is the safest abortion

The later in pregnancy the abortion is performed, the greater the risk of complication. On the other hand, when performed before the eighth week of pregnancy, it is one of the safest of all surgical procedures. Abortion only becomes dangerous when indecision, fear, or misinformation delay it. *So don't wait.*

ABORTION COMPLICATIONS

35. Major complications of abortion

Most serious complications occur in later abortions. These include:

a. *Hemorrhage.* There can be several causes for a postabortion hemorrhage: the tissues of conception have not been completely evacuated, and the remainder is delivered with a lot of bleeding afterward; the uterus has not completely contracted after the abortion, causing sudden severe bleeding; or lacerations or perforations of the uterus have occurred without anyone noticing.

The symptom of hemorrhage is heavy bleeding that persists; *if it occurs, don't wait to reach a doctor by phone; go to the doctor or to the nearest emergency room immediately.*

In an early abortion, excess bleeding will be detected more frequently while the woman is still in the clinic: in later abortions, hemorrhage generally occurs after the woman has gone home. Hemorrhage is much more likely after a late abortion than after an early one.

b. *Infection* of the uterine lining, or endometritis, (en-doh-mee-TRY-tis) occurs in about 2–3 per cent or all abortions, but is more frequent in procedures after twelve weeks. The symptoms are:

1. A foul-smelling vaginal discharge
2. Persistent lower abdominal pain or cramping
3. Fever

See a doctor immediately if you suspect infection. Antibiotics will be prescribed which should arrest the infection within twenty-four hours; generally they should be taken for seven to ten days. In severe cases, hospitalization may be in order.

Extension of the infection to the Fallopian tubes and general abdomen is very rare in legal abortions—although it was fearfully frequent with illegal abortions.

c. *Perforation of the uterus* is a complication of suction abortions which again increases in incidence as the pregnancy increases in duration. It occurs in about one in five hundred abortions. It is usually caused when an instrument used in the procedure (either a dilator or suction curette) accidentally pierces the upper part of the uterus. With a perforation in the uterus the woman will be observed for signs of bleeding into the abdomen and excess vaginal bleeding. Many physicians will recommend laparoscopy (la-par-OS-co-py) for women in whom uterine perforation is suspected. (See p. 105) In this operation, the doctor inserts a scope through the navel to view the uterus directly and see whether there is a hole, and significant bleeding, in which case there would have to be further repair. If perforations are not detected at the time of the procedure, later signs could be severe abdominal pain and bleeding into the abdomen. Before nine weeks of pregnancy, this complication is very rare.

d. *Cervical lacerations* can occur in both early and late abortions. In the suction procedures, these are usually caused by the tenaculum tearing through the soft cervix, or by dilators, and can almost always be repaired easily, with little long-term problem. In the later procedures (especially with prostaglandin abortions) severe cervical lacerations can occur with very forceful contractions working against a cervix that is very tightly closed. If the lacerations are severe, a complicated repair may be needed. Laminaria (see ✗29 above) inserted into the cervix before the abortion procedure may reduce this complication. Cervical lacerations occur in one of every 100–200 procedures. (Ref. 6)

e. *Injection of solution into a vein during instillation*

This can sometimes occur *during* the saline or urea instillation procedure or, when blood absorbs the solution, in the hours immediately afterward. It will be detected by blood tests showing increased salt or urea in the blood. Early symptoms will be severe headache, thirst, dizziness, nausea, and abdominal pain. The nurse or doctor should be notified if you have these symptoms so that a doctor can treat it immediately.

f. *Blood-clotting disorders* are *rare* complications of abortion, mainly reported in association with saline instillation but also reported with urea and suction procedures. Some women, during the process of the abortion or shortly thereafter, develop a disorder called *disseminated intravascular coagulation* (DIC) in which small clots occur in the blood vessels, and all the substances important for blood clotting are used up. The symptoms are uncontrollable bleeding from the uterus as well as the gums and nose in some cases. The treatment is the administration of plasma or fresh blood and the rapid delivery of the fetus.

g. *Allergic reaction to local anesthesia.* This often can be avoided by careful attention to pre-existing allergies and medical history before the procedure begins.

h. *Failure to discontinue the pregnancy.* In 1–5 per cent of menstrual extractions and suction abortions, the pregnancy is not ended and a very disappointed woman will have to return for another procedure. In saline procedures, 3–5 per cent of women will have to receive a repeat injection of saline because they do not go into labor within twenty-four to forty-eight hours.

36. Can a woman die from an abortion?

You are in less mortal danger with a legal abortion than with a normal, term delivery.

Data from a very large sample of abortions performed in 1972–76 before eight weeks of pregnancy, show a death rate of 1/100,000. Between nine and ten weeks, the risk is 2.8/100,000 and between eleven and twelve weeks, 4.7/100,000. After twelve weeks, the mortality rate becomes much higher; 13.0 deaths per 100,000 women having abortions between thirteen and fifteen weeks; 26.8 deaths per 100,000 women having abortions between sixteen and twenty weeks. At 21 weeks or more the death rate was 44.7/100,000. (Ref. 2)

It is only when the abortions of over twelve weeks are encountered that the death rate exceeds the death rate for childbirth. In 1975, 10.8 women died per every 100,000 live births. (Ref. 7) This figure refers to *all* deaths due to *all* complications in pregnant or recently pregnant women. *So in the first three months of pregnancy, abortion is safer than giving birth.* Thereafter, it becomes an increasingly dangerous procedure which should be avoided if at all possible by early action. Each year that abortion has been legal, the death rate has gone down. This is probably because women are obtaining earlier abortions.

37. Long-term effects of abortion

a. Uncomplicated abortions probably have no effect on a woman's ability to conceive or bear children in the future. However, if the procedure is complicated by uterine and tubal infection, infertility may result as from other pelvic infections. (See pp. 96–97)

b. There is some evidence that *repeated abortions* can cause a higher incidence of premature deliveries in future pregnancies. Some Eastern European countries where abortion is widely used as a method of birth control, show much higher prematurity rates than the rest of Europe. (Ref. 8) This has *not* been confirmed by studies made in this country and in Britain.

38. Emotional effects of abortion

The major emotional effect of abortion is relief at the safe end of an unwanted pregnancy and at this proof that a woman can control the course of her own life.

Those women who go into the abortion with severe, unresolved doubts may come out of it with feelings of guilt and depression that can last for weeks. Sometimes women who thought they were sure about the abortion are plagued by depression afterward. This may be more likely to occur after late abortions, when a woman has had time to feel and look pregnant, and the abortion itself has been so similar to delivery.

These feelings of depression generally pass quickly.

They have to do as much with the emotional shock of discovering you are pregnant when you don't want to be as with the abortion itself.

Postabortion depression is not punishment for a crime! It is just a depression, the aftereffect of a harrowing experience, supported by endocrine changes that affect your mood. Treat it the way you would treat a depression for any other reason—with a change of scene or a change of pace, lots of company or pleasant solitude, a little self-indulgence, the distractions of work and entertainment.

It is important to remember that the loss of a pregnancy, whether by therapeutic abortion or spontaneous abortion may produce a reaction similar to mourning. For this reason it is important to be able to remind yourself that you did not want the pregnancy, could not have continued it—and abortion was the only way to end it.

In the event that depression continues and becomes more severe, seek help from a qualified psychiatrist, psychologist, or family counselor.

39. How to choose a safe abortion clinic

a. If a woman has any doubt at all about her private doctor's ability to perform an effective, safe abortion (bad word-of-mouth is as good a deterrent as any), she should go to a clinic which specializes in abortion.

b. Abortion is now a business—and women must watch out for unscrupulous operators. Abortion clinics recommending some unusual procedures should be avoided. (Many women who submitted to the unusual "supercoil" abortions by Dr. Harvey Karman wound up with infected abortions; at least one woman was rendered permanently sterile.)

c. When choosing a clinic:

Make sure the physicians on staff there are certified by the American Board of Obstetrics and Gynecology by checking on them with your local medical society.

Call the city or state board of health, give the name of the clinic and verify that it is operating within the criteria set for public safety.

Do not go to a clinic which is *not* affiliated with a nearby hospital. Many clinics operate on independent premises—but all the good ones are associated with hospitals so that in case of any emergency, a woman can be transferred to hospital care immediately.

Planned Parenthood or other non-profit abortion-referral services in your community can be called for an opinion on the clinic and physicians you are considering.

Try to get several opinions from women who have used the clinic in the past.

No matter what wonderful things you have heard about the clinic, do not accept answers to questions about the credentials of the place and the staff from the clinic itself. *Always verify your choice* with reliable outside sources—the local medical society, local board of health, local Planned Parenthood, women who have used the facility previously.

40. The out-of-town abortion

If you have to leave your home locale to have the abortion:

a. Check out the clinic you are going to in the same thorough way you would check out a local clinic.

b. Try not to go alone or return alone—company is comforting when you're in a strange town.

c. Tell someone in your home town where you are going and how they can reach you.

d. Do not make a long return trip the same day as the abortion; try to arrange to stay over at least one night—if the clinic cannot suggest a nice place within your means, try the Y.

ILLUSTRATIONS

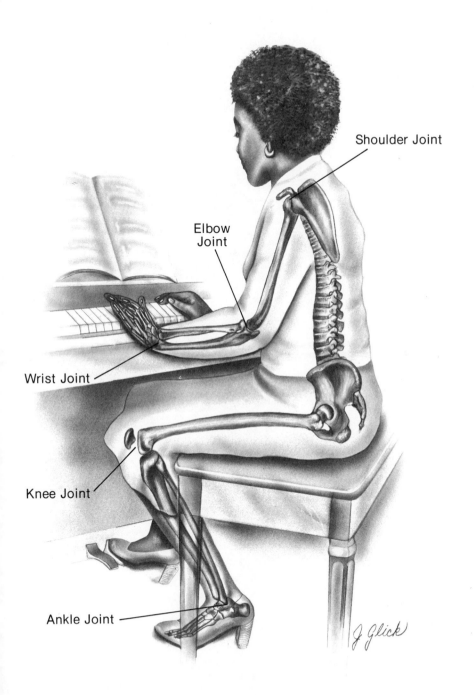

Shoulder Joint

Elbow Joint

Wrist Joint

Knee Joint

Ankle Joint

J. Glick

BONES AND JOINTS

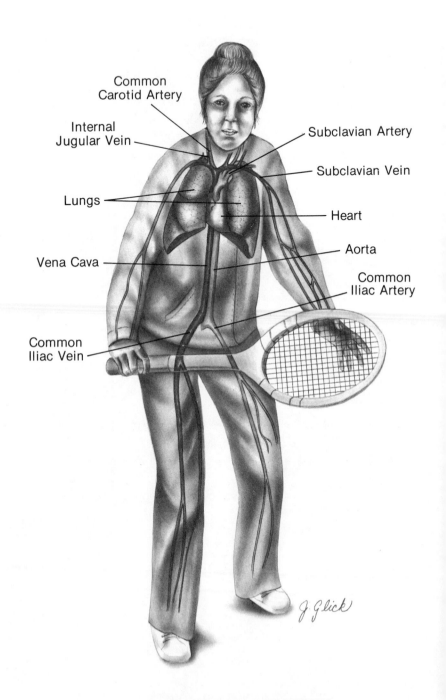

Common
Carotid Artery

Internal
Jugular Vein

Lungs

Vena Cava

Common
Iliac Vein

Subclavian Artery

Subclavian Vein

Heart

Aorta

Common
Iliac Artery

J. Glick

THE CARDIOVASCULAR SYSTEM

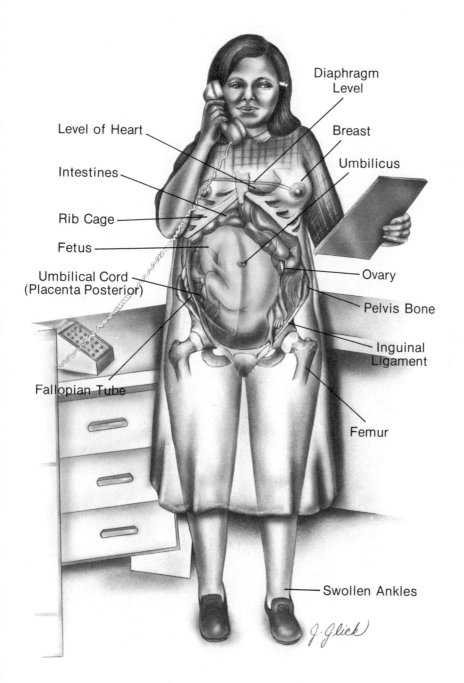

Diaphragm
Level

Level of Heart

Breast

Intestines

Umbilicus

Rib Cage

Fetus

Umbilical Cord
(Placenta Posterior)

Ovary

Pelvis Bone

Inguinal
Ligament

Fallopian Tube

Femur

Swollen Ankles

J. Glick

PREGNANCY AT ADVANCED STAGE

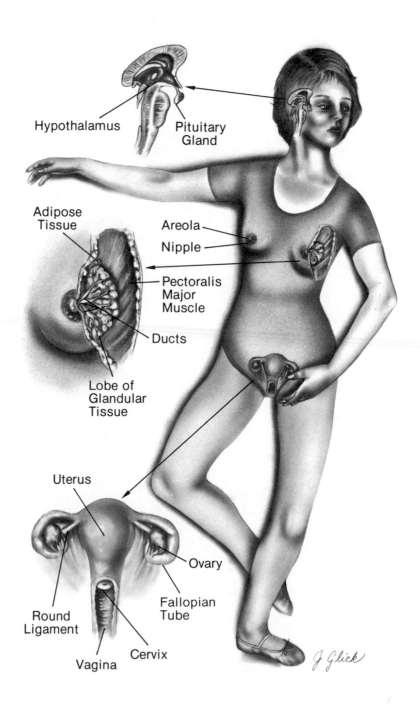

Hypothalamus

Pituitary
Gland

Adipose
Tissue

Areola

Nipple

Pectoralis
Major
Muscle

Ducts

Lobe of
Glandular
Tissue

Uterus

Ovary

Fallopian
Tube

Round
Ligament

Cervix

Vagina

J. Glick

THE REPRODUCTIVE SYSTEM

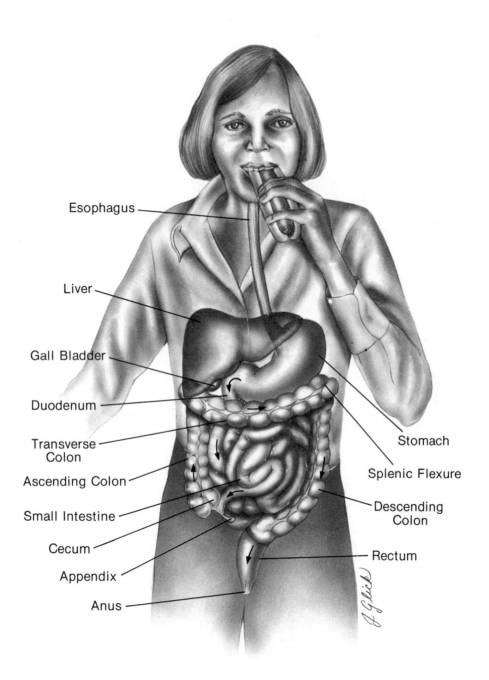

Esophagus

Liver

Gall Bladder

Duodenum

Transverse
Colon

Ascending Colon

Small Intestine

Cecum

Appendix

Anus

Stomach

Splenic Flexure

Descending
Colon

Rectum

THE DIGESTIVE SYSTEM

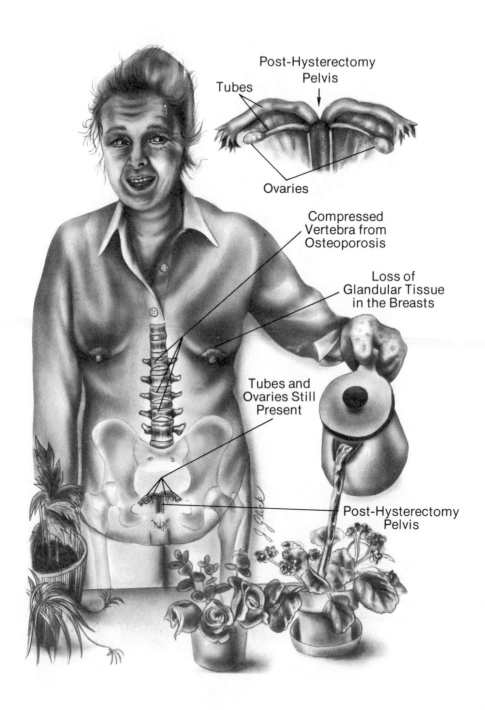

Post-Hysterectomy
Pelvis

Tubes

Ovaries

Compressed
Vertebra from
Osteoporosis

Loss of
Glandular Tissue
in the Breasts

Tubes and
Ovaries Still
Present

Post-Hysterectomy
Pelvis

POST-MENOPAUSAL WOMAN

e. Make sure you return home with all the prescriptions you may need, including written advice on over-the-counter drugs and postabortion care. That will save you long-distance phone calls later on.

f. See a local physician not later than three weeks after returning home.

As with abortions in your own locality, make sure you know the *full name* of the doctor or doctors attending at your abortion.

41. Never have an abortion in secret

Even though abortion is a woman's legal right, many women—especially young girls—do not want to tell anyone they are pregnant and go into the abortion procedure in secret. This is foolish and unnecessary and immeasurably increases the emotional wear and tear on the woman.

If you cannot tell your parents, tell a trusted friend.

If you cannot tell anyone you know, go to Planned Parenthood or other abortion-counseling agencies and tell someone there. Your confidence will be respected. Frequently you can walk into the local hospital and ask to see a social worker—you should be able to get good advice and strictest confidence here. Also consider talking to clergy.

It is vital not to have any operation in secret because complications may arise which must be taken care of immediately, and which you cannot treat yourself.

Also, there is no comfort to match the comfort of a friend when you are in a tight spot, when you are worried and tense, facing a new experience and wrestling with unfamiliar fears.

42. Counseling comes with abortion

Any accredited clinic or hospital which provides abortion services provides counseling of some sort.

At worst, you will be asked some questions about why you want the abortion, how many other children you have, etc., which waste your time and seem more like the collection of material for a school term paper than a real effort at guidance. At best, you can find yourself provided with a wise and sympathetic counselor at a time when many women really need one.

If you have serious doubts about the abortion, don't rely on the counselors at the abortion agency. They are on staff; if you need to be sent home, they cannot realistically be expected to stress that possibility; *they are there to calm you down, not change your mind.* In exactly the same way, a visit to an antiabortion counseling agency, or some clergy, will get you the same sort of one-sided advice. If a woman is married and able to provide a familial home for her child—many counselors who would otherwise recommend abortion will try to dissuade her. This variety of biases will be apparent if you look hard at the prospective counselor. Try to see people who are not likely to impose *external social criteria* on your personal situation.

You can get good counseling from friends, from your local family service, from a consciousness-raising group, from clergy—especially clergy who have *not* known you since you were a little girl, who did not perform your wedding ceremony or officiate at your oldest girl's christening or your youngest boy's bar mitzvah. It is a fact that because of the newness of the legality of abortion, many women do not know what they think about it—and counseling can help a woman think through her ideas on abortion and come to a conclusion that is right for her.

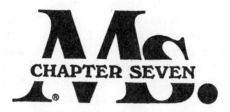

CHAPTER SEVEN

GENETICS and PRENATAL DIAGNOSIS

Genetics—the science of heredity—will provide us with some of our most brilliant medical advances and some of our most excruciating moral dilemmas in the coming decades. New discoveries in genetics and related fields such as eugenics (you-GEN-ics), molecular biology (mo-LEK-u-lar), environmental medicine, and biophysics are coming thick and fast. Eugenics is the science of making improvements in the genetic inheritance of people; molecular biology, the study of the microscopic particles that make up the cells of life, may be used to affect the cells that control inheritance; environmental medicine is the study of how factors like sunlight and pollution affect our health, including the health of our unborn children and grandchildren; biophysics applies what physicists know about matter and energy to the human body; the ultrasound (see p. 186), which uses sound waves to assess the health of a fetus, is an invention of biophysics. All these fields, now in their flowering, feed the study of heredity. Their technology is often baffling to the non-scientist; *however we must understand something about that technology if we are to keep control of our own lives.*

The questions asked of genetic research often sound like science fiction (remember, visiting Mars sounded like science fiction a few years ago). Ask yourself this: What will happen to society if children can be created routinely by the union of sperm and egg in a laboratory? What will happen to the human species if human beings can be created *without* sexual union—by making an egg reproduce itself without a sperm, so that it becomes an exact duplicate of its parent? (This is called *cloning;* it has already been accomplished with small organisms. (See p. 114)

If genetically inherited disease can be wiped out by genetic medicine, can *any* inherited quality be bred in or out? For example, can we breed for blue eyes or musical talent? When technology makes the production of "perfect" people possible, what will happen to those of us who are "imperfect"? And who will control the definition of perfection?

If molecular biologists create new forms of life by recombining the genetic material of different organisms, will these new forms be good for humanity or will they destroy us all? (Ref. 1) How is it possible even to *experiment* with these new forms of knowledge and keep the world safe from biological disaster either through accident (read *The*

Andromeda Strain by Michael Crichton) or through design (read *Mein Kampf* by Adolf Hitler)?

In days gone by, poor women were wet nurses for rich women who didn't wish to be bothered suckling a child. Genetic engineering allows us to envisage the day when a woman who doesn't want to be bothered *carrying* a child can allow her egg to be fertilized in a laboratory and implanted in another woman, whom she has hired to carry the baby for her.

And what will happen, in a world where most people still prefer sons, when genetic technology allows us to predict *and control* the sex of our unborn children?

It is not possible to consider these questions in this chapter, which confines itself to genetic technology that specifically affects the health of women and their unborn children.

But it would be wise for women to read further in this field, which promises so much and threatens so much and about which we must all be educated enough to make *personal* decisions, so that the final decisions will not be entirely out of our hands.

NORMAL DEVELOPMENT— THE ROLE OF CHROMOSOMES

1. Chromosomes and their component genes contain the genetic material that determines individual characteristics

A chromosome (CROW-ma-soame) is a human cell part made up of long strands of DNA (deoxyribonucleic acid), and protein. DNA is the material of inheritance. Each person has twenty-three pairs of chromosomes, twenty-two pairs to control all physical and (to a degree) mental characteristics; the twenty-third pair determining which sex a person will be.

Genes are the tiny components of the chromosomes that control each individual characteristic that is inherited. There are one or more genes for virtually everything in the human body—blood, bones, hair, skin coloring—everything.

Chromosomes have two functions.

a. They control individual heredity.

b. They regulate *differentiation* (See ⌗6, 7 below), the process by which the fertilized egg grows and develops into different kinds of cells forming the different parts of the body.

2. Mutation: a change in chromosomal pattern

A mutation is a change in the pattern of heredity, leading to the development of a new characteristic—or the absence of an old characteristic—in a new generation. For millions of years, mutations could only be caused gradually by such things as environmental pressures and natural accident; the patterns of dappling, for example, that occur in nature evolved over time—in zebras, in poppies, in the infinite colorations of fish.

In recent years, especially since the industrial revolution and its pollutants and the great breakthroughs in physics that led to the harnessing of atomic energy, mutations—usually rare in the physical world—have become more frequent. Frighteningly so. It is now quite likely that man will injure nature through environmental pollution so that the injury is passed on to future generations, if not in humans, then in the other plants and animals with which we share this planet.

For example, radiation and food additives are known to cause genetic mutations and cancer in laboratory bacteria and small animals, and potentially have the same effects on humans.

3. How the pattern of chromosomes is studied

a. A sample of tissue scraped from the inside of the mouth will yield a picture of the sex chromosomes in an adult. This is a rapid test, (though not entirely accurate) sometimes used to determine the sex of athletes.

b. Lymphocytes (LIM-foh-sites)—white blood cells taken from a blood sample, are grown in cell culture and then analyzed for their total chromosomal pattern. This is the test commonly used to test the parents of an abnormal child to determine whether one or both of them is a carrier of the abnormal genes, and is more accurate than the smear test. This test can also be used to determine the true sex of a child who has abnormal genitals. (See p. 273)

c. Cells from the fetus, obtained in a sample of amniotic fluid, can also be grown in cell culture and analyzed. The cells can be studied for chromosome patterns as well as for enzymes and chemicals which indicate certain diseases.

4. How sex is determined

The sex chromosomes for men and women show a differing pattern. Most females have two X chromosomes and most males one X and a smaller Y chromosome.

Each sperm and each egg have twenty-three chromosomes. When they combine at fertilization, they become a union with forty-six chromosomes—twenty-three from the mother and twenty-three from the father. Since a woman has two X chromosomes, she can only produce eggs with X chromosomes. Since a man has one X and one Y chromosome, he can produce either kind of cell as his sperm. *Thus, the father determines the sex of the baby.* If he sends along an X sperm that fertilizes the egg, that will create an XX fetus—a girl. If he sends along a Y sperm, that will create an XY fetus—a boy.

5. Cell division immediately after fertilization

After the sperm fertilizes the egg in the Fallopian tube, the cells rapidly divide and multiply. By the time the conceptus (con-SEP-tus) reaches the uterus, there are about eight to sixteen cells in it, all born of the original two cells (sperm and egg) that created the original fifty-fifty chromosomal split between mother and father, all mirroring the original genetic pattern set by the sperm and the egg. Implantation in the uterus should be complete by the seventeeth day after fertilization.

6. How cells differentiate after conception

From the time of implantation (day seventeen) to the fifty-fifth day after conception, the cells are differentiating. Initially all the cells have the same chromosomal pattern, but soon they change (differentiation), some of them becoming the heart; some becoming the fingernails, etc. Some people believe that the process of differentiation begins as early as the stage when the conceptus consists of only four cells. (Ref. 2) The chromosomes have a major role in controlling differentiation, but how they do this is not completely understood.

7. Induction: the geography of differentiation

Very little is known about how differentiation starts. However, it *is* known that once this process begins, an *orderly* arrangement of cells is necessary for differentiation to continue normally. Certain kinds of cells must be arranged next to certain other kinds of cells; *their effect on each other* allows them to develop properly. This is called *induction.* Anything that disorders the placement of the cells is a threat to proper differentiation: *thalidomide* was an example. (See ※9 below)

8. Birth assets: the overwhelming majority of inherited characteristics

The overwhelming majority of inherited characteristics are for the good of the child, and women who are expecting children should be sure to keep this in mind. The word "genius" is related to the word "gene" because it is known to be caused by a miraculous admixture of inheritance and environmental conditioning.

Generally, the human species has improved over the generations: through improved nutrition, improved medicine, improved environment (particularly political environments that allow talent to express itself), and *outbreeding,* that mixing of communities which prevents so much of the damage that inbreeding (breeding among closely related people) can cause.

For example, if a mutation has caused a defect in a family and one or two generations later, cousins from that family have a child, the child is more likely to inherit the defect than if her parents had not been related. (See ⚡10 below)

Most of us never think about it, but from the point of view of genetic health, it is good for humankind to have opened its borders, paved its roads. In all the races of humanity, in every family in the world, there is the potential for genetic defect and genetic asset. In America, where today's children are so likely to have inherited traits from many ancestors of differing national backgrounds, the potential for inherited genetic assets is greater than any potential for damage.

9. Birth defects: congenital or inherited

a. *Defects caused by outside influences in early pregnancy* Up to fifty-five days after conception, a number of factors may interfere with the chemical messages among the dividing cells of the fetus and affect differentiation and induction, leading to birth defects.

Thalidomide is a *drug* which interferes with the induction of the cells that form the arms and legs.

Rubella is a *virus* that interferes with differentiation of cells that form many body parts including brain, eyes, and heart.

High-dose radiation is an *environmental factor* which can interfere with any group of cells in the body, causing defects that are obvious when the baby is born or which show up later in life (for example, a late-developing cancer).

Such birth defects are *congenital.*

The child is *born* with them but has *not inherited* them from previous generations.

b. *Defects caused by outside influences later in pregnancy* After fifty-five days of gestation, the fetus is less vulnerable to substances affecting differentiation and induction. The kinds of birth defects that can be caused at this time are often more insidious in that they affect the *rate of growth* of certain body parts or the body as a whole. Malnutrition of the mother, for example, may lead to an underweight baby with higher risk of infant death or small brain size. Maternal diseases that interfere with the blood supply to the fetus (such as high blood pressure, kidney disease, and excess smoking) may cause brain damage by impairing oxygen flow to the brain. Damage to the fetus during labor and delivery would be included in this group of defects.

Again, birth defects of this kind are *congenital.*

The child is *born* with them but has *not inherited* them from previous generations.

c. *Birth defects caused by abnormal genes or chromosomes* Some birth defects are caused by disordered messages from abnormal genes or chromosomes. Many of these disorders can be passed on from generation to generation.

Tay-Sachs disease, sickle-cell anemia, and cystic fibrosis are passed on this way, along with other relatively rare conditions (see below). Sometimes, the defect is unimportant—for example, color blindness, or oddly shaped fingers. Sometimes it is very severe—for example, hemophilia (bleeder's disease), caused by the inherited absence of the clotting factor in the blood.

These birth defects are *congenital,* in that the child is born with them. *They are also inherited,* in that the child has *inherited* them from previous generations.

Prenatal testing and amniocentesis have been most useful for detecting some inherited disorders, much less so for other congenital defects.

10. Recessive genes: the source of most inherited diseases

All chromosomes are present in pairs, so all genes are paired as well. This means that two genes, one from the father and one from the mother, determine each characteristic. Some genes are *dominant,* and the traits which derive from them are *dominant traits.*

For example, the gene for brown eyes is stronger than that for blue eyes. Thus, if a child has a blue-eyed parent and a brown-eyed parent, the child will most likely express the dominant trait—and have brown eyes. (See ✗13 below)

Most abnormal genes exist in "carrier state." This means that some people carry an abnormal gene which is masked by the normal gene of the pair. The abnormal gene is called *recessive;* the trait which derives from it is called a *recessive trait.* The abnormality can only express itself in a child who has two carrier parents.

If both parents carry the recessive gene for the abnormality, 75 per cent of their children will be normal, or at worst be carriers of the gene, 25 per cent of the children will express the abnormality.

Most recessive genes are associated with particular ethnic or family groups. Between 5 and 10 per cent of American blacks of West African parentage carry the recessive gene for sickle-cell anemia. If two people who carry the gene have a child, there is a 25 per cent chance that the child will be stricken with sickle-cell disease; that is, one out of four children born to such a couple will have the disease. (See p. 370)

Similarly, cystic fibrosis, a genetic respiratory ailment, affects children of families which originated in northern Europe, but does not turn up in Italian families, for example. European Jews must watch out for Tay-Sachs disease, a neurological degeneration of young children leading to loss of brain function and death. Jewish people from the Middle East are generally not affected.

11. How recessive-gene diseases originate

Most recessive-gene diseases are clouded in history; they probably originated through a mutation in a particular family in a particular locality. In fact, the mutation may have occurred originally because it was *needed;* it was *selected for* in the evolutionary process. For instance, part of the persistence of the gene for sickle-cell anemia is attributed to the fact that people who were carriers of this disease were more resistant to malaria, which is endemic in West Africa.

These recessive genes are passed on to descendants, and when two people who somewhere in generations past were touched by those descendants have children together, there is a one-in-four chance that the offspring can inherit two of the recessive genes and the disease can appear again.

12. Sex-linked genetic disorders

Sometimes, a recessive gene for a disease is present on the X chromosome. In girls, if one X chromosome carries the defective gene and the other X chromosome is normal, the disease will not show up. However, the woman who carries the disease recessively on one of her X chromosomes will pass the disease on to *half* of her sons. This is because half of her eggs will contain the abnormal gene, and the genes on the Y chromosome are not strong enough to counteract the effect. Hemophilia and muscular dystrophy are the major sex-linked recessive-gene diseases.

13. Dominant-gene diseases

Dominant genes are expressed in either one of the parents, and can be expected in 50 per cent of the children, regardless of the fact that one parent may be entirely healthy. Therefore, in the case of severe diseases, there are usually no children, and most dominant-gene diseases are simply not transmitted through the generations. An exception is Huntington's Chorea, a disease characterized by spasmodic movements of the face and hands gradually leading to loss of mental abilities and death; this is probably a dominant-gene disease, a very rare disorder that unfortunately does not express itself until late in life (between thirty and fifty). Woody Guthrie, the great American composer, suffered and died from this disease *after* he had had his children. They are still young and must simply wait to discover whether they fall into the fated 50 per cent.

14. Diseases associated with abnormal numbers of chromosomes

In recessive and other gene diseases, the chromosomes remain normal in number and appearance. However, there are some birth defects which are caused by chromosomal disorders; usually these can be detected prenatally by checking the chromosomes in a sample of amniotic fluid cells (amniocentesis).

Chromosomal anomalies in a fetus are usually accidental; they do not pass from generation to generation. Most are caused by an accident during division of the germ cells (the cells which produce the egg and sperm). If a sperm has too many or too few chromosomes, it is usually unable to fertilize an egg and just dies. If an egg has too many or too few chromosomes, a severe chromosomal disorder may be passed on to the fetus.

If the chromosomal miscount is too great, the fetus usually dies before birth, as in the case of *triploidy,* in which the fetus has chromosomes in triplicate, not duplicate (sixty-nine instead of forty-six).

If the chromosomal miscount is not too severe (for example, one extra chromosome or one too few), then the resulting child may live to be born, with a gross abnormality.

15. Non-disjunction: the cause of most chromosomal abnormalities which the fetus can survive

Non-disjunction describes the situation in which, when germ cells divide, one set of chromosomes sticks together. Therefore, after union with the egg, the two-by-two division does not apply for all twenty-three sets of chromosomes. One set of chromosomes may be a triplet; or one set may be a single.

16. Diseases caused by non-disjunction

The most frequent variety of non-disjunction is *mongolism,* in which three chromosomes are present on the twenty-first set.

Trisomy 18 (multiple congenital defects) is another variety; it occurs when three chromosomes are present on the eighteenth set.

Klinefelter's Syndrome is a case of non-disjunction in which a male child has an extra X chromosome in the twenty-third set determining sex. Instead of being XY, he is XXY. Such a boy will have underdeveloped testicles and several other developmental problems.

17. Mongolism: a form of retardation that can be lessened with prenatal testing

a. Mongolism or Down's Syndrome is a kind of retardation that is responsible for almost 30 per cent of all the severely retarded children in the United States and Western Europe. (Ref. 3)

Mongolism (and all other disorders caused by non-disjunction) occurs in greater frequency among the pregnancies of older women. The approximate risk of mongolism is as follows:

up to age 35:	1–2 in 1,000 pregnancies
age 35–40:	3–11 in 1,000 pregnancies
age 41–42:	1–2 per cent
age 43–45:	3 per cent
age 45+:	3–5 per cent

In short, a woman under age thirty-five has a slight risk of having a child with Down's Syndrome; over age thirty-five, the risk is significant.

Women who are over age thirty-five may choose to have amniocentesis (am-ne-o-sen-TEE-sis) for genetic testing, to rule out mongolism or other chromosomal disease. If abnormality is discovered, abortion is an option. If no abnormality in the chromosomes is found, that will be most comforting to women who may have been very worried over the possibility. (See ✕19 below)

b. Another less frequent type of mongolism occurs in children of younger women; in these cases, some genetic material from one of the twenty-first set of chromosomes (either the one from the father or the one from the mother) is displaced onto another chromosome. When the cells divide, one of them has more genetic material than the rest, and the result is a mongoloid child. This type of disorder can also be detected prenatally. There is a 5–10 per cent chance that if it happens once, it will be repeated. This is higher than the chance of repetition with the mongolism that occurs with older women (see above).

GENETIC TESTING AND AMNIOCENTESIS

---

18. Genetic testing and amniocentesis: ways to test for and prevent birth defects

a. Genetic testing is the testing of mother and father for genetic traits which might, in combination, damage the child. Some recessive-gene diseases, e.g., sickle-cell disease, Tay-Sachs, affecting particular ethnic groups can now be tested for and discovered, so that men and women who find that they are carrying the disease traits can rethink whether they wish to have children together or plan for further testing after conception.

b. The chromosomes of the fetus can be checked by testing some amniotic fluid cells, obtained by amniocentesis. This prenatal test will discover most major chromosomal anomalies early enough in pregnancy for the mother of an afflicted child to have an abortion, if she chooses.

c. Amniotic fluid cells can be tested for substances that indicate recessive diseases which involve abnormal metabolism such as Tay-Sachs disease. It can also detect some physical abnormalities such as spinal-column defects.

d. Other procedures such as ultrasound and amniography (see ≠29 below) may detect structural defects in later pregnancy.

19. Amniocentesis

Amniocentesis is a simple test by which some of the amniotic fluid around the fetus is drawn off between fourteen and sixteen weeks of gestation, and the cells tested for chromosomal patterns and other substances. Generally, an ultrasound (see ≠29 below) is performed first to locate the placenta so that the practitioner who inserts the needle to withdraw the fluid may avoid it. Thereafter, 10–20 ccs of amniotic fluid is withdrawn and placed in a culture medium in the laboratory, where the cells grow. Within two to four weeks, the chromosomal pattern (and any abnormalities in it) can be detected and various specific chemicals can be identified in metabolic disorders. The test must be performed under sterile conditions in a hospital or office. In 90 per cent of cases, an adequate number of cells for testing can be grown. In the remaining 10 per cent, the test may not work and may have to be repeated.

20. The risks of amniocentesis

As with other specialized procedures, it is best to go to a center where amniocentesis is performed frequently and where the practitioners and the labs are experienced. There is very little risk in this test for the mother (very rare cases of infection, bleeding, fainting, and amniotic-fluid leak). The risks for the fetus are more severe, but still *very rare:* for example, the needle might go through a part of the fetus. Another risk is that the test may cause early labor, but, when done by experienced people, this risk is probably only a little greater than for pregnancies without amniocentesis. (Ref. 4, 5, 6, 7)

21. The limits of amniocentesis

At present amniocentesis can only discover chromosomal abnormalities and some inherited metabolic diseases and structural defects of the spine. *It cannot discover damage to the fetus that is caused by virus, X ray, drugs, and thousands of other factors that could conceivably cause a birth defect.*

22. Who should consider having amniocentesis?

a. Women over thirty-five.

Many American women are putting off having children until later in life in order to establish careers. Since chromosomal abnormalities increase dramatically after age thirty-five, women over this age should avail themselves of the test if they are willing to abort an abnormal fetus. (Younger women may consider amniocentesis, but the risk of mongolism for them is less than the risk of the procedure causing a miscarriage, at present.)

b. Younger women who have previously borne a mongoloid child or a child with some other chromosomal abnormality.

c. Women with a high possibility of a specific inherited metabolic disease.

This includes, for example, the woman who along with her husband, carries the trait for Tay-Sachs, or a woman who has previously borne a child with some other inherited metabolic disorder. If a couple has a family history of any rare disease, they should check with a genetics testing center to determine their risk for having a child with a similar problem.

d. Women who are carriers of sex-linked disorders (like hemophilia).

e. Women who have had children with spinal cord or skull defects.

23. Tay-Sachs disease can be controlled by genetic testing and amniocentesis

The gene for Tay-Sachs disease occurs in one in thirty Ashkenazi Jews (Jews from families that originated in Central and Eastern Europe) in America. Carriers can be detected by a simple blood test which will discover the level of the enzyme hexosaminidase A in the blood. If two carriers have children, one in four of those children will die of Tay-Sachs. If parents know themselves to be carriers, they can conceive a child and then resort to amniocentesis, to check for a deficiency of the enzyme in the amniotic fluid or in the cells derived from it. High-risk couples whose religious observance normally prohibits abortion should seek counseling with rabbinic authorities before proceeding with the amniocentesis. An alternative way to prevent the disease is to use artificial insemination. (See p. 112)

Do not wait until you are pregnant to find out if you and your man are carriers. Have yourself tested before you decide to have children. Know what risks you are—and are not—running when you conceive a child.

24. Amniocentesis as a test for sex-linked genetic disorders

Amniocentesis can determine the sex of the child: if this is the only information being sought, the test is certainly not worth the trouble, with one medical exception: women who carry the trait for sex-linked genetic disorders, such as muscular dystrophy or hemophilia, may expect 50 per cent of their sons to be affected. In this case, a woman might not wish to carry a male fetus to term and amniocentesis is probably in order. Women who are carriers usually know who they are because the disease is in the immediate family. Watch for news of prenatal diagnosis of hemophilia.

25. Amniocentesis for alpha-fetoprotein and prenatal diagnosis of brain and spinal cord defects

Alpha-fetoprotein is a substance present in the amniotic fluid during the first ten to twelve weeks of gestation; thereafter it declines rapidly if the fetus is normal. However, in cases of some spinal and brain defects in the infant, the level of alpha-fetoprotein remains high; amniocentesis will verify a high concentration after twelve weeks, thus forewarning the parents of a serious problem to come.

Defects which can be detected in this manner are anacephaly (in which the infant has no head), spina bifida with meningomyelocele (me-NING-go-my-ell-o-seel) (a structural defect in the spinal column in which some vertebral arches may be missing and some of the spinal cord tissue may protrude). *These are the only structural defects which can currently be predetermined by amniocentesis.*

Women who have previously had children with these disorders run a risk of recurrence and should be tested. *The test for alpha-fetoprotein is performed routinely, even when the amniocentesis is done for another reason.*

WATCH FOR NEWS: Since 90 per cent of the cases of spinal and brain defects occur in the children of couples with no family history of these problems, until now, they usually had to wait until they had an affected child to know whether further pregnancies should be tested. A screening test on the mother's blood during pregnancy may soon be widely available to detect which women might be at higher risk for carrying an abnormal fetus, and thus amniocentesis would be strongly suggested in these women, to detect the spinal and brain defects.

26. Amniocentesis for sickle-cell anemia

Americans who think that their ancestors may have originated in West Africa should have themselves tested for sickle-cell trait (a simple blood test) before they have children.

Once a child is conceived, prenatal diagnosis of whether that child will suffer from sickle-cell anemia is not yet widely available, but probably will be in the next year or so. Watch for news of this or consult your nearest genetics counseling center.

27. Amniocentesis for cystic fibrosis

Cystic fibrosis is a severe, chronic respiratory disease caused by recessive genes which occurs mainly in people with northern European ancestry. At present it cannot be determined whether a man or woman is a carrier of the disease. If a couple has had a previously affected child, they should contact a genetics counseling center. Amniocentesis may soon be able to detect whether a fetus is affected by this disease.

28. Fetoscopy: a form of prenatal testing

Fetoscopy requires the insertion of a scope into the uterus to look directly at the fetus and at times to obtain a small amount of fetal blood for laboratory evaluation. This is difficult for several reasons:

a. A rather large hole has to be made in the uterus and amniotic sac to extract the blood, with a danger of complications for mother and child.

b. When the blood is extracted, the mother's blood may also be present, confusing the sample and preventing an accurate lab reading.

Fetoscopy can also be an important detector of structural defects in the infant, such as meningomyelocele (see ※25 above)—an outpouching of the lower spinal cord—because these can be directly visualized. However, these defects can usually be detected more safely by ultrasound and amniocentesis.

29. Ultrasound and amniography can be used to detect some structural defects in the fetus

An ultrasound (see p. 186) is a test by which sound waves are bounced off the fetal sac to indicate the shape of the baby. An abnormal pattern of waves will indicate a structural defect. In amniography, a small amount of dye that will not harm the fetus is injected into the amniotic fluid and then an X ray is taken; the dye will outline the shape of the fetus on the picture, showing if there are any structural defects. Amniography is generally not done until late in the pregnancy, when there is less danger to the fetus from the X ray; it is much more difficult at this point to end the pregnancy if the fetus is severely misformed. Amniography has a limited role in modern obstetrics.

30. Counseling is an important part of genetic testing programs

Couples who participate in genetic testing for potential defects in their children can anticipate severe emotional strain. If an abnormal fetus is detected, this may have a devastating effect on the individuals or their relationship. Marriage or psychological counseling is a must at this time. Most good genetic counseling centers will provide expert advice and support.

INFECTIONS AND BIRTH DEFECTS

---

31. Rubella and prenatal testing

Rubella—German measles—is a virus which, if contracted by the mother early in her pregnancy, causes severe or minor malformations, including retardation, in 50 per cent of affected pregnancies.

Thus it is absolutely essential for every woman to be vaccinated against rubella if she has not had the disease in childhood and developed a natural immunity to it.

If you are not certain whether you have had rubella, get a blood test for it. If the results show a high level of antibody, then you can be assured that you have had the disease and are immune. If the antibody count is low get vaccinated.

If you are pregnant and think that you may have had contact with rubella, and are unsure whether you had the disease or vaccination before, get a blood test immediately. Generally if the antibody count is high, you're safe; there is no need for worry or for further testing. If the antibody count is low, a second test should be taken about three weeks later. If the titers are higher in this second test then this is proof that a woman has recently had the disease. Consult a doctor early in pregnancy.

If the blood test shows that you have contracted rubella, you may wish to consider abortion. *If you are less than fifty-five days from conception when the infection occurred, the chances are very high that the infant is damaged (about 30–50 per cent).*

Prenatal diagnosis is not able to determine fetal damage by viruses.

Other viruses which may damage the fetus if infection is in the early stages are listed in Table 3. These viruses usually do not affect the fetus so virulently as rubella, but counseling should be sought if you are infected during pregnancy.

32. The symptoms of rubella

These include a fine rash over the chest and back and swollen glands in the back of the neck. Even if a woman does not develop these symptoms, she should be tested if there is contact with any other person with the symptoms.

33. When to be vaccinated against rubella

The best time to be vaccinated is before pregnancy is even a remote possibility. Since you must wait two to three months after the vaccination to become pregnant, consider being vaccinated immediately *after* giving birth.

Most reports now say that it is safe to be vaccinated during breast-feeding, the vaccine does not appear to cause any problems for the newborn.

34. Warning: Avoid vaccinations with live virus during pregnancy

Some immunizations involve the injection of a very low dose of live virus to allow the person to build up immunity to the virus as protection. The live vaccines include rubella, smallpox, oral polio, and yellow fever. Routine vaccinations should be avoided during pregnancy because the live virus can infect the fetus. However, if there is an epidemic of a disease, the vaccination may be safer than risking the infection. Consult *public health* officials in these cases.

OTHER CAUSES OF BIRTH DEFECTS

35. Radiation exposure and prenatal testing

No one really knows what dosage of radiation can cause fetal damage during pregnancy. In general, the risk of single films or diagnostic X rays is very low. If X-ray treatment for diseases such as cancer is given to the pelvic area in early pregnancy, the risk is very high.

Fetal damage by X rays cannot be determined by prenatal testing.

36. Warning: Avoid radiation if you are pregnant

Even though the *exact* risk is unknown, the *potential* for radiation damage should lead pregnant women to avoid any unnecessary X rays. If chest X rays or dental X rays, for instance, are absolutely necessary, the abdomen should be shielded with a lead apron.

37. Warning: Any drug given in pregnancy may potentially damage the fetus

Table 4 lists the drugs that are known or suspected to cause damage, but the wise woman will avoid *any* medication not absolutely essential for her well-being. *Damage by drugs cannot routinely be detected by genetic testing.*

38. Choosing the sex of your baby: the Shettles theory

Dr. L. B. Shettles has propounded a theory, for which he claims 80 per cent success, to help parents get the baby of the sex they want. There is no guarantee of success in this procedure, but it is probably harmless enough, and those who wish to try it need fear nothing more than the arrival of a bouncing baby of the sex they didn't want.

Shettles claims that, by altering the times of coitus and using acid or basic douches, his patients have much success in getting children of the sex they prefer. (Ref. 8) Other physicians have not been able to duplicate these results, but at present, there is no danger in trying this method.

TABLE 3

INFECTIONS WHICH MAY CAUSE DAMAGE TO A FETUS

Chicken pox
Coxsackie B
Cytomegalovirus
Hepatitis
Herpes simplex
Influenza
Rubella (German measles)
Smallpox (now apparently eradicated)
Syphilis
Toxoplasmosis
Vaccinia (from smallpox immunization)
Venezuelan equine encephalitis

TABLE 4
DRUGS KNOWN TO CAUSE FETAL DAMAGE

Alcohol
Androgens (male hormones)
Anticancer drugs
Antiseizure drugs (phenytoin, trimethadione)
Coumadin or warfarin
Estrogen (DES)
Heroin
Methadone
Nicotine
Thalidomide

SUSPECT, BUT NOT PROVEN CONCLUSIVELY

Antibiotics (tetracycline, chloramphenicol,
   novobiocin, streptomycin)
Aspirin
Diuretics
Hexachlorophene
Iodine in high doses
Lithium
LSD
Marijuana
Oral drugs for diabetes
Phenylmercuric acetate (PMA)
Progestins (synthetic progesterones)
Sulfa drugs
Thiouracil
Tranquilizers (diazepam, meprobamate, chlordiazepoxide)

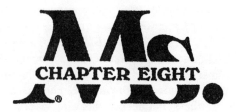

CHAPTER EIGHT

EVERYDAY
GOOD HEALTH

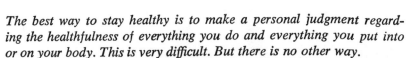

The best way to stay healthy is to make a personal judgment regarding the healthfulness of everything you do and everything you put into or on your body. This is very difficult. But there is no other way.

Starting from childhood, someone has to decide which foods are good, which cosmetics are good, which social habits are healthful, which hygiene regimens are worthwhile. A parent cannot just trundle down the aisles of the supermarket throwing everything the children want into the cart; many of the things they want are at best non-nutritious and at worst harmful to the body, even though they may be delicious and brilliantly advertised and packaged. A woman cannot accept the notion that if a product is on the shelves of her drugstore, it is *ipso facto* safe. It may not be safe *for her*. It may be safe for her—but it may be ineffective and a waste of her money. A woman must judge the air she breathes for its healthfulness; the water she drinks for its healthfulness. If all citizens concerned themselves with the healthfulness of the everyday environment, and took action both as consumers and voters to protect it, the environment would be cleaner and more healthful; there is no doubt of that.

Everyday good health is created by the individual woman, rendering judgments on every single aspect of her daily life and that of her family. Though everyone else may be mad for a fad in diet or cosmetics, though everyone else may be smoking, drinking liquor, wearing six-inch heels, rushing onto the tennis courts despite decades of previous inactivity, the individual woman must stand aside, make her own decisions and join the crowd *only* when it suits her personally.

As a general rule, the movement toward a more natural, untreated, undrugged existence is a good one. *It can be a grave mistake to underestimate how healthy you are normally;* to weaken your legs by driving when you are strong enough to walk; to weaken your gut by taking laxatives when your body is strong enough to eliminate on its own; to take medications for colds that your system could fight off independently. A healthy body stays healthier if it is used; underuse may be tantamount to misuse.

The environment both inside and outside the body is up for grabs today, by every economic and political interest in the country. The consumer, who is also the patient, who is also the voter, who is also the parent must try with all the self-knowledge and power at her command to make her own grab for the environment, to control it, and decide what sort of life is healthy *for herself.*

RECOMMENDED HYGIENE

1. Recommendation: Preferred hygiene is plain soap and water

Hygiene is understood in the traditional sense as cleanliness, which a great American ethic places next to godliness. Today, *cleanliness sometimes goes beyond what is actually healthful;* we are encouraged to eradicate every odor from our bodies, and in so doing we sometimes eradicate the odor-causing bacteria which are natural to our bodies and protect our general health. We wash our hair so much that we dry it out beyond repair. We wipe the hair off our bodies with products that sometimes irritate the skin. We use easy-drying fabrics because we are always washing our clothing; yet for many women, these fabrics are not as healthful as natural fibers which may take longer to dry and sometimes don't come as clean. We endured phosphates in our detergents in order to have cleaner clothes, only to find we were destroying our fresh-water lakes with them and depleting our fish supply. Since fish is the high-protein, low-calorie, low-cholesterol staple of a well-balanced diet, we were in fact buying bad nutrition with extraordinary cleanliness.

A woman who is simply trying to keep clean and feel fresh can do so with plain soap and water. *She must make a critical judgment about every additional product she uses to keep herself, her house and her clothes clean.* In general, it can be said that not much besides soap and water is actually needed.

2. Natural bacteria are essential to good health

A healthy body is covered with friendly bacteria. Bacteria which endanger are usually picked up by the hands, transported to the mouth and on to the gut, or picked up from the air and absorbed into the respiratory system. The purpose of bathing is to protect the body from unfriendly bacteria without killing off the natural bacteria that live on the body and in many cases protect its normal functioning.

3. Sensible bathing

A daily bath or shower will control body odor and make a woman feel good—but she does not have to bathe her entire body *every day* without fail to maintain good health.

Hands and lower arms, the areas most exposed to outside dirt and bacteria, should be washed frequently during the day; before every meal; and after every trip to the bathroom.

It is important to wash out the mouth frequently, if only with plain water, and, ideally, to brush teeth after every meal to prevent accumulations of food that cause odor and decay.

Wash underarms and the pubic and vaginal area daily to prevent odor. The face is washed mainly to remove dirt and excess oily secretions. It is quite normal for a woman to find that soap dries her skin more than she likes and to choose instead plain water and/or cleansing cream.

4. Vaginal hygiene

The vagina is a clean place; normal urine does not make it dirty, for urine is sterile; normal semen does not make it dirty, for it also is sterile. The national advertising campaigns on vaginal hygiene products might make a woman think that her vagina is a hotbed of soil to be washed and perfumed away incessantly. A mature woman should know better and should inform her daughters. The natural secretions of the vagina are there to protect a woman's health, and too much scrubbing and douching (see ⅟7 below) may actually wash away her defense against outside infection.

The bowel contents are not sterile—and it is very important to wipe the anus from behind, so as not to draw bowel contents toward the vagina, inviting cystitis and vaginitis. (See p. 316) This habit should be taught to young girls when they are toilet-trained. It will protect them for a lifetime. In addition, the urethra and vagina should be wiped after urination from front to back.

5. Vaginal odor is usually held not by the vagina but by the pubic hair: wash it away

If you are bothered by vaginal odor, wash the outer pubic area; in most cases, it is the hair that catches and holds the odor. Wash the hair and labia and you clean the odor away. In addition, try natural-fiber cotton underpants which are more absorbent and deodorizing than synthetics. If these methods do not work, check with a doctor, for odor may be an early sign of vaginal infection. (See p. 299)

6. Avoid perfumed products for vaginal hygiene

Perfume may cause irritation; it is not a necessary part of vaginal hygiene and may give some women trouble. *It is nice to smell nice, but it is better for general health not to smell at all.* And remember, a foul vaginal odor may be a sign of infection. By perfuming the vagina regularly, with sweet-smelling soaps, douches, or vaginal sprays, you may be concealing an odor which is a vital early warning signal of a problem.

7. Routine douching is not necessary for good health

Douching (doosh-ing) is the flushing of water up into the vagina with a thin hose or syringe to clean the vaginal canal. This job can also be done by the upward spurting water of a bidet (bee-day), a special tub for cleaning the vaginal and rectal areas found often in bathrooms abroad.

Many women have never douched; others do so routinely after intercourse and after each monthly period. So long as you use mild ingredients such as warm water or water and white vinegar, or baking soda, there is probably no harm to even daily douching. However, this is not *necessary* for good hygiene. WARNING: Don't use caustic materials such as Lysol; these can cause severe irritations to the lining of the vagina.

If a woman decides to douche, she should buy an ordinary douche bag. It will last for years. Most bags hold about a quart of water. Just fill the bag with warm water or water mixed with one or two tablespoons of white vinegar or baking soda, insert the syringe about two to three inches into the vagina and allow the solution to flow in and out. A woman may douche in the bathtub or on the toilet, whichever is more convenient. The bag should never be more than three feet above the level of the vagina so that excess pressure does not develop.

The bag should be rinsed with warm water and dried by hanging upside down. The tubing should also be allowed to drain.

RECOMMENDATION: *Do not close the lips of the vagina while douching; this is now a discredited method.* It may allow the pressure of the water to build up inside and force some water up into the cervix and Fallopian tubes, where it could cause infection. If you use a bulb syringe, don't squeeze the plastic bottle too firmly, to avoid similar excess pressure.

If a woman has a vaginal infection, her physician may recommend daily douching, along with therapy for the infection. Usually a dilute solution of white vinegar is recommended, for it makes the vagina slightly acidic and helps to clear some abnormal bacteria and monilia. (See p. 300)

RECOMMENDATION: It is much easier for the solution to get into the uterus during pregnancy and in the postpartum period. *So do not douche during pregnancy or for three to four weeks after a delivery or abortion unless specifically instructed to do so by your physician.* If you are so instructed, keep the bag very low to limit the pressure in the vagina. If irritation or pain develops after frequent douching, stop douching. If these continue, see a doctor.

8. Assume that all foreign chemicals placed in the vagina are absorbed into the body—and choose carefully

The Food and Drug Administration has investigated all the ingredients in douches and feminine hygiene products. Probably, most are safe; but why take a chance? And why spend your money needlessly?

a. Prepacked or premixed douches are not proven dangerous, except to women who happen to be allergic to the perfume in them. However, they usually hold a pint or less of liquid, which is not enough volume to do much cleaning; they are not more effective in any way than plain water, or water and vinegar; and they are much more expensive.

b. Disposable douching equipment is not dangerous, but it is an unnecessary expense. A syringe does not become permanently soiled because it has been used to clean a vagina; it does not have to be thrown away like plastic gloves after surgery. The vagina is a clean place to begin with and one douche bag for a few dollars can keep it perfectly clean for many many years.

c. OPINION: Do not use "feminine hygiene sprays." They contain perfuming agents which frequently cause allergic reactions. In the past, some contained hexachlorophene, causing both allergic reactions and potential fetal damage in pregnancy, so they are now banned. *If you find a vaginal spray with hexachlorophene on the shelves where you shop, tell the store manager to get rid of it.* WARNING: Pregnant women should avoid hexachlorophene soaps completely. They may be associated with increased birth defects.

9. Body odor

Most body odor comes from perspiration and the growth of bacteria in the armpits and pubic area. Soap and water will help in eliminating the bacteria and excess perspiration. Shaving the hair will also help. Deodorants for the armpits are safe, *but don't use them in the pubic area.*

Tight-fitting clothing, clinging, synthetic fiber undergarments and slacks aggravate body odor, especially in hot weather. Try not to wrap up so tightly in the summertime and choose clothes of *natural* fibers.

10. Bad breath

Bad breath usually comes from food left over in the mouth, deteriorating under the impact of natural salivary juices, or from the leftover odor of strong foods, liquor, tobacco. Brushing teeth and rinsing the mouth will usually wash it away. Mouthwashes are fine but not necessary. Many people find that plain water is just as good.

Persistent bad breath may be a sign of serious dental decay. Sometimes generalized disease will cause it as well; a woman may notice that when she has a bad cold or sinus infection, her breath will smell bad. If your breath smells foul, and repeated rinsing and brushing cannot control it, see a dentist or doctor.

11. Hair removal is a cosmetic decision, not a health matter

Hair does not make a woman's body dirty. Whether she removes it, from her legs or armpits, for example, is entirely a *cosmetic* decision, unrelated to good health.

a. *Hair may trap perspiration and its odor.* The areas of the body most thickly covered with sweat glands also tend to be covered with hair. So in hot weather particularly, hair may trap perspiration and the natural odor it causes. Many women remove underarm and pubic hair in the summer to avoid this. However, hair removal does not solve an odor problem completely; *you still have to wash.*

b. OPINION: *Shaving is the safest method of hair removal.* A light lathering with soap before shaving will make the blade run more smoothly. An electric razor is fine as well. *Make sure you're dry when you use it.* When hair is shaved, its early regrowth looks dark and stubby; it only looks that way; in fact the Old Wives' Tales (OWTs) that say shaved hair grows back darker or more thickly are quite wrong. Bleaching, tweezing or electrolysis (see ⚥11f below) for unwanted hair on your face tends to be more effective.

c. OPINION: *Depilatories (chemical hair-removers) should only be used on the legs.* Most depilatories (de-PILL-a-tories) can irritate skin, eyes and/or nostrils. Therefore, use them only on your legs and test a small area first for allergic reaction. If the skin puffs up, or a rash develops, go back to shaving.

d. *Waxing is a more permanent way to remove hair from legs.* A woman can do it at home or have it done professionally. Wax is melted, cooled a little so that it does not burn, then smeared on the legs. Pieces of cloth are placed on it. The wax dries. Then cloths and wax are ripped off, pulling the hair out with them. The hair does not grow back for quite some time and women who use wax for years may find eventually that it does not grow back at all. Waxing is uncomfortable; imagine an adhesive bandage being pulled off the hairy side of your arm.

e. *Facial hair should only be removed by bleaching, tweezing or electrolysis.* The first order of treatment is bleaching with plain hydrogen peroxide. Plucking the darkest hairs with a tweezer is also effective and harmless (after years of tweezing, these hairs may not come back).

Shaving is safe but not permanent. WARNING: *Do not use depilatories or hot wax around your eyes.*

f. *Electrolysis is the most permanent type of hair removal.* A needle is touched to the hair follicle, a tiny electrical current is applied, destroying the hair base, then the hair itself is tweezed out. Electrolysis hurts. Most women cannot take too much of it at one time and must go back for repeated short appointments. This can become enormously expensive (in 1976 in New York City, about $18.00 for twenty minutes). A new alternative to electrolysis is a process by which the hair is grasped with an electrified tweezer that kills the hair base without touching the skin. This is a much less painful process but even more expensive ($15.00 for fifteen minutes).

OPINION: Generally, permanent hair removal is so protracted, expensive, and uncomfortable that only women who feel *severely disfigured* by excess hair should consider it.

g. *Sudden new growth of hair in unexpected areas should take a woman to her physician.* This may be caused by a hormone imbalance or other illness. It should be checked. Don't try to remove the hair until the reason for the growth has been discovered.

DRUGS AND COSMETICS

---

12. When is a cosmetic a drug?

There are two kinds of "cosmetics."

Those that have ingredients that are absorbed into the body causing body changes are considered drugs under the law and are regulated by the Food and Drug Administration for safety *and* effectiveness. A hormone face cream would be an example.

Those cosmetics with no ingredients which are significantly absorbed into the body, or which alter body function, can be regulated *only* for safety and *not* for effectiveness.

13. Cosmetics may legally make any non-medical claim

As long as it is not medical, a cosmetic may claim to do anything for a woman in its advertising and not have to prove it. This is why cosmetic advertising is so fantasmagoric, promising to make you breathtaking, younger, sexier, everything that a copywriter can imagine women want to be.

If cosmetic advertising can actually make you believe these outlandish things and buy the product, then it is quite a miraculous achievement and you probably deserve to be parted from your hard-earned money. Cosmetics make many women look and feel much better; for many others, they do absolutely nothing. The government does not interfere with the individual's right to choose in this instance; you're on your own.

14. Allergic reaction is frequent with cosmetics

Many women react badly to ingredients in cosmetics such as perfumes, hair dyes, and mascara, usually by itching and swelling or redness in the area. Because of these reactions, as of September 1976, all cosmetics were required to list all their ingredients on the label. *Read the label.* Read the notations regarding possible irritation or allergy; use the product on a small area first to see if it affects you badly.

If it does, look for a product with different ingredients. *Report the reaction to the FDA* and to the manufacturer. (See ✕18 below for the address)

Some face make-up seems to aggravate acne: this is the reason so many actors who wear heavy stage make-up end up with rutted skin. If you are having trouble with acne, and wear face make-up routinely, shop around for another product and/or get a medical opinion. (See p. 31)

WARNING: *Never try to cover a skin condition with a cosmetic without asking medical advice first.* You may need medication.

15. Preferred hair care

Many young girls have oily hair that requires frequent washing to keep it looking clean and fresh. The same people may grow up into women who have hopelessly dry hair that splits at the ends, breaks off, even falls out—because by that time they may have bleached it, dyed it repeatedly, use a blower to dry and curl it, a curling iron to iron it, all of which slowly but surely hurt the hair. There are an enormous number of hair products to choose from, and as with other cosmetics, a woman should be wary of advertising. *Remember: Any claim can be made legally if there is no medical aspect to it.* Several things should be kept in mind:

a. No product will increase the actual *volume* of hair. A body wave and some shampoos and rinses may add a *feeling* of thickness.

b. Protein conditioners do help to make damaged hair more manageable.

c. Some postshampoo acidic rinses eliminate knots and make it easier to comb through hair when it is wet.

d. Comb—do not brush—your hair when it is wet. Brushing may damage the hair.

e. "Baby shampoo" lacks the hard washing ingredients that make eyes sting; therefore, it is excellent for little children whose hair tends to be thinner and easier to clean anyway. Older women may find that baby shampoo cannot get their hair as clean as they wish.

f. In general, a detergent shampoo washes the hair cleaner than an acid shampoo.

g. Lemon juice makes oily hair more manageable. Use actual lemon juice, not the reconstituted type.

h. The aniline (ANN-ih-line) in hair dye and rinses may create allergic reactions in some women. Before dyeing either at home or in the beauty shop, do a patch test. Apply a small amount of the dye solution with a cotton swab to a patch of hair behind your ear or on the skin inside the crook of your elbow. In the case of dye, two solutions must be mixed together; use the combined solution, not each of the two separately. Wait twenty-four hours. If any red blotches appear, do not use the product. (Ref. 1)

WARNING: Avoid products containing dye substances, 2,4-diaminoanisole (2,4-DAA), and 4-methoxy-m-phenylenediamine (4-MMPD). These have been shown to cause cancer in lab animals.

Concern about these products has increased, with recent studies that show beauticians have an increased risk for lung cancer.

These conclusions are not definitive, because none of the studies have taken into consideration the smoking habits of the subjects (see pp. 260–61; Ref. 2 and 3) or the possibility that hair sprays may be a factor.

While waiting for further studies women should use dyes containing other compounds—henna is a good alternative.

Never apply dye or tint to your eyebrows, for your eyes may be sensitive to the fumes of the solution (not to speak of accidental direct application) even if your skin is not.

i. Some women find they are much more sensitive to the chemical in hair dye when they are pregnant. In general, it is a good idea to avoid hair coloring at this time.

j. If your hair is falling out, breaking off without end, don't just experiment with different products infinitely. Seek professional advice from a cosmetologist or dermatologist.

k. *Hair sprays are on their way out.* A warning has been issued on hydrocarbon propellants used in these products, for they may be dangerous if inhaled and environmentalists have concluded that their widespread use may damage the very atmosphere of the earth. All manufacturers will soon be switching to squirts. You can hasten the process by switching to hair squirts yourself, and asking your beauty shop to do the same.

16. Deodorants and antiperspirants

A *deodorant* does not stop wetness. It may mask perspiration odor by killing or limiting the natural bacteria that create the odor, or by merely adding a fragrance to conceal the odor that gets by. A deodorant is classified by the FDA as a *cosmetic*.

An *antiperspirant* is classified as a *drug*. It contains aluminum salts which temporarily close the openings of the sweat glands and stop wetness. In addition, it may contain an antibacterial agent to fight odor —causing bacteria.

An FDA-American Academy of Dermatology Study in 1975 shows that of all toiletries on the market, deodorants and antiperspirants produce the most adverse reactions. Some women find they are allergic to the aluminum salts, some to the perfume. If redness or swollen glands develop under the arms, switch to a brand without perfume. If redness continues, stop using the product altogether. Frequent washing and the application of non-irritating powder will do just as well for many people. (Ref. 4)

OPINION: For dollar value, the roll-on and stick deodorants are the best. Most manufacturers will begin to push these now, reacting to the drive to remove propellant sprays from the market.

17. Perfume and contact dermatitis

Contact dermatitis (dur-ma-TYE-tis) is a general term for reactions of the skin to substances applied to it. Perfume is perhaps the most common substance to cause contact dermatitis. Many women develop reactions to perfume in the form of an itch, a rash, stinging or red blotches. If you experience these reactions, switch to non-perfumed products (soaps, toilet paper, tampons, deodorants, douches, etc.). In addition, oil of bergamot—an ingredient of some perfumes—can cause a photosensitive reaction (dark skin blotches) if worn in the bright sun. *Be careful.* Don't wear perfume while sunbathing.

18. Mascara and eye infections

Eyes are very sensitive, easily infected by small numbers of bacteria which would not hurt the body elsewhere. In order to prevent infection with *pseudomonas* (soo-do-MOAN-as), which can grow in eye products, the FDA allows manufacturers to include an antibacterial mercury substance, to keep the products (and therefore the eyes) sterile. *Other than this, mercury compounds are not allowed in cosmetics.*

A recent study on five hundred women showed that mascara can also become contaminated with *staphylococcus epidermidis,* which can cause chronic lid infections called *bacterial blepharitis* (bleh-far-EYE-tiss). (Ref. 5) The trouble arises mainly because water-based mascaras do not contain adequate preservatives to keep out bacteria. Bacterial blepharitis symptoms are: redness along the eyelid, eye irritation, loss of lashes. If you experience these symptoms, stop using your mascara and see your doctor. If you scratch your eye with a mascara brush and pain or redness persists more than twenty-four hours, get to your physician. If the mascara was infected, fast treatment can save you from severe eye problems.

Any trouble with mascara or any other cosmetic products should prompt you to write to the Food and Drug Administration, 5600 Fishers Lane, Rockville, MD 20852, *and* to the manufacturer. Look AHEAD: Consumers are pressing for laws to *require* inclusion of small amounts of mercury and preservatives such as *parabens* to prevent these infections. In the meantime, read labels; use only products which contain these ingredients; or use those which *do not* have water as an ingredient.

19. Nail polish is fine, but give your nails an occasional rest from it

Polishing nails in and of itself is not dangerous, but some women find that if they leave polish on all the time, the nails get brittle and crack easily.

20. Infections and psoriasis in the finger and toenails

The fingers come in contact with more dirt and more moisture than any other part of the body; it is logical therefore that fungus infections, which thrive in moist places, should easily lodge around and under the fingernails. Treat these with local applications of medicine your physician or pharmacist recommends.

Psoriasis (sore-EYE-a-siss) is a skin disease often affecting the scalp, elbow, and knee areas, and occasionally causing an inflammation of the nails which is very similar in appearance to fungal infection.

Assume that any recurrent or long-term scaling and itching around the nails is worth checking with a doctor.

OVER-THE-COUNTER DRUGS

21. The FDA and the regulation of over-the-counter drugs

An over-the-counter drug is different from a prescription drug in one regard; it is considered to be a drug, in that it is absorbed by the body, has an effect on the body, *but the government deems that it can be safely taken at the discretion of the consumer without the guidance of a physician.*

Prior to 1962, an American drug manufacturer could, essentially, market any product that he could manufacture. It didn't make much difference whether the over-the-counter product was actually *effective* or not, so long as it was fairly safe.

After 1962, every drug product had to pass certain more stringent guidelines to control safety *and* effectiveness. And in the years since then, the FDA has been slowly and laboriously examining over-the-counter products for both safety *and* efficacy. As the test results accrue, the regulations become more stringent; the labels on drugs become more complex, more worth reading.

Today, several rules should be followed in the purchase of any over-the-counter drug.

a. *Read the label before buying—the whole label.* Take seriously every direction; it has been placed there for your safety; it is based on thorough evaluation of the method of action of the drug. This evaluation is costing the taxpayer large amounts of money, so use what you have dearly purchased.

b. *Do not take any drug, even an over-the-counter drug, in early pregnancy if not absolutely needed.*

c. Every ingredient in over-the-counter drugs has probably been evaluated by the FDA, or soon will be, so the formulations of some products are changing. If you find that an over-the-counter drug has, in your estimation, seriously misrepresented what it can accomplish in its advertising, call that fact to the attention of the FDA. And if you suffer any adverse effect from the drug, stop taking it; write the FDA and the manufacturer. You may be wrong; that is, you may think the drug is doing something to you that is actually caused by something else entirely. *But be suspicious.* In a free market, the testimony of consumers is a vital guide, both to the government regulatory agencies and to the manufacturers themselves.

d. When buying over-the-counter drugs, compare the ingredients. When faced with two products which have the same ingredients in the same quantities, *buy the cheaper.* They have all been regulated in exactly the same way, and if they say they are the same, then they are the same. The name brand in this case gives no advantage over the store brand, for example.

e. *Look ahead* to the time when you will be able to buy prescription and some over-the-counter drugs by their *generic* names. This is already being considered by some state health insurance bodies. It means that the consumer would be able to buy a drug in its original form, much as the pharmacist does, without the additional dress-up of manufacturers' names and packaging, and without the additional cost. This depends, of course, on close FDA regulation of quality control in the manufacturing process.

22. Over-the-counter pain-killers: aspirin, acetaminophen, and phenacetin

a. Aspirin is quite safe if used in moderation. It should always be taken with milk, antacids, or food so that it will not irritate the stomach lining. *It should not be taken during late pregnancy.* (See pp. 138–39)

b. Acetaminophen (a-SEET-a-meen-o-fen) is also affective against pain and does not irritate the stomach lining as aspirin may. However, it doesn't work against arthritic pain as well as aspirin. (See pp. 373–74)

c. Combination pain-killers usually have aspirin as their major ingredient but may have substances like antacids to make them more palatable. Check the labels *and* the prices! OPINION: Aspirin taken with milk is usually a cheaper, equally effective combination.

d. WARNING: If you use pain-killers regularly, avoid those with phenacetin (feen-a-SEET-in). This compound in chronic high doses causes kidney disease. (Acetaminophen and aspirin in high doses may have a similar effect, *especially when used with laxatives.* (See ⚡27 below)

e. Overdoses of aspirin and acetaminophen are both dangerous, especially for children. Keep these and all other drugs out of reach.

23. For sleeplessness, exercise is the best medicine

Some people feel refreshed with four hours' sleep; some need a full eight to ten hours; some are satisfied with frequent catnaps. However you get your rest, it is vital to your health that you get it *regularly.*

a. Accumulated tension often causes sleeplessness; a tranquilizer may relax you temporarily, but it won't relieve the underlying tension that made you wakeful in the first place. For tension and resultant sleeplessness, the very best medicine is exercise. *Try exercise first.* USE SLEEPING MEDICATIONS WITH THE UTMOST CAUTION AND GREATEST POSSIBLE INFREQUENCY!

b. Try these time-honored methods repeatedly before indulging in a sedative:

—Take a hot bath before retiring.

—Drink a glass of warm milk. Avoid coffee or tea in the evening.

—Exercise strenuously, then wait an hour or so before going to sleep.

—Do not eat immediately before retiring. Leave a couple of hours between your last meal and sleep.

c. The major causes of disturbed sleep are:

—Situational stress (ongoing problems)

—Specific stress (something you're worried about)

—Physical pain (a toothache is worse at night when nothing distracts you from it)

—Circadian Phase Shift (otherwise known as "jet lag")

—Increasing age (older people sleep lightly and fitfully; this is *normal*)

—Medical problems such as angina, asthma, and duodenal ulcers may display their symptoms more boldly at night.

d. *Depression* affects the body's metabolism as well as its sleep patterns. A depressed person may sleep excessively because she feels tired all the time or because she's so blue that she would rather not be awake. Another sign of depression is a pattern of waking up at three or four o'clock every morning.

24. Recent guidelines on sleeping medications

The FDA panel on sleeping medications made the following recommendations in its report in the Federal Register, December 8, 1975.

a. Bromides should be removed from all sleeping medications because they have tended to produce a cumulative effect and may result in mental disturbances, irritability, memory difficulty and skin rashes. WARNING: *It may take some time to get bromide drugs off the market; the customer should always pass up these medications.*

b. Avoid products with *scopolamine,* also for reasons of safety.

c. Antihistamines which also have a sedative effect have been allowed to remain in sleeping medications pending further proof of their effectiveness. These include compounds such as diphenhydramine (dye-fenn-HIGH-dra-mean) and pyrilamine (pie-RILL-a-mean). (Ref. 6)

25. Preferred care of the bowels

Early in this century, it became a popularly accepted notion that a daily bowel movement was necessary; children were taught to move their bowels at the same time every day, without fail. Otherwise, it was supposed that the uneliminated waste products in the bowel would poison the body.

Of course, regular elimination is essential to good health. But "regular" does not mean every day, or the same time every day. "Regular" means "at regular intervals": a bowel movement every other day, every two or three days may be perfectly sufficient.

26. Over-the-counter laxatives

Because the rigid definitions of regularity have such a hold on our people, we, as a nation, take too many laxatives. Laxatives are fine occasionally, to relieve the discomforts of constipation. But when taken regularly, they encourage dependence; the bowel loses its natural strength, and the cycle may perpetuate itself.

Keep several things in mind when using a laxative.

a. Know when you are really constipated. If stool is anything short of rock-hard, then you are probably not constipated.

b. If you are constipated, try a combination of bran cereal, fresh fruit, leafy vegetables, and lots of water to relieve the diet. Exercise will help too—for it improves circulation and food metabolism. *If you have a laxative habit,* try the same regimen. It may take a few days for your body to adjust, you may experience some assorted discomforts with withdrawal, but the changeover is vital to your good health.

Worrisome signs such as narrowing of stools and blood in stools should prompt a physician's examination. Some medications may cause constipation, such as, narcotics, oral contraceptives, iron, and some antacids.

c. If constipation persists, try a *bulk stool softener.* These are usually seed preparations with psyllium or cellulose which create a bulkier, softer stool. They draw water into the stool, putting greater pressure on the bowel, encouraging it to move naturally. WARNING: Bulk laxatives tend to interfere with the body's metabolism of drugs such as salicylates and digitalis, so that the drugs are absorbed less effectively and the dosages have to be increased. WARNING: *If you are on any prescription drug, check with your pharmacist about possible interference from a non-prescription drug such as a laxative or stool softener.*

d. Most laxatives on the market are safe (Ref. 7) but every effort should be made not to rely on them for a bowel movement, for in the long run, laxative dependency weakens the bowel and general health.

27. Laxatives, pain-killers, and kidney disease

Recent reports say the incidence of kidney disease may be higher in people who take large amounts of aspirin, acetaminophen or phenacetin, especially when the same people are chronic users of laxatives. (Ref. 8) Avoid as many medications as possible!

28. Gas pains, one of the most common everyday afflictions

Most people occasionally suffer from gas pains, and learn from experience that they will eventually pass. The symptoms of gas are usually pain in the lower abdomen or under the rib cage. Typically, the pains move around in the abdomen and are accompanied by excessive belching or passing gas from the rectum.

Sometimes a particular food causes gas. If you're suffering, avoid leafy vegetables, onions, spicy foods, carbonated beverages, beer.

Another frequent cause is air-swallowing. Many people, when they are nervous, tend to swallow repeatedly and since there is nothing in the mouth, most of what they swallow is air. You may be able to control this if you are *conscious* of the way you react to tension.

Several products on the market containing simethicone (sim-ETH-ih-cone) or charcoal are good absorbers of gas. Or try lying on a firm surface and rubbing your stomach clockwise to relieve the pain. Stool softeners may help if constipation is also present.

Persistent pain, fever, or bleeding should take you to a doctor.

29. Over-the-counter drugs for allergy

Millions of Americans suffer from allergies to pollen or to air pollution and occasionally require antihistamines and decongestants to relieve runny nose and itching eyes. These complaints are so frequent that the consumption of this class of drugs is enormous; in fact, many people take them on a continuing basis. RECOMMENDATION: If you plan to take allergy drugs more than once in a while, consult a doctor. You may need stronger medications than those available over-the-counter; you may require allergy testing and desensitization shots.

WARNING: *Wheezing* is not a normal symptom of everyday allergy; it may indicate asthma, or heart disease and should not be treated without a doctor's supervision.

30. How to use an over-the-counter drug

a. *As infrequently as possible.* A drug is defined as a drug because it is absorbed into the blood stream and affects the body. A healthy person who eats and exercises properly should have need for drugs only occasionally, and should not make a habit of taking any medication. Avoid *all* drugs in pregnancy.

b. Ask your *pharmacist* any questions about any drug which you may have forgotten to ask your doctor. A pharmacist knows about any possible side effects and any possible bad reactions from the interaction of several drugs being taken simultaneously. This is especially true if you are taking medications prescribed *by several different doctors.* RECOMMENDATION: If you are taking a number of drugs, keep all your records at one pharmacy where the pharmacist can immediately detect a possible interaction between drugs by checking your file. If your pharmacist doesn't keep such records find one who does.

c. Many over-the-counter drugs have package inserts which are vital reading for the well-informed consumer.

d. If you want additional information about any drug you are taking, consult a pharmacology text in your local library or buy *The Physician's Desk Reference,* published by Medical Economics, Oradell, NJ 07649.

e. If you have any adverse or unusual reaction to any drug, write both to the manufacturer and the FDA, 5600 Fishers Lane, Rockville, MD 20852. Both parties must be informed by the public if they are to improve and control the everyday products we use.

f. The FDA is reasonably thorough in its rulings, but enforcement takes a long time, and there really isn't enough staff to enforce the rules in local areas all over the country. *Consumers must help* by reporting adverse reactions and apparent infractions in labeling rules. NEVER BUY A PRODUCT IN WHICH ALL THE INGREDIENTS ARE NOT LISTED ON THE PACKAGE, WHETHER IT BE A DRUG OR A COSMETIC. It may be a product which has been on the shelf for a long time, which has not been redesigned yet to comply with FDA regulations.

g. *Do not use over-the-counter drugs instead of doctors.* Many people use a variety of different products over prolonged time periods, trying to avoid the cost of a medical visit. *If any symptoms occur for which drugs of any kind are needed for more than one week, a doctor should be consulted.* In the long run, you may save money, for most drugs are not cheap. In addition, the persistence of a symptom may signify a serious problem that you should check more thoroughly.

MENSTRUAL HYGIENE

31. Hygiene during menstruation: some innovations

In addition to the traditional belt-with-pad and cardboard-encased tampon, there are now some new items on the market:

a. *Beltless sanitary napkins* have a strip of adhesive on the underside which sticks to underpants or pantyhose and holds the pad in place without a belt. If you wear loose underwear, these won't work.

b. *Very small pads* are advertised as useful for the few days of extremely light flow. However, they were undoubtedly developed because millions of women on the pill normally experience very light flow. They tend to fold on the sides.

c. *Plastic-encased tampons* work exactly the same as the cardboard-encased variety. *Keep in mind, however, that the plastic is not biode-gradable.* It does not break up into natural components and disappear back into the earth when discarded, and so it eventually pollutes the environment. Thus, ocean bathing beaches are often littered with plastic tampon containers, disposed of at sea and washed up intact on the shore. Even the rolling, salty oceans cannot destroy them. OPINION: If tampons are all the same to you—*and they should be*—opt for those which have biodegradable casings, or no casings at all.

d. *Perfumed tampons and artificial fibers in pads* are irritating to some women, can cause contact dermatitis, redness and itching around the vulva. If this happens, switch to other products. Perfumed pads and tampons are unnecessary to combat odor during menstruation anyway. Washing is preferable.

32. Over-the-counter drugs for menstrual discomfort

The main compound in these is aspirin or salicylimide (sal-ih-SILL-ih-mide), which is very much like aspirin. More expensive than ordinary aspirin, *they are no more effective* for the average woman. Avoid those containing phenacetin. (See ✕22d above)

Some contain *mild* diuretics, such as parabrom or ammonium chloride, whose effectiveness has not yet been proven.

COSMETIC SURGERY

33. Voluntary cosmetic surgery

Surgery is "voluntary" when it is not needed for reasons of health but is desired nonetheless by the patient. Although unnecessary surgery should be avoided as a rule, some women feel so disfigured by a particular feature that they opt for this alternative; the cosmetic and psychological benefits can be very considerable. However, it is important to remember that a nose job—for example—will not solve all your social problems; it will just straighten your nose. (NOTE: Since it is medically irrelevant, *most* health insurance plans do not cover cosmetic surgery.)

34. Who is a qualified cosmetic surgeon?

Plastic surgeons go through a four-to-five-year residency in general surgery after internship and medical school; then they train another two to three years in cosmetic surgery. Their fees are high, but those few who stick it out and make the grade can generally be relied upon to do a good job. If a woman cannot afford the prices she can go to a clinic which is training plastic surgeons: the procedure she desires will be done by a resident (who has already been trained in general surgery) and supervised by a plastic surgeon. Check into a plastic surgeon's credentials with the medical society to make sure that a less-qualified surgeon is not performing the procedure. Choose a doctor who is Board-certified in plastic surgery.

35. Nasoplasty ("nose job")

This is the most common kind of cosmetic surgery. The nose is broken and the cartilage is reshaped under local anesthesia with medicine given for sedation. The patient is usually in the hospital three to five days, and will have severe bruising, black eyes, and swelling around the nose and cheeks for two to three weeks thereafter. When this heals, there will be no visible scar. There are a few complications to this procedure: rarely, an infection or scarring inside the passage. Sometimes, the "new" nose does not come out exactly as expected and this possibility must be anticipated. However, in most cases, the result is very satisfactory.

36. Wrinkles

The skin wrinkles because it has been weathered and stretched and used with time. The only way to get rid of wrinkles is by cosmetic surgery or by covering them up with make-up. Some things do contribute to faster aging of the skin:

a. Heredity;

b. Too much exposure to sun and wind, particularly ocean wind;

c. Excessive drinking, for alcohol dries the skin;

d. Heavy smoking, which impairs circulation in the skin of the face (as well as the hands and feet);

e. Excess creaming and massaging of the face (this is a relatively new theory; see ✕37 below) and

f. Frequent weight gain and loss (the weight gain stretches the skin; when the weight is lost, the skin sags and wrinkles over the diminished flesh).

It is unfortunate that in our youth-oriented culture, wrinkles, which express the character and personality of a person so well, must be viewed as things to be eliminated. Try to stand by yourself and leave your wrinkles alone.

37. Massage and facial exercise may actually lead to wrinkles

Although facial massage and exercises have been heralded for years as a way to keep the skin looking young, it is now thought to promote wrinkles. (Ref. 9) The theory is that collagen fibers in the skin are responsible for skin tone and that massage and exercise break it down, causing the skin to sag and wrinkle. Collagen is a protein that helps to hold tissue, cartilage and bone in shape (the word itself comes from the Greek root *koila,* meaning glue). Wrinkles appear where the face moves the most, where movement has damaged the collagen so that it cannot replenish itself fast enough and do its work of holding the facial tissues in shape. This theory, if it is true, means that the least wrinkled face is the one that never moves, never laughs or suffers or feels the blast of a fresh wind.

Surely, it is better to be wrinkled.

38. Rhytidectomy ("face lift") (rye-tih-DECK-toe-me)

This operation is usually performed because the patient thinks he or she is excessively wrinkled and has too much overfolding tissue under the chin (double chin). An incision is made across the top of the scalp, behind the ears and under the chin. Local anesthesia is generally used. A rim of tissue is removed all around. The skin is attached again, more tautly than before. There will be no visible scar. This operation keeps a woman in the hospital four to five days; three weeks or more are required before the swelling and the bruising clears up.

39. What can be expected from a face lift?

Anyone who has a face lift looks better for a while. However, natural aging processes will eventually begin to wrinkle the newly smooth face again and many people who are desperate about their wrinkles will have the face lift more than once. *It is vital to remember* that a face lift makes *only* the face look more youthful. The rest of the body is sagging and wrinkling normally.

40. Opinion: Estrogen creams do little to fade wrinkles, and are to be avoided

Estrogen face creams make wrinkles fade a little, temporarily, because they force the skin to hold more moisture, to swell up and press out the wrinkles. They must be used continuously to have any significant effect and may cause estrogen to build up in the body, creating unpleasant side effects. (See p. 290) They are best avoided. Other moisturizing creams without estrogen will have essentially the same effect. Mask applications also make the face tissues retain water temporarily. The high-dose estrogen creams have now been taken off the over-the-counter market for safety's sake and are available only by prescription.

41. Facial discolorations

As a woman gets older, her body has undergone many endocrine cyclic changes: years and years of menstruation; pregnancies; climacteric. These hormone cycles sometimes have an effect on the pigment cells in the skin so that freckles, "liver spots," and other small discolorations may appear. If these grow unsightly, some may be removed by a dermatologist with local anesthetic in the office. If you have them removed and they grow back, don't have them removed again—use make-up to cover them. Creams that are available over-the-counter which claim to fade these spots and freckles are generally not effective. The best and cheapest answer is make-up.

42. Blepharoplasty (eyelid repair) (BLEFF-ah-roe-plass-tee)

A small piece of skin is removed from each upper and lower lid so that the remaining skin will stretch more tautly. Vision is not impaired; the eyelid crease hides the scars. Frequently, this procedure is done in conjunction with a face lift.

43. Breast surgery

Women increasingly seek cosmetic surgery to increase or decrease breast size, to even out the size or to replace a breast lost by mastectomy. This highly complicated surgery should not be undertaken lightly, either from a medical or psychological point of view. Some women should seek counseling before embarking upon this route.

44. Warning: Never accept silicone injections in the breast!

In the 1960s, when female nudity became so prominent in magazines and in "topless" nightclubs, women, their managers and physicians began experimenting with injection of silicone into breast tissue to increase the size of the breasts and offset natural sagging. *This was a catastrophe!* Infections, poisoning, and necrosis (tissue death) of breast cells, even cancerous growths resulted in many cases. *Never* use this procedure, and if you know anyone who is considering it, *warn her off!*

45. Solid silicone implant to increase breast size

The only relatively safe procedure to increase breast size today is *implantation of a solid chunk of silicone* in the base of the breast, where it will not interfere with breast function, including breast-feeding. The implant can be made with local or general anesthesia; the incision is relatively simple. In a few cases, there are complications: hematoma (blood clot) or infection, or, at a later date, formation of a capsule around the implant. *The procedure should only be contemplated by a woman*

    a. after mastectomy, or

    b. when breasts vary greatly in size one from the other.

46. Breast reduction is more complex than breast enlargement

Breast reduction surgery takes two to three hours in the operating room, sometimes requires blood transfusions, and leaves rather large scars under the breasts. The *only* women who should consider it are

    a. those with grossly large breasts which create serious secondary discomforts—trouble in breathing, chronic backache; irritation from pulling bra straps; or

    b. women with one breast which is much larger than the other.

47. A developing procedure: breast augmentation after mastectomy (see page 354)

Artificial prostheses to make breasts look normal in her clothes are widely available and very satisfactory for many women who have undergone mastectomy. However, women who are not content with the prosthesis may wish to consider silicone implants. *At present, there is no indication that these implants spur any recurrence of malignancy.*

The implant can be done at the time of surgery itself (especially if the tumor is very small and a simple mastectomy or subcutaneous mastectomy is possible). Not all surgeons are willing to perform this replacement if a radical mastectomy is needed. (See p. 349)

The implant can also be done in women who had mastectomy in the past. Consult a plastic surgeon.

Remember that the replacement breast will not look just like the other breast. However, techniques are improving and there are now even ways of simulating a nipple by tattooing or by grafting skin from the vulva or remaining nipple onto the new breast.

DENTAL CARE

---

48. Tooth decay: a preventable epidemic

Ninety-five per cent of Americans suffer from tooth decay, and 50 per cent have lost their teeth by the time they are sixty—an incredibly high figure which could be dramatically reduced simply by improved diet and regular fluoridation.

49. What causes tooth decay?

a. Plaque (pronounced "plack") is a thick gel formed by saliva and bacteria combining in the mouth. As the bacteria digest sugar, an acid is formed which eats away at the enamel of the tooth. If the plaque stays on the tooth and hardens, it forms calculus (a calcium substance, so hard it has to be chipped and scraped away). Calculus can cause irritation and infection of the gums.

b. Sugar (carbohydrate), especially the "free" sugar in candy and cakes, causes bacteria in the mouth to thrive, encouraging plaque formation. The more sugar in the diet the more bacteria to digest it, the more acid forming to destroy tooth enamel. Americans have one of the highest free-sugar consumption rates in the world; one survey estimated that the average American eats about *125 pounds* of refined sugar each year! That is dental suicide.

c. Heredity determines the innate strength of tooth enamel to a very great degree. *Know your family's dental history*. If it is bad, take every step to protect yourself and your children.

50. Preferred dental hygiene

a. Virtually all medical and dental authorities now agree that fluoride in a community water supply can help prevent cavities—people living in fluoridated communities experience 60 per cent less tooth decay in the first twelve years of their lives. If the water in your area is not fluoridated, get fluoride treatments at your dentist yearly; brush with a fluoridated toothpaste. Children in such areas should take vitamins with fluoride in them daily for the first twelve to fourteen years. (Fluoride in water may also help prevent osteoporosis in later life, see p. 293)

b. Avoid the candy-type vitamins for children. They contain sugar. If you cannot find unsugared vitamins because of the current fad to the contrary, give your kids an ordinary combined vitamin *plus* a fluoride pill. Either the pediatrician or the dentist can prescribe this.

c. Brush after every meal; this helps prevent plaque buildup.

d. Don't use a very hard toothbrush; it may hurt your gums.

e. Use non-waxed dental floss daily to prevent food that is caught between the teeth from rotting and causing decay.

f. RECOMMENDATION: Do not use toothpastes with whiteners routinely. The whiteners may be abrasive to tooth enamel. Remember: absolutely white teeth look crazy, false, and abnormal. There is nothing unhealthy about slightly yellow teeth; if you want your teeth to look whiter, try a different color lipstick; white often looks brighter or duller depending on the color that is around it.

g. RECOMMENDATION: Avoid toothpastes with chloroform and formaldehyde in them. These are dangerous substances even in low concentrations.

h. See a dentist at least once a year; twice a year before age thirty. The process of decay seems to stabilize with most people at this age.

i. There are now tablets which can be taken which discolor the areas of plaque and enable a woman to brush away plaque more efficiently. If you are bothered by constant decay, try them.

j. Don't smoke. It will turn your teeth yellow; maybe brown and causes gum infections.

k. If you have teeth removed, see that you *hasten* to have the appropriate bridgework done. The teeth hold each other in place; when one goes, all the rest weaken, may change position and get loose. Bridgework must be done by highly qualified people who have been recommended to you by other dentists and by other patients as well as your local dental school. If your bridge doesn't seem to fit, or is irritating you, have it refitted immediately. Badly-fitting bridges that irritate the gums can cause much more serious infection and illness.

l. Calculus should be removed regularly by the dentist or hygienist.

m. If you have bad teeth, with lots of cavities and an obvious tendency toward decay, have your teeth X-rayed yearly. If you have good teeth, avoid the X rays or have them infrequently; they are an unnecessary risk to you. If you're pregnant, try to avoid dental X rays. If you must have them, make sure your abdomen is completely screened. Dental treatment during pregnancy is now considered safe provided you have approval of your obstetrician.

51. Gingivitis and pyorrhea: common gum ailments

When plaque along the gum line calcifies, it can cause an inflammation called gingivitis. This should be treated immediately by removal of the calculus and medication to relieve the inflammation. Sometimes, the plaque and calculus creep around between the gum and the teeth; the constant irritation can lead to pyorrhea, a more serious gum inflammation, and loosening of the teeth, sometimes loss of them.

52. Smoking is terrible for your teeth

Smoking discolors your teeth and discolors calculus, which starts off white. It increases the risk of gum disease, especially in young women, so that *smokers are twice as likely to lose their teeth as are nonsmokers of the same age.*

53. Dental anesthetics

Most oral surgeons have had some months of training in anesthesiology and may well be qualified to administer general anesthesia, for example, for tooth extractions. *Make sure* your oral surgeon has been trained before accepting the notion of general anesthetic outside a hospital. *Make sure* that your blood pressure will be monitored during the procedure. If you have any medical problems of any sort, do not allow yourself to be put out in the dentist's office; you can have your tooth extracted in the hospital or under local anesthesia. Sniffs of nitrous oxide, which do not induce sleep, are much safer than general anesthesia.

The safest recourse is in local anesthetics; a dentist can numb your mouth totally without the risk and complexity of general anesthesia. WARNING: *Never have a general anesthetic for dental work during pregnancy*—because you run the risk of decreasing the oxygen supply to your baby.

THE IMPORTANCE OF PROPER DIET

54. A nutritious diet is rarely followed in America

Very few people in the United States now follow a basic, nutritious diet without excess calories or junk food. Advertising has done a job on Americans: snacks are in, good food is out. The table of basic food substances found in the Appendix (Table 6) shows the average need of an adult. If you do heavy work, you need more calories and nutrition; if you do sedentary work, you need less.

The way a woman eats as an adult derives partially from patterns set in childhood (e.g., not liking spinach) and partially from adult conditioning patterns (e.g., eating very fast). Individual metabolic rates vary, so that the same diet and same exercise pattern will result in different body weights for different individuals. A woman should embark on a well-balanced diet for herself, and if she has children should discourage non-nutritious foods which add nothing but fat or carbohydrates to the body. *Exercise must go together with diet.* If you don't develop a good exercise pattern, you cannot eat as much as you want; it's as simple as that.

55. Nutritional values

A calorie is a unit of energy supplied to the body by food. The body burns calories as it moves and metabolizes. There are three categories of foods:

    a. Fats
    b. Proteins
    c. Carbohydrates

Carbohydrate calories burn off the fastest; fat calories more slowly; protein calories least quickly. Most reducing diets therefore suggest a decrease in fats and carbohydrates and maintenance of proteins. A body which does not receive enough protein will suffer from malnutrition. Thus, some of the fattest people who look quite well-nourished are actually malnourished, because their diet is overrich in fat and carbohydrate and deficient in protein, and some people who are slender and appear to be in great shape are actually malnourished because they are not receiving enough calories of all the different food groups. For example, a person who *looks* thin can have an excess of cholesterol in her system from excess saturated fat consumption.

56. Healthful shopping and cooking

Health foods are neither processed, preserved, or recolored; they *may* be healthier than processed foods because they are more natural, but one does wonder why they should be so much more expensive.

a. One excellent, and less expensive, way to put "health foods" into your daily diet is to cook. Cook the broccoli fresh instead of buying it frozen. Cook the chicken yourself instead of buying it prefried. Make the cookies yourself instead of buying them packaged, with all their preservatives, sweetenings and processing. You may not get fewer calories with your own baking—but you'll get fewer chemicals.

b. When you buy fresh produce, wash it *very well*. There's no sense eating the spray that kept the aphids away.

c. Powdered non-fat dry milk is just as nutritious as any other milk on the market and much cheaper. In addition, it lacks the butter fat which adds calories and cholesterol to your diet.

d. Fish is high in protein, low in calories, and can be the staple of a well-balanced diet. Try to cultivate a taste for fish and eat it several times a week. Cook it plain, avoid caloric sauces and frying techniques.

e. Trim the fat off beef and lamb before cooking; there's enough fat inlaid in a good piece of meat to keep the flavor.

f. There is considerable worry about the cancer-causing potential of the nitrites used to prevent botulism in processed meats such as hot dogs, cold cuts, and bacon. Try to avoid these meats. Encourage the development of safe alternatives.

g. Most bread is re-enriched with the vitamins and minerals which were otherwise processed out. Thus, white bread is generally just as nutritious as other kinds, although it may lack fiber of whole grains.

h. "Fast foods" imply fast service; too often, they also imply fast consumption—and resulting improper digestion. If you're going out to eat, try to linger over your food as you would at home. Eating out should be at least as much fun as eating in, even when it's cheap.

i. Among the most dangerous food additives are those we put in ourselves—salt and sugar. Salt augments retention of water, and this may be particularly dangerous to people with a personal or family history of hypertension. Train yourself—and your children—not to add extra salt to food that has already been prepared with salt.

Free sugar (that is, not occurring naturally in fruit, for example) has very little nutritive value except for supplying fast-burning calories. It contributes greatly to obesity and to tooth decay. (See #49 above)

Avoid presweetened breakfast cereals.

Avoid fruit or fruit juices that are canned with extra sugar.

Drink coffee or tea without sugar.

Eat protein snacks rather than sugary or salty ones.

57. The use of sugar substitutes such as saccharin is still debatable

Sugar is bad for you and saccharin is bad for you (studies show the potential to cause cancer, at least in animals), so at present, the best policy is to use both as sparingly as possible. The data currently available shows that small amounts of both substances are reasonably safe. Watch for further news. (Ref. 10)

VITAMINS

58. Opinion: Healthy women should avoid megavitamin therapy.

Ever since Linus Pauling, who received the Nobel Prize for chemistry and not for nutrition, suggested that large doses of Vitamin C could prevent the common cold, people have been infatuated with the notion that vitamins—truly a natural medicine—could be used to create good health. There is no proof that they will—and some evidence that overdosing on vitamins can hamper good health.

Overdosing on Vitamin A can cause mental disorientation, skin disorders; growth retardation in children.

Overdosing on Vitamin D can put too much calcium in the blood.

Overdosing on Vitamin C is thought to aggravate gout, kidney stones and to lower fertility.

Vitamin E is sold for everything from smooth skin to increased energy and control of hot flashes in menopause. *No one has proven that it works for anything,* except as an antioxidant which *may* help to keep the body's oxygen supply steady.

Do not overdose on any vitamins. Take the recommended daily allowance only. (See p. 268) Today, the regulatory situation is this: when sold without prescription, no vitamin can exceed more than one and one half times the RDA. High-potency fat-soluble and D vitamins are now sold only by prescription. Of course you can take ten pills a day on your own recognizance, government regulation or no—but as researches reveal the wide variety of disorders caused by megavitamin doses, that would seem a very unwise course.

(Megavitamin therapy to cure mentally and physically ill people is another, still experimental, matter.) (Ref. 11 and 12)

59. Vitamin deficiency and the oral contraceptives

Some studies have shown that the blood levels of several vitamins go down when a woman is on the pill—Vitamins B-6, C, and folic acid in particular. (Ref. 13) A woman should make sure she eats foods high in these vitamins or takes the vitamins supplementally while she is on the pill. Vitamin B-6 deficiency is believed to cause mood changes among women on the pill, so supplements of two to ten times the normal daily amounts should be taken. (See p. 46)

OBESITY

60. How obesity threatens good health

At least 10–20 per cent of Americans are 25 per cent or more over their ideal weight. This makes them more susceptible to:

a. Endocrine disorders (including irregular menses, infertility)

b. Elevated blood sugar (diabetes is four times as common in overweight people)

c. Increased incidence of breast and endometrial cancer. (See pp. 346–47, 364)

d. Lung disorders

e. Osteoarthritis (see pp. 377–78)

f. Heart attack; stroke; other cardiovascular illness such as hypertension

g. Gall-bladder disease

h. Complicated pregnancy and delivery

i. Psychologic disorders, including depression

61. Psychological aspects of overeating

Many people overeat because of tension, emotional problems, boredom, or unhappiness (for example, prolonged grieving). In fact, some people overeat *in order to* get fat: fatness is psychologically *useful* to them. It may help them avoid situations which they fear—for example, athletic or social competition. It may provide them with the isolation they desire—in that case, fatness may be the secondary armor of a person who really just wants to be alone. In a society which preferred fat women, it would be normal for women to seek to be fat. Older women of the generation that immigrated from Europe and the Middle East often comment on how shocking it was to find that plump girls, considered so desirable in Italy, for example, or Poland, were not preferred in America.

Counselors have long been accustomed to advising women that being fat is a kind of social cop-out, indicating at the worst sexual coldness and at the least poor mental adjustment.

In fact, there may be *excellent* reasons that a person should wish to be out of the social or sexual mainstream. But even if a woman thinks her psychiatrist is wrong, even if she has gone through much consciousness-raising to not hate herself because she is overweight, *she must never forget that it is unhealthy to be fat.* You can adjust psychologically to overweight—but you should still try to lose the excess, because undoubtedly it is shortening your life.

62. Opinion: Diets and diet doctors—consult the nutritionist.

Most people get fat from underexercising *and* overeating. Very few people get fat from glandular malfunction or "sluggish thyroid": in fact, such people are usually very sick in other ways as well and overweight is often the least of their problems.

Too many people who seek out diet doctors harbor some mystical belief in a magic formula or pill that will make them lose weight and still be able to eat whatever they want. *This just isn't possible.*

Although many physicians specialize in diet, there is no actual medical specialty, complete with board examinations, in this field. This means that *anyone* with a theory can qualify, and books on diet by all kinds of doctors have been proliferating. Their evaluation is entirely up to the reader. If any advice can be given at all, it *is probably that a book about nutrition—not about dieting—will serve you best.* (Jean Mayer's work is recommended.)

Here are some general guidelines about diets and diet doctors:

a. *Liquid-protein diets may be dangerous to your health.* The very popular "last chance diet" has, indeed, proved to be the last chance for many women. There have now been many reports of sudden deaths in women using these diets. Their use is now under review by the FDA and medical experts. (Ref. 14, 15) At present, women should avoid these diets unless under very rigid medical supervision.

b. WARNING: *Avoid taking medications for dieting.* Will power doesn't come in a bottle or hypodermic. Amphetamines, which take away your appetite, also make you nervous, sleepless, unable to concentrate. If your diet doctor prescribes them, get another doctor, for this is now considered bad medicine. The only exception to this rule is a case of massive obesity, a health emergency. (See ✻63 below)

c. WARNING: *Do not accept HCG (Human Chorionic Gonadotropin) injections for weight loss. They have not been proven effective, and HCG is too powerful a drug to use in this way.* Many weight-control clinics and doctors are now using this hormone, which is produced by the placenta in normal pregnancy, as an assistance with a low-calorie diet. Some doctors claim that this redistributes the fat of the body. The FDA is so concerned that it has mandated a statement about HCG's ineffectiveness. There is to date no evidence of serious side effects, but this is a powerful hormone, so beware. (See p. 121)

d. Do not go on a one-food or fad diet. All types of food are needed for good nutrition.

e. Do not go on a crash diet. Rapid weight loss is dangerous to your health. *Three pounds a week is the most that a healthy woman should lose.*

f. Never go on a diet without an appropriate companion plan of exercise. As you lose weight, this will keep your skin and muscles in good shape: it will also speed the weight-loss process.

g. With increased understanding of the way foods work *in combination with each other* to burn calories, some recent diets have appeared which emphasize what you eat rather than the quantity. The "Scarsdale Diet" is a case in point. These diets may work well for some women but it's vital not to stay on them for more than two weeks, and stop them sooner if constipation or other digestive problems result.

h. OPINION: Use one of the following two methods as an aid in sensible weight reduction:

1. Group plans such as Weight Watchers work for many people. The advantage of these plans is that they advocate good, nutritious diets and slow, steady weight loss, rather than medications and rapid weight loss. Besides, some women find it easier to diet with the help of others in the same situation.

2. Behavior-modification plans work well for some people. Basically, these programs hope to change eating habits so that food is eaten more slowly and under better conditions (e.g. early in the day, when metabolism is faster).

TABLE 5
HEIGHT/WEIGHT CHART FOR WOMEN

HEIGHT	AVERAGE HEALTHFUL WEIGHT +/−10%	DANGEROUS WEIGHT— MORE THAN 25% OVERWEIGHT
6'	165	205
5'10"	155	195
5'8"	145	185
5'6"	140	175
5'4"	135	165
5'2"	130	155
5'	125	150

63. Massive obesity: a health emergency (See Table 5 for ideal height/ weight)

If you weigh twice as much as you should for your height, you have a problem which should be treated as an emergency. No leisurely experimenting with diets will do in this case. You are in great danger and must act now.

a. Consult a specialist in endocrinology and metabolism.

b. Have all the appropriate blood tests to determine, scientifically, which specific diet plan you require.

c. Lose weight under carefully controlled medical conditions. These should be set only by endocrine specialists in conjunction with an extensive weight reduction program.

d. The doctor may hospitalize you. Check that your insurance covers this mode of treatment.

e. "Fat farms"—special resorts where diet and exercise are carefully controlled—often succeed in getting their guests to lose weight. They must be supervised by physicians whose credentials you have checked widely—and you must leave them with a program of weight maintenance to which you are prepared to adhere.

64. Calculate the risk: the intestinal bypass operation to prevent obesity

If all other methods fail for the massively obese person, a surgical procedure is possible in which a section of the small intestine is eliminated from the normal flow. This should be used only as a last resort, for risk of the complications is high. A significant number of people do not survive the operation (from 1.4 to 14 per cent in various studies). Diarrhea and frequent bowel movements may persist more than six months afterward; liver disease has also been reported. A woman who has this surgery should only do so on the advice of both an endocrinologist and a surgeon and should go to a hospital center which does the procedure frequently. (Ref. 16) An alternative surgical procedure which may be safer is stomach stapling. (Ref. 17) Watch for news.

65. Involuntary weight loss may indicate ill health

Weight gain may or may not mean you are sick—but *involuntary weight loss means that something is wrong*. Get a medical examination, especially if you have any other abnormal symptoms.

66. Coffee, tea, soda: caffeine and tension

Caffeine is a relatively powerful stimulant which occurs naturally in coffee, tea, and the cocoa bean from which soda (including diet soda) is made. WARNING: Each cup of coffee contains between 100 and 125 mg of caffeine; if you drink coffee after every meal, you are getting a lot of caffeine; if you drink two or three cups after every meal and a couple more during the day, you may be overdosing with caffeine.

Symptoms of excess caffeine may be extreme nervousness, heartburn, heart palpitations, and diarrhea. It was believed for some time that caffeine caused ulcers, colitis, and heart disease. However, a recent study showed that even *decaffeinated* coffee is associated with ulcers. (Ref. 18) And no good evidence has confirmed an association between caffeine and heart disease. (Ref. 19) At present, all we can say is that caffeine is a powerful stimulant which may cause some medical problems in susceptible people. (Ref. 20) It should not be used excessively.

67. Cholesterol is not a great danger to most women before menopause

Cholesterol is a kind of fat, present in butter, and other saturated fats and oils, high-fat meats such as pork, untrimmed beef and lamb, whole milk, and eggs. In the body it is manufactured in the liver and is then metabolized into steroids, hormones, and bile acids and is present in cell membranes. If cholesterol and other lipids are present in the blood stream in high levels, they may build up in the interior of the arteries, causing a narrowing of the passage. This process is called arteriosclerosis or hardening of the arteries.

Women seem to have a lower risk of arteriosclerosis before the age of menopause. It now appears that an important factor in determining whether a person is adversely affected by cholesterol buildup is the type of complex molecule by which the cholesterol is carried in the blood stream. Some of the cholesterol is carried as high-density lipoproteins

(HDL) which are large molecules, high in protein, low in cholesterol. The rest is carried in low-density lipoproteins (LDL) which are high in cholesterol, low in protein. The HDLs appear to have a protective effect on cardiovascular disease; the higher the HDL/LDL ratio, the less the risk of cardiovascular disease, such as heart attack and stroke. Things which increase HDL levels are decreased dietary intake of saturated fats and strenuous exercise. Women, premenopausally, seem to have higher HDL levels and therefore less risk of cardiovascular disease. This protection is decreased by obesity, smoking, use of estrogens, and a diet high in fat. Women should have their cholesterol levels measured periodically—especially over age forty. Values less than 200 mg/cc of blood are normal. Watch for further news in this area. Some physicians are encouraging the routine determination of the HDL/LDL levels, especially in high-risk people. (Ref. 21, 22)

68. High-fiber foods and cancer of the colon

It has not been proven conclusively that high-fiber foods, like vegetables, salads, whole-grain breads, and unprocessed cereal grains, will prevent cancer of the colon—but they will make your intestine work better by helping the waste move faster through it, and may save you from the discomfort of constipation. (Ref. 23)

69. The case for and against food additives and preservatives

Look ahead! Watch the newspapers! Preservatives and food additives are now under scrutiny by the FDA and health groups, and several may soon be outlawed.

a. Some red dyes used in food colorings have already been banned because of their potential to cause cancer.

b. DES (see pp. 366–67) has been found to cause vaginal cancer in the daughters of women who took it during pregnancy. However, it is still added to animal feeds to fatten poultry and cattle. OPINION: The FDA seems unduly hesitant in ruling that this substance be removed from animal feed. Do everything you can as a consumer, a voter, and a taxpayer to speed the process.

Some food additives however are beneficial to general health.

c. Thirty years ago, stomach cancer was extremely common among American men; it is the only form of cancer that has *declined* dramatically in recent years. One theory to explain this decline is that *antioxidants* in the *preservatives* now put into foods prevent the formation of peroxides that are created in fats when they become rancid. These peroxides are considered a leading cause of stomach cancer.

d. Other preservatives prevent the formation of molds, which, when formed on unpreserved foods, are powerful carcinogens. Dr. Jean Mayer suggests that the very low rate of liver cancer in this country, as compared to the very high rates in the less-developed world, is attributable to the prevention of mold-formation by preservatives in food. (Ref. 24, 25)

70. Lactose intolerance

Lactose is a natural sugar occurring in milk and milk products. Many people find that after babyhood (and sometimes during infancy), they are unable to digest milk. A glassful gives them a stomach ache, nausea and diarrhea. Cheese and yogurt, which are lower in lactose content, are better tolerated. These people have a deficiency in the intestinal enzyme, *lactase,* which might be added to milk before drinking. Watch for developments in this area. If you suffer from excess gas and colitis, consider that lactose intolerance may be the cause. People with southern European and African ancestry seem to be the most affected.

71. Acidophilus replacement

Lactobacillus acidophilus is a bacteria normally present in the colon where it assists in digestion of milk products. (This is very similar to the lactobacillus normally present in the vagina.) Under certain circumstances such as prolonged antibiotic usage, the normal bacteria of the colon are killed off and some people believe that for good digestion to continue, the acidophilus must be replaced. Special milk with acidophilus is sold at rather high prices: yogurt, which contains another lactobacillus, probably works just as well.

72. Exercise is essential for good health throughout life

It is incontrovertible that people who exercise regularly look better, live longer, and stay healthier.

a. *Calisthenics* done regularly every day keep your body in shape, assist body systems in functioning, and clear your head. An excellent all-round system is that recommended by the Royal Canadian Air Force; a woman may select any system depending on what is best for her. (For example, a pianist or typist will prefer different exercises from those needed by a saleswoman or cook, because the first may suffer from cramped back muscles, the second may suffer from aching legs and feet.) Diplomats and homemakers who must work under chronic severe tension may prefer a system like yoga, which stretches the muscles while relaxing the mind as well. Many women find that it is helpful to learn the exercises in weekly or twice-weekly classes, (e.g. ballet, oriental systems), and continue practicing at home.

b. *Avoid now-and-then strenuous exercise.*

If you have stopped exercising for some time, don't leap into strenuous exercise suddenly. Too many tennis players and joggers have been stricken by heart attacks because they did not build up to this particularly strenuous form of exercise; because they overestimated their strength or, rather, underestimated their accumulated weakness. See your doctor before undertaking strenuous exercise if you are over forty. Do not do any strenuous exercise in the midday sun if you are out of shape.

c. Swimming is a good all-around exercise for everyone. You don't have to swim fast or with perfect form to enjoy the benefits of relaxation and improved muscle tone that come with swimming.

d. Exercise prevents or alleviates many of the conditions that chronically make women feel ill; for example, it helps to prevent osteoporosis; alleviates dysmenorrhea and constipation; by strengthening muscles, it makes childbirth easier.

SMOKING AND HOW TO QUIT

73. Smoking is terrible for your health

It is almost ludicrous and trite to mention that smoking is bad for you. Everyone over age three knows that! Smoking is just about the worst thing a woman can do to herself, other than allow herself to become grossly obese. Smoking is the major factor in the development of lung cancer, bronchitis, emphysema, heart attack, hypertension, stroke, severe gum disease and loss of teeth, early menopause, bladder cancer, and bad facial wrinkles. (Refs. 26–30) Women who smoke and who take the oral contraceptives are at much greater risk than non-smokers for heart attack and stroke. (See p. 47) However, the smoking is a greater factor than the pill. Women who smoke and who do not take the pill are at greater risk for these problems than are non-smoking pill takers.

There is no getting around the fact that smokers are voluntarily doing irreparable harm to their bodies. Pregnant women who smoke are voluntarily exposing their babies to great danger, including fetal death. (See pp. 182–83) It is truly a futile exercise for a woman to follow all of the other advice in this book and then continue to smoke.

Economic factors should also be considered. In this time of worrying about the huge costs of health care, it is tragic to see that "self-inflicted" illnesses such as smoking and alcoholism (see below) now consume an astounding estimated 20 per cent of the direct-service health costs in this country. (Ref. 30, 31)

Women must at least cut back in their smoking, to no more than ten cigarettes a day. Stopping altogether would be far better.

74. Women are smoking more than ever today

Since the warnings about cigarette smoking were placed on packaging and in advertising, there has been a small decline in smoking—but the incidence of smoking among women has risen especially among teen-agers. One reason may be that some advertisers have successfully equated smoking with liberation. Another reason is that women, with all they have to do and want to be today, are just plain tense. Smoking is an inappropriate and dangerous way to reduce tension.

75. How to stop smoking

A number of good products may help you stop smoking, including very-low-tar-and-nicotine cigarettes which generally taste so bad to to-bacco lovers that they kill the desire for cigarettes. Smoke Enders, like Weight Watchers, employs group therapy to help kick the habit. Chil-dren are very useful in the fight to stop, for they have been convinced by school propaganda that smoking will kill their parents and feel justified in tearing up and throwing away cigarettes. The protesting adult feels foolish struggling with a six-year-old for possession of a tube of tobacco which the adult knows full well is poisonous to the system. Hence, the final reason for a halt to smoking is simple shame.

No pill now on the market is useful in helping a smoker stop. Taste-distorting lozenges can be of assistance, since they ruin the taste of the cigarette and most smokers smoke for taste. For example, very strong mints, strong cinnamon candies, are quite good. If you are a person who smokes most when you are under a lot of tension, substitute an-other oral satisfaction. Chew on something. People who thought they smoked to *relieve* tension find very often that the smoking itself caused them to be more tense than they had to be. As with dieting, there is no medical subspecialty in smoking; doctors who claim to have a system that will make you stop can be tried at the shopper's risk. Many people find that after they stop smoking, they gain weight (because they are compensating their oral needs by eating more). Many find that they are constipated for a while. Although smoking does loosen the bowel in some cases, it is no better at this job than a bowl of bran flakes and much worse for general health.

See reference section for list of pamphlets available on how to stop smoking.

ALCOHOL AND ITS DANGERS

76. Alcoholic beverages in moderation are not medically dangerous

At present, well-nourished people who have a drink or two a day seem to show no adverse medical effects. Some studies have actually shown that they live longer than non-drinkers. The key word, of course, is moderation.

77. How to avoid getting drunk

If you want to drink to be social, but don't want to get intoxicated or suffer too much the following day, consider these ideas:

a. Eat while you drink. It makes the drink last longer—and also dulls the effect of the alcohol entering your blood stream.

b. Sip your drink slowly; nurse it; make it last; then your body can absorb the alcohol more effectively.

c. If you anticipate a hangover, drink several glasses of milk and juice before bed to replenish fluids and soothe the stomach, or take several mutivitamin pills. Analgesics may help, but chances are that nothing will prevent hangover entirely.

78. How to know if you are an alcoholic

Ask yourself the following questions, and answer them *honestly:*

a. Do you take a drink in the morning?

b. Do you drink at lunch every day without fail?

c. Do you get high every night, or do you absolutely need to drink to get to sleep?

If the answer to any one of these questions is "yes," you may be on your way to a drinking problem. *If the answer to two or more is "yes," you are already an alcoholic. Seek help immediately!*

79. The medical risks of alcoholism

The most serious medical problems caused by alcoholism are:

a. Cirrhosis of the liver (destruction of the liver cells—often fatal)

b. Peptic ulcer (with bleeding into the bowel)

c. Malnutrition and vitamin deficiency

d. Severe anemia

e. Heart disease (damage to the heart muscle)

f. Severe mental disorders (hallucinations, loss of memory, and actual destruction of brain cells)

g. Seizures (often associated with withdrawal from alcohol)

h. Babies born to mothers who are alcoholics inherit the fetal alcohol syndrome. (See p. 182)

80. Organizations that help alcoholics

a. A general medical practitioner can start therapy for an alcohol problem but will probably eventually refer the patient to an alcoholics' organization for maintenance and further help.

b. Alcoholics Anonymous has been most successful in helping alcoholics stay away from liquor, curing each other with understanding and a mutual sharing of a terrible problem.

c. Al-Anon provides counseling for family and friends of alcoholics; Alateen deals with the problems of teen-age alcoholics.

d. There are many alcoholic treatment centers throughout the country funded by the federal government for both inpatient and outpatient therapy. Usually the treatment begins with several weeks' hospitalization, followed by ongoing therapy. Women alcoholics have received very little attention by these facilities, which mainly treat males as the "more important" members of society to be rehabilitated. (This holds true for rehabilitation of prisoners too.) Women who need treatment should call their county health departments or the regional offices of HEW to get information. Many times a referral from a physician is needed, so see your family doctor.

TRANQUILIZERS

81. Warning: Tranquilizers and other drugs affecting the emotions are dangerously overprescribed and overused by women

Tranquilizers (anti-anxiety drugs) are the most commonly prescribed drugs in this country. (See Table 7) These drugs, while very effective in relieving anxiety, are very powerful and potentially addictive. If high doses are taken, withdrawal symptoms may occur when a woman tries to stop the drugs.

Women receive the bulk of the prescriptions for tranquilizers, not only for anxiety, but for a myriad of complaints which may or may not be related to anxiety. There is a prevailing bias among physicians that women's disorders are far more likely to be "psychoneurotic" than men's, and for this reason the drugs are overprescribed. Frequently, they are prescribed when the doctor doesn't take the time to discuss the woman's problem fully or to do a complete examination. *Don't let this happen to you.*

We live in an anxiety-ridden, violent age, and many women (and men) have times when they are overwrought and tense. When a woman feels nervous, she should attempt to determine why. What in her life situation is causing the problem? If she has increasing tension and sleeplessness, then she may need professional counseling with a psychiatrist, psychologist or marriage counselor to aid in determining the cause of the problem. In the long run, counseling is far better for a woman's health than drugs. It is important that a woman learn to deal with her problems rather than become dependent on long-term therapy with potentially addictive medications. *Don't accept tranquilizers just to mask anxiety without determining the cause.*

If tranquilizers are absolutely necessary for treatment of severe anxiety attacks, they should be taken in low doses only and for short periods of time *unless* they are prescribed in combination with ongoing psychotherapy.

82. Calculate the risk: Drink carefully if you are taking tranquilizers or barbiturates

The combination of alcohol and tranquilizers is dangerous to your health; excesses of the two can cause blackouts or have other severe potentially lethal effects on your nervous system. *NEVER COMBINE THE TWO!*

83. Marijuana

An estimated 13 million people smoke marijuana regularly in America—it provides a mild "high" without the hangover and ill health associated with heavy drinking.

Attempts to find some terrible effect of marijuana to discourage pot-smokers have failed generally. There are some reports of acute psychosis; fast heart rate; impaired coordination because of adverse effect on the brain. Some tests in tissue culture show that marijuana smoke can cause malignancies, just like tobacco smoke—but this remains to be proven by incidence among people. Reports of genetic damage because of marijuana smoking by pregnant women remain unproven too. *However, marijuana is a drug and it certainly is a good idea not to use it, or any other drug, during early pregnancy.* (Ref. 32)

A new development: Recently, there have been some reports that marijuana has good effects on the disease glaucoma, in which pressure builds up in the eye because of poor drainage of internal optic fluids. If you suffer from glaucoma and other treatments have failed, ask your doctor about marijuana.

Reports that sex is "better" when the partners are under the influence of marijuana are yet to be proven by the sexologists; individuals can judge for themselves whether they prefer to be more, or less, bereft of their senses when making love.

Other "hard" drugs are disastrous for a woman's health. Avoid them at all cost!

84. Energy, stress, and fatigue

Energy is a natural endowment: good nutrition, adequate exercise, and enough satisfying sleep will maintain it in full measure. Yet few women (or men) receive these simple basic ingredients, and as more women go to work and suffer the extraordinary stress of the American workday, fatigue—lack of energy—becomes a great problem.

"Quick energy" is that extra little burst of steam you can get from a candy bar (fast-burning carbohydrate) or from emotional stimulation which causes the release of adrenaline. This kind of energy is vital—but you can't live on it.

85. Poor nutrition may cause fatigue

A breakfast of coffee alone, which constitutes no nutrition, will eventually contribute to fatigue. The caffeine, and the sugar, in the coffee may provide quick energy. But the protein in whole wheat bread or whole grain cereal or an egg or a glass of unsweetened orange juice provides the energy that the body needs *all day*.

86. Lack of exercise may cause fatigue

It is almost axiomatic that the people who feel the most tired are those who have worked for years in an office or factory, at a sedentary job. Exercise renews the body's oxygen supply by increasing the flow of oxygen through the circulatory system: thus, if you can't get any exercise on the job, run in the morning or play tennis at night or get out and garden at lunchtime.

87. Stress may cause fatigue; prolonged stress may cause disease

When you are under a lot of stress, your body reacts to help you cope with it: your muscles tighten; your mind races; your blood pressure and cholesterol levels rise. Over time, stress of this kind can predispose the body to serious disease—heart trouble and ulcers, for example. WARNING: *Fatigue is the first signal that you may be under too much stress for your own health.* If you are exhausted every day after work, curtailing your social life, unable to read or enjoy a movie, then maybe the fatigue you are suffering from should be regarded as a warning—and you should take a second look at your work. The Na-

TABLE 6

FOOD SUBSTANCES—RECOMMENDED DAILY ALLOWANCES

	ADULT WOMEN	PREGNANCY AND LACTATION	BODY FUNCTION	FOOD SOURCES
Carbohydrates	4–7 g	4–7 g	Main source of energy—excess stored as fat (cellulose-bulk)	breads, sugar, cereals (cellulose—dried fruits, grains, nuts, vegetables)
Fats	No more than 35% of diet—polyunsaturated oils better		energy, fatty insulation of the body	eggs, liver, kidney, sweetbreads, whole milk, oils
Protein	46–50 g	76–80 g	body structure	meat, poultry, fish, milk, cheese, eggs, soybeans
Minerals *Calcium*	800 mg	1200 mg	bones and teeth, regulators of muscle contraction, blood clotting and nerve function	milk and milk products
Phosphorus	800 mg	1200 mg	bones and teeth, coenzymes in metabolic pathways	meat, poultry, fish and eggs
Magnesium	300 mg	450 mg	coenzyme in metabolic pathways	leafy green vegetables, nuts, soybeans (average diet deficient)

	ADULT WOMEN	PREGNANCY AND LACTATION	BODY FUNCTION	FOOD SOURCES
Iron	18 mg	18 mg+ (must take supplements)	blood cells	liver, meats, egg yolks, leafy vegetables, raisins, prunes, apricots
Iodine	100 mcg	125–150 mcg	part of thyroid hormone	seafood and seaweed, iodized salt
Zinc	15 mg	20–25 mg	coenzyme, hair, bones and male sex gland function	animal protein

Fat-soluble Vitamins—Avoid excess intake—these are stored in body if present in excess

	ADULT WOMEN	PREGNANCY AND LACTATION	BODY FUNCTION	FOOD SOURCES
Vitamin A	5000 IU	8000 IU	visual pigments, skin and mucus membranes	whole milk, butter, egg yolks, liver, kidney, yellow fruits and vegetables
Vitamin D	400 IU	400 IU	calcium absorption and bone metabolism	egg yolk, milk, butter, liver (exposure to sunlight allows body to manufacture its own supply)
Vitamin E	30 IU	30 IU	inhibits oxidation of unsaturated fatty acids—rest of activity not proven	vegetable oils, leafy vegetables, whole grain cereals

Water Soluble Vitamins—excess is excreted

	ADULT WOMEN	PREGNANCY AND LACTATION	BODY FUNCTION	FOOD SOURCES
Vitamin C	60 mg	60 mg	formation of connective tissue and adrenal gland function	citrus fruits, berries, melons, leafy green vegetables
Folic Acid	0.4 mg	0.8 mg	coenzyme in synthesis of nucleic acids—deficiency=anemia	whole grain cereals, leafy green vegetables, meats, milk (supplements needed in pregnancy and if on the pill)
Niacin (nicotinic acid)	20 mg	20 mg	coenzyme in fat metabolism	liver, kidney, brewer's yeast, tuna, muscle meats, poultry, peanuts
Riboflavin	1.7 mg	2.0 mg	coenzyme in metabolism of carbohydrates, fats, and proteins	brewer's yeast, glandular meats, milk, cheese, eggs, veal, beef, leafy green vegetables
Thiamine	1.5 mg	1.7 mg	coenzyme and important in nerve function	brewer's yeast, wheat germ, whole grain cereals, pork, nuts
Vitamin B-6	2.0 mg	2.5 mg	coenzyme especially in protein metabolism. Needed for chemical reactions in brain.	muscle meats, liver, vegetables and whole grain cereals (may need to be supplemented if on the pill)
Vitamin B-12	6.0 mcg	8 mcg	red-cell production, coenzyme in many cell processes	animal foods, especially liver, brewer's yeast (vegetarians may need supplements)

(Ref. 12, 34)

TABLE 7

MOST FREQUENTLY PRESCRIBED TRANQUILIZERS

GENERIC NAME	MAJOR BRAND NAMES	USUAL DOSE (total/day)
Chlordiazepoxide	Librium	20–40 mg
Clorazepate dipotassium	Tranxene	30 mg
Diazepam	Valium	8–30 mg
Doxepin HCL	Sinequan	up to 150 mg
	Adapin	
Hydroxyzine	Atarax	75–300 mg
	Vistaril	
Meprobamate	Equanil	1,200–1,600 mg
	Miltown	
Oxazepam	Serax	40–60 mg

tional Institute of Occupational Safety and Health reports that people in the following jobs are under the most stress:

a. Assembly-line inspectors
b. Health-care technicians
c. Clinical lab technicians
d. Miners
e. Assembly-line workers
f. Warehouse workers
g. Middle-level executives
h. Public relations people
i. Practical nurses
j. Waiters and waitresses
(Ref. 33)

Research during International Women's Year (1976) showed that the hardest-working person IN THE ENTIRE WORLD is the woman who works a full day and then comes home to cook, clean, and otherwise care for house, children, and husband.

Do not accept crippling fatigue due to stress as the sine qua non *of your everyday life.* Depending on your personality and your individual circumstances, you may be able to relocate to a less stressful situation and get your energy, and your good health, back.

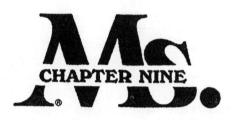

CHAPTER NINE

LITTLE GIRLS

The vast majority of young children are healthy and, fortunately, most pediatric practice involves taking care of them *when they are healthy,* with routine examinations, immunizations, etc. Thus, children do not generally associate their pediatricians with dangerous illness or fierce pain. Most pediatricians do everything they can to win the trust of their patients. They fill their waiting rooms with toys and picture books, paint cartoon murals on their walls, distribute balloons.

The environment of a "grown-up" doctor has none of these charming amenities; to a child, a gynecologist's office may look like a Frankensteinian torture chamber. A long, thin table; stirrups, plastic gloves. (In fact, you don't have to be a child to have your hangups about stirrups.)

If a little girl does have to deal with vaginal infection or other genital problems, the pediatrician she knows and trusts has a better chance of getting her through it without distress than the gynecologist—and is usually just as well qualified medically to handle the problem.

So if your little girl has a gynecological problem, take her to the pediatrician. Try to keep the gynecologist out of her life until she becomes a teen-ager or sexually active. Some gynecologists specialize in pediatric gynecology and would be appropriate physicians for special problems.

1. Breast enlargement is normal in newborn infants

Up until two to three weeks of age, a newborn female infant may have breast enlargement due to high levels of female hormones present during pregnancy. There may be a small amount of cloudy secretion from the nipples, known as "witch's milk." By three weeks, the maternal hormone levels no longer affect the baby's body. Very frequently, boy babies will show exactly the same breast enlargement, and this is normal.

2. Genital swelling and discharge is normal in newborn girls

When a baby is born, the genitals frequently appear swollen; the clitoris may seem to be very large; the vaginal wall may appear swollen. Often, a mucus discharge comes from the vagina. Like breast enlargement in infants, this comes from the effect of the maternal hormones. The internal organs, including the uterus, are slightly larger at birth as well. As the hormone levels fall, there may be a few drops of blood from the shrinking uterus and this appears as vaginal bleeding. At three weeks, when maternal hormones no longer achieve high levels in the baby's blood stream these effects will disappear. They are perfectly normal, indicating a healthy body that is responsive to hormone stimulation.

DEVELOPMENTAL PROBLEMS

3. Imperforate hymen

The hymen is the thin membrane that partly covers the entrance to the vagina. It has a hole in it normally. Shortly after birth, the girl should be examined by a pediatrician or obstetrician to make sure that an opening is present—that the hymen is not imperforate (im-PER-for-it). Ask the examining physician to check this—it is not always routine and there have been some cases in which a girl got all the way to puberty before imperforate hymen was detected. Imperforate hymen will not cause any pain or any difficulty except that as puberty approaches, the normal discharges of the vagina may be caught behind the hymen, creating secondary problems of pain and swelling in the lower abdomen.

If the hymen is imperforate, it must be surgically opened in the hospital. This involves one or two days hospitalization and is a simple procedure causing very little discomfort for the child.

4. Confusion as to the sex of a baby

In *extremely rare* cases, the clitoris of a newborn female infant seems almost as large as a penis; or in boys, the scrotum is not completely fused in the midline, creating a vaginalike cavity. In these circumstances there may be real confusion as to the sex of the child.

A scraping of cells from inside the cheek can be checked for chromosome count or a test on white blood cells can be done to prove the sex of the child. (See p. 210) Thereafter, appropriate surgery can be done to establish genital sex and create a more normal life for the infant. If any such confusion exists, have it cleared up with a chromosome test immediately, and thereafter with the appropriate surgery. Occasionally, a child has been reared as the wrong sex—and it has been shown that after two to three years of age it is psychologically impossible to successfully reverse the gender identity of the child. (Ref. 1)

5. Premature development of breasts and pubic hair

Very often little girls (three to six years old) will develop small amounts of pubic hair and breast tissue. *This is almost always nothing to worry about.* A fast, simple vaginal smear can be taken by the pediatrician to check if female hormones are actually elevated, and premature puberty is taking place. Most often, the hormone levels are normal for the age of the child. If the smear is normal and the general physical examination is normal, forget it. There is nothing to worry about. The breast growth and pubic hair growth will limit itself, and normal puberty will occur later on.

If the tests are not normal, see an endocrinologist (a physician specializing in body chemistry and hormones) recommended by your pediatrician.

The biggest problem with this self-limiting, early development is that parents become terribly anxious about it, constantly examining their daughter, and making her feel self-conscious and deformed. Try not to let your girl see that you are worried, so the episode can pass—as it probably will—without abiding trauma.

WARNING: *Make sure your daughter has not taken your birth-control pills or other hormonal medication, for these can cause breast changes.*

VAGINAL DISCHARGE AND RELATED PROBLEMS

---

6. Vulvovaginitis: the most common gynecological problem of little girls

Irritation of the vulva and vagina is common in little girls aged two to six. Most often it is caused by:

a. Contamination of the vagina by organisms from the bowel. Teach your girl to wipe from front to back, so that she does not wipe bowel contents toward the vagina. If you find any bowel stains on her underwear, suspect that she is not wiping herself completely and correct the situation. The vagina of a little girl is thinner than that of an adult woman and therefore more susceptible to this kind of infection.

Other causes of vaginitis symptoms—itching, odor, and discharge—are

b. Pinworms

c. Viruses and bacteria which normally infect the throat and lungs;

d. Monilia—a less frequent cause in little girls;

e. trichomonas and gonorrhea—almost never contracted unless the child has been sexually assaulted;

f. and occasionally, foreign bodies which the child herself has placed in the vagina. (See ⚹7 below)

If a child complains of itching and the vulva appears red or irritated

g. suspect bubble baths, detergents used to wash clothes, or harsh, perfumed soaps.

In the summertime,

h. the chemicals in swimming pools or the damp and grit of sand-boxes can also cause the symptoms of vulvovaginitis.

7. It is normal for a little girl to place something in her vagina, sometimes

Between the ages of four and six, little girls are sometimes very curious about their genitals and may place something in the vagina—usually toilet paper or tissue but sometimes a paper clip; a peanut; a piece of crayon—as part of the exploration. (Does this hole in me have a bottom? Does it go all the way through me?) A foreign body placed in the vagina will usually cause heavy discharge and a very foul odor; the odor will differentiate for the parent between this cause and, say, a bubble-bath-induced vaginitis.

8. Treatment for foreign objects in the vagina

If a very foul odor makes you suspect that your daughter has placed something in her vagina, see the pediatrician. The doctor should be able to wash it out painlessly at the office. She will have to be examined by the pediatrician—but this will not be painful; a tiny speculum will be used, if any is at all. A large foreign body which has lodged well up into the vagina may have to be removed under anesthesia.

As preventive medicine, talk to your little girl and assuage her curiosity about her vagina and simply tell her calmly but firmly, not to put anything into it because this will hurt her.

9. Treatment for vulvovaginitis in little girls

Eighty per cent of cases are caused by fecal contamination. Assume this is the cause and start treating it yourself. Having the child soak three or four times a day in a warm water bath for ten to twenty minutes will clear the irritation. Use *only* a mild soap without perfume. After she has a bowel movement, wash her yourself with soap and warm water. Plain petroleum jelly will soothe a lot of irritation on the outside of the vagina.

If the symptoms persist for more than two days, or if there is any bleeding or pain consult a pediatrician. Meanwhile, as preventive medicine, get rid of the bubble bath for good; use only mild soaps all the time; use a gentle detergent on her clothes, even if you have to wash them separately from everyone else's.

For other infections, such as monilia, special medications will be given by the doctor. If there is any chance at all that your girl has been molested (a trichomonas or gonorrhea infection is a sure sign), seek professional psychological and legal aid immediately.

10. Labial agglutination (closing of the lips of the vagina)

Related to vaginal infections in children is labial agglutination or fusion (ag-GLUE-tin-ation) in which the small lips of the vagina seem to get stuck together so that the vagina looks as though it has closed up.

This is not serious: it is a side effect of vulvovaginitis, and is only cause for alarm if accompanied by bleeding or if the child has difficulty urinating.

Try sitz-bath treatments; dry your daughter after each one; and apply petroleum jelly. After a few days, try to *gently* separate the lips. If these do not separate, consult a pediatrician who may prescribe a steroid or estrogen cream to thicken the lips and make them more resistant to infection. Estrogen should be used only in very small doses and for short periods of time. Applied lightly for one to two weeks, the cream should make the lips part by themselves.

In severe cases, the doctor may have to part the lips of the vagina. *This should be the last resort because it is painful to the child.* Never let a doctor do this as a first step, and if it is suggested as a first step, get another opinion.

11. Urinary infections

These are common in young girls, caused generally by fecal contamination and irritating soaps and bubble baths. The symptoms are plain: pain on urination and frequency. The diagnosis and treatment involve a urinalysis and if positive, treatment with sulfa drugs or some other antibiotic.

Sometimes, pediatricians suggest dilation of the urethra. This is a painful treatment, potentially traumatic psychologically, usually unnecessary. If your pediatrician suggests it, get a second opinion.

12. Vaginal bleeding in little girls calls for prompt medical attention

This can be caused by injury (a fall off a bike), infection, a foreign body, serious illness such as a tumor, or sexual assault. It should take you to the doctor right away, for diagnosis and treatment.

13. How to prevent vulvovaginitis and urinary tract infections in little girls

a. Teach your girl to wipe from front to back after a bowel movement, and teach her to keep wiping with successive pieces of paper until the paper is clean.

b. Don't use harsh detergents on her laundry.

c. Don't allow her to use strong, perfumed soap. Stick to the mildest soap available. Don't use bubble bath or bath oils.

d. Don't let her sit around in a wet bathing suit. Make sure that she washes herself in plain water after swimming in a chlorinated pool.

e. Make sure she wears cotton underpants. If she wears tights or stockings, make sure she wears them *over* her underpants.

f. Teach her not to put things inside her vagina, if she has done so in the past. If she has never done so, don't give her the idea by bringing up the subject.

14. Virginity

Virginity is a very vague and unimportant concept, notwithstanding the great obsession which male-dominated cultures have had with it over the centuries.

Physically, a girl is a virgin until her hymen is broken. This usually happens either through the use of tampons or by sexual intercourse. The size of the opening in the vagina varies, so bleeding does not always occur at the time the hymen is broken. Excess physical activity does not cause the hymen to be broken.

Experientially, a girl is a virgin until she has had sex. It is best not to burden your little girl with any notion of the importance of physical virginity. It should be her sexual activity, not the state of her hymen, that should be of interest to her.

15. Masturbation is common among young girls

Masturbation affords sexual pleasure, if not full orgasm, to young girls and many of them do it. There is nothing abnormal about this. There is nothing abnormal if they don't do it. Masturbation may cause irritation of the genitals. Treat it as you would vulvitis, with vaseline and sitz baths, but don't make too much of it or you may be inviting your daughter to continue with her masturbation obsessively, just because she gets so much attention that way.

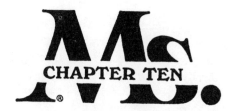

CHAPTER TEN

CHANGE OF LIFE

The word "menopause" is commonly misused to refer to all the symptoms, side effects, crises, and discomforts associated with that time in her life when a woman's ovaries cease to produce eggs and she stops menstruating. Specifically, *menopause* refers only to the end of the menstrual flow—which is but one aspect of a time more properly called *climacteric* (kly-MAC-teric) or change of life.

Change of life can occur normally in women between the ages of forty-three and fifty-five; normal cases exist beyond that range. Some physicians and women think of change of life as "ovarian deficiency disease" and medicate it indefinitely from the time it starts. They are overstating the case quite excessively. *Change of life is not a sickness.* It is a normal process through which all women pass.

Much of the anxiety about change of life is due not to its actual physiological effects but to the deep-rooted, negative attitudes we have toward aging in this country. People who overtreat change of life as though it were a sickness are often treating nothing more than their own fears of growing older. In cultures where the elderly are revered—for example, in China—change of life produces little concern. In our own country, where close to 20 per cent of the population will be over sixty-five by 1980, it should be a national priority to develop a new attitude about aging. Change of life does not finish a woman any more than some company rule about mandatory retirement actually ends the working capacity of any individual. In fact, women who manage *to listen to their bodies* rather than the propaganda of the youth culture may feel better *after* change of life than they did before.

Remember that the men around you are growing older too; remember that if you were twenty-two again, you wouldn't know anywhere near as much as you do now; remember that the average American woman lives to be seventy-seven years old and that at least one third of your life is still ahead of you.

In fact, even with symptoms and discomforts, change of life is a sign of good health and normal progress—just as menarche was when you were a girl.

BIOLOGICAL CHANGES
DURING CHANGE OF LIFE

1. Normal change of life

Biologically, during the last four or five years of menstruation, the menstrual cycle gradually comes to a halt. The eggs in the ovaries lose their responsiveness to the gonadotropins, so that no follicles develop and no ovulation occurs. The ebb and flow of estrogen and progesterone production stops. The hypothalamus and pituitary continue functioning, however, producing the releasing hormones and follicle stimulating hormone (FSH) and luteinizing hormone (LH). These latter two hormones are secreted in very high levels after menopause. (See pp. 16–17)

The common menstrual pattern, in change of life, is this; gradually, the number of days between menstrual periods increases, interspersed with regular cycles of normal length. *Most women cease ovulating gradually: you cannot be sure of your infertility until menstruation has ceased for good.* Sometimes, menstrual bleeding is normal; sometimes light, next to nothing. Menopause occurs when the monthly flow ceases.

Usually, the whole change-of-life process takes a year or two. Some women have discomforting symptoms because of the new hormonal supply pattern that is establishing itself—*but only 10 per cent have severe symptoms of any kind.*

At their worst, the discomforts of change of life can be very unsettling—but like dysmenorrhea, they are the upsetting side effects of a *normal* process. Even when you are suffering from bad hot flashes, for example, *you are still healthy. These are not symptoms of disease.*

2. New hormone production system at change of life

Change-of-life discomforts are caused by hormonal changes, particularly estrogen loss. But the body anticipates these, and has other machinery to *naturally* replace the hormones that are no longer being produced in as great quantity by the ovaries.

a. *The adrenal glands* continue to produce some estrogen as well as larger amounts of androgen (male hormone) which are converted to estrogen in fatty tissue and other parts of the body.

b. *The ovaries themselves* continue to produce very small amounts of estrogen as well as androgen that is converted to estrogen.

What makes women differ so greatly in their physiological reaction to change of life is that *the capacity to metabolize androgen into estrogen varies widely among individuals.* About 40 per cent of postmenopausal women have blood levels of estrogen which are just as high as the levels in the first half of their menstrual cycles before change of life. (Ref. 1)

3. Physical symptoms of estrogen decline which may occur at change of life

These include:
a. Hot flashes;
b. Thinning of the vaginal lining.

The physical symptoms of estrogen decline *do not* include such problems as hypertension, heart attacks, obesity, reduced vision or hearing, and the many other diseases which increase with age, not just with menopause.

4. Hot flashes

A hot flash or hot flush is a discomforting sensation of being suddenly roasted, heated up from within. The hot flash usually begins in the chest, spreads to the neck and head; it will make a woman turn very red, and may make her perspire heavily. Sometimes a hot flash begins in the toes and spreads over the entire body. It lasts from several seconds to several minutes, and may leave the woman with a chilled feeling. Hot flashes may start before menopause but more frequently begin in the years afterward. At least 75 per cent of women have some hot flashes during change of life, but in only 10–20 per cent are these so severe that treatment is needed.

5. What causes hot flashes?

No one really knows. For no apparent physiological reason, the blood vessels have suddenly become much more sensitive to changes in the nervous system. They dilate involuntarily; blood rushes to the skin surface, heating up the body; then the vessels revert to normal size. Some say this is due to estrogen deficiency; others say it is due to high levels of FSH and LH.

6. Treatment of hot flashes

Unless the hot flashes are very severe, prolonged, or frequent, there should be no treatment. In time, they will end—and most women learn to cope with them until they do.

Try to avoid stressful situations, for these aggravate the condition. By this time, you're old enough to know if city traffic or contract negotiations or your son's rock group try your nerves in the best of times. Change of life may be the best of times, therefore, to avoid them.

If you are bothered by frequent, prolonged, extremely severe hot flashes, or if your sleep is being disturbed mercilessly, you may consider medical treatment, which will usually relieve the symptoms. (See ⚹23 below)

7. Thinning of the vaginal lining

Normally at change of life, the vaginal surface, which formerly consisted of ten to twelve layers of cells, begins thinning to about two to three layers, a symptom of estrogen decline. Previously, the thick vaginal lining supplied lubrication during intercourse and protected the vagina from infection. If this thinning is severe, a woman may experience pain or burning during intercourse, vaginal discharge, and a tight feeling in the vaginal area. These symptoms, if they occur at all, do not usually occur until several years after the periods have stopped.

Only 25–35 per cent of women experience so much thinning in vaginal lining that they are made uncomfortable. Sometimes the thinning can lead to *pelvic relaxation*—cystocele or rectocele. (See p. 321)

8. Diagnosis of thinning in the vaginal lining

A vaginal Pap smear, and in some cases, just a look at the vagina, will suffice to diagnose whether severe thinning has occurred. Physicians may use the terms *senile vaginitis* or *atrophic vaginitis* in making the diagnosis; these sound terrible, because they imply that the woman is atrophied or senile (which is ridiculous) and that she has vaginitis, a disease which she usually does not have. If your physician uses these terms, don't let them frighten you. They are merely typical of medical hyperbole.

9. Treatment of thinning in the vaginal lining

Treatment can begin with the over-the-counter lubricating jellies often used during intercourse. If these don't relieve the symptoms, small amounts of estrogen cream may be prescribed. These creams, applied directly to the vagina, act to thicken the lining. Since the estrogen is absorbed into the body through the vagina, only *the minimum amount* needed to keep the symptoms under control should be used. Usually the woman applies the cream daily for a week; then she can cut back gradually to as little as once or twice a week. (See ⚹23 below)

10. Pelvic relaxation symptoms often appear after menopause

With the thinning of the vaginal mucosa after menopause, some women may experience symptoms of pelvic relaxation for the first time, or the symptoms may become severe. These include cystocele and rectocele and the loss of urine during coughing and sneezing. (See p. 321) Frequency and urgency of urination may also occur. In many cases, vaginal estrogen creams and exercises to improve vaginal tone (see p. 321) will greatly alleviate these symptoms. Try these methods before considering surgical repair and/or hysterectomy, which may be suggested.

11. Skin changes at change of life

After menopause, estrogen decline *may* contribute to a thinning and drying of the skin all over the body, most notably on the face, arms, and breasts. It is very hard indeed to tell what part of the skin change is actually due to change-of-life hormone cycles, and what part is due to the simple passage of time; to weathering. Women who have spent a lieftime in the sun and/or the wind and those who smoke a lot tend to become more wrinkled than other women as they grow older.

OPINION: Because of fanaticism about youth and beauty, which has little to do with health, estrogenic compounds may be prescribed for these normal skin changes. *Don't use them! Estrogen-replacement therapy is not a safe treatment for wrinkles!* Even estrogen-containing creams may be dangerous if used excessively, since estrogen is absorbed through the skin into the body. And in most cases, the estrogen has little effect on the skin.

Remember: you are old enough now to deserve a mature redefinition of beauty—and it starts, as always, with your own acceptance of your own particular flesh.

12. Glandular tissue of the breasts diminishes during change of life

This may mean that your breasts will lose some of their fullness, and firmness and may change shape. Hormone treatments will not help. Now as always breast shape depends on good posture, regular exercise, good muscle tone, and the distant signals of heredity.

13. Hair changes during change of life

Some women experience thinning of the pubic hair as well as the hair on their heads, or may note a slight increase in body hair, especially on the face. This is due to the relative increase in androgens; don't worry about it. If you have a few more hairs on your face because of androgen increase, remember that much of that same androgen supply is being turned into estrogen, thereby naturally replacing that critical female hormone you may have lost when you stopped ovulating.

If hair growth is excessive (on the chest, or all over the face), then the woman should be examined for some other endocrine disorder. *This is not normal* for menopausal women.

14. Weight gain is not a side effect of change of life

The biological processes of change of life *do not* cause the weight gain many women experience in these years. What creates the weight gain is a decrease in activity with no concurrent decrease in food intake. Exercise is very important in retarding osteoporosis, among other medical problems. (See ⚡36, ⚡38 below) and should be continued indefinitely.

A woman at this time may not experience a gain in pounds but rather a change in body proportions, making her *look* fatter even if she doesn't weigh more. For example, the upper arm may grow heavier; the waistline may thicken. If you are not actually gaining weight, don't worry about these changing proportions; regular exercise will go far to control them, *especially if you have been doing it all along.* A new, change-of-life calisthenics routine is great for your circulation, but don't expect it to reverse the proportions of your body back in time.

15. Sex drive and sexual activity in change of life

Men—not women—have the greatest problems with decreased sex drive with aging. There is no physiological reason for a woman to experience a letdown in libido or sexual pleasure; estrogens have little effect on sex drive; *the major hormonal factors in sex drive are the androgens, which continue to be produced by a woman's body in sufficient quantity well into old age.*

Many women note an *increase* in sex drive after menopause, when pregnancy is no longer a risk. (This is comparable to the soaring libido some women report after surgical sterilization, for exactly the same reason.)

Psychological problems with sex at this time are often caused by men, who may be bewildered at their loss of power and somehow shift the blame onto partners; and by women who allow themselves to be traumatized by feelings that they are no longer attractive because they are no longer menstruating and cannot have children. As in most things, love and understanding are the sure cures; if they are not present, the best psychological counseling will probably not help.

16. Severe premenstrual syndrome is a sign of progesterone deficiency at change of life

During the years immediately prior to menopause, many women experience a severe increase in premenstrual syndrome, including breast tenderness, a feeling of fullness in the pelvis and lower abdomen, and weight gain. This has nothing to do with estrogen decline. It occurs because of *progesterone* decline, and if it is very bothersome, can be treated with progesterone given during the second half of the cycle. (See pp. 327–28)

17. Normal patterns of menstrual bleeding during change of life

There are two *normal* patterns:

a. A gradual decrease in the amount of flow; gradually longer times between periods, interspersed with regular periods; occasional skipping of a period until, gradually, it just doesn't come back.

b. Regular menstruation straight through to a total stop.

18. Suspicious patterns of menstrual bleeding during change of life

a. Women should not experience heavy or gushing flows;

b. The period should not last *longer* than usual;

c. Periods should not occur any more frequently than every twenty-one days;

d. Once bleeding has ceased for twelve months it should not recur.

Any of the above patterns may indicate just an unusual hitch in normal menopause. However, these patterns may also suggest a problem—so a woman should have herself checked.

19. Diagnosis and treatment of unusual bleeding patterns around the change of life

If an unusual pattern occurs, a D & C (see p. 329) is the best course for diagnosing the cause and, in 80–90 per cent of cases, eliminating it. Some of the more serious causes, *occurring in a minority of cases,* are hyperplasia of the endometrium, and cancer of the endometrium, cervix, or ovary. (See p. 364) A Pap smear should always be done before a D & C, to diagnose or rule out cervical cancer.

Endometrial biopsy and endometrial washings are procedures performed in the physician's office, to obtain small samples of the uterine lining in cases of minor bleeding problems around the time of menopause. If the washings or biopsy show no abnormality, if the bleeding problem is minor and if bleeding patterns subsequently return to normal, a D & C can sometimes be avoided. (See pp. 364–65)

20. Other symptoms of menopause

Some nonspecific problems such as dizziness, headaches, nervousness, numbness in the fingers are commonly attributed to change of life. Some studies show that these symptoms are more common during change of life, others show that they are not. (Ref. 2, 3) *There is absolutely no proof that these symptoms are caused by estrogen decline, so estrogen is not an appropriate treatment.*

Don't blame everything on change of life! You may succeed in convincing yourself that it is making you sick when it is not; you may end up taking drugs which are worse for you than change of life itself, drugs which may not alleviate your symptoms in any case.

21. Premature change of life

In a very few women, menopause occurs at an early age—in the twenties or thirties—for several reasons:

a. *Heredity.* In this case the menopause is not a sign of ill health but simply due to genetic predilection.

b. *Ovarian failure.* There are a *few* alarming reports of ovarian failure among women who have taken birth-control pills and after discontinuing, have ceased ovulating and experience change of life at an unusually young age. (Ref. 4, and see p. 53) Other reports also suggest that mumps infection of the ovaries may be another cause of premature menopause. (Ref. 5) Still other women may develop antibodies to ovarian tissue, in an autoimmune reaction as in rheumatoid arthritis (Ref. 6 and see p. 372)

c. *Surgical removal of the ovaries.* This is the most common cause of premature menopause. Loss of *one* ovary will not lead to change of life, but removal of both will cause this. *In young women, removal of both ovaries should be carefully guarded against unless absolutely necessary!* (See p. 333) Premature menopause can be differentiated from other causes of amenorrhea (loss of periods) by a test for blood FSH and LH levels. These are elevated after menopause.

22. Menopause and estrogen withdrawal are more bothersome for young women

The metabolism of androgen into estrogen happens naturally in older women who have *gradually* approached change of life. But this form of estrogen replacement is nowhere near as reliable among young women who have *suddenly* encountered change of life because of castration (surgical removal of the ovaries) or ovarian failure. The resultant sudden estrogen loss may inflict severe symptoms, through aggravated forms of all the ordinary side effects.

RECOMMENDATION: *Therefore, premature menopause is one of the very few situations in which estrogen-replacement therapy is recommended routinely.* A woman should continue the therapy until she is forty-five to fifty years of age and then gradually wean herself away.

(See ✳26) By this time the body's auxiliary hormone-supply systems may catch up with her situation. Another reason for estrogen-replacement therapy in this instance is that prematurely menopausal women who do not receive it seem to experience a greater tendency toward osteoporosis and heart attacks. (Ref. 1, 7)

ESTROGEN-REPLACEMENT THERAPY

23. Opinion: Estrogen-replacement therapy (ERT) is a dangerously overused treatment

Avoid it if at all possible.

Like hysterectomy and general anesthesia for normal childbirth, estrogen-replacement therapy is a dangerously overused gynecologic treatment. In the past twenty years, this therapy has become almost routine in parts of the country; in some localities an estimated 50 per cent (!) of older women had been on estrogen or were currently receiving it. (Ref. 8)

This incredible overuse of hormones will taper off rapidly in the next few years because of the recent frightening discovery: the incidence of endometrial cancer in postmenopausal women has risen dramatically in the last two decades and is apparently related to the widespread use of estrogen-replacement therapy. (Refs. 9–15) One study debates this point, (Ref. 16) but the great bulk of evidence supports the association. Already the number of cases has begun to decrease with the decline in use of estrogen. (Ref. 15) There is also concern, but not yet proof, that improper administration of estrogen may increase growth of breast cancers. (See p. 345)

Physicians are partly motivated to dispense this treatment so freely because of the self-hatred of aging women who demand a magic potion to make them young again. Women are reinforced in their foolishness, and doctors in their laxity, by wealthy and creative cosmetic companies, as well as drug companies and their public relations campaigns.

A woman facing change of life should not accept estrogen therapy for routine treatment or for any minor discomforts.

24. Warning! Accept temporary estrogen-replacement therapy only for:

a. Severe, prolonged hot flashes;

b. In cream form, for severe vaginal dryness and thinning after menopause;

c. For premature menopause, resulting from surgical castration or ovarian failure before age forty (to be taken only until age forty-five to fifty)

25. The safest method of taking estrogen, for women who must have it

a. Always take the lowest possible dose which will relieve the symptoms (this applies to pills and creams).

b. Take the therapy for the shortest time possible.

c. Take the oral doses in a cyclic fashion with progestogen.

These rules should be followed whether the woman has her uterus or not. The major reason for the cyclic administration is to avoid continuous unopposed estrogen effects on the endometrium and the breasts. Estrogen alone, continuously given, is more likely to be a cause of endometrial cancer and may have a similar effect on the breasts.

RECOMMENDATION: One of the best methods of estrogen replacement is to take estrogen daily for the first two weeks of the month and then take a progestogen tablet each day during the third week. The last week of the month, take nothing. This method of taking the pills may help to reverse any changes which the estrogen may have caused in the endometrium on breasts. Discuss this cyclic method of taking the estrogen with your doctor.

26. After symptoms are under control, start decreasing the estrogen dosage

Women taking estrogen to alleviate hot flashes should usually start on a fairly high dose and gradually cut back; after being on the drugs one month, *at the most two months,* take a lower dose or take the pill every other day. Let your physician know you are doing this. Always go one week a month without any estrogen at all. After several months, you should be able to withdraw from the treatment completely. Try not to use it for more than six months except in premature menopause.

27. Recommendation: which type of estrogen to use—ethinyl estradiol preferable to conjugated estrogens

Various types of estrogen are used to treat these symptoms. The most widely used have been the conjugated estrogens (isolated from mare urine); these are the substances associated with endometrial cancer in the recent studies. Whether the major problem is method of administration (daily vs. cyclically) or the particular drug itself is not yet clear. *However, at present, the use of other types of estrogen such as ethinyl estradiol (a common estrogen used in the birth-control pill) seems safer.* LOOK AHEAD: Some reports show good results with long-acting estrogen shots in controlling menopausal symptoms. However, the risks of this treatment have yet to be determined. Watch the news for further reports.

28. Alternatives to estrogen in the control of hot flashes

Options do exist for women who are severely bothered by hot flashes.

a. If the symptoms are particularly severe at certain times of the day or under certain stressful conditions, *sedatives* or *mild tranquilizers* may be helpful for *short* periods of time.

b. *Some drugs which act to stabilize the nerve* endings around the *blood vessels* are suggested by some, but they are not terribly effective.

c. *Progestogens frequently control hot flashes* to a large extent and are probably much safer for many women, especially those with complicating problems such as obesity, hypertension, cystic breasts, heart disease, and diabetes. Norethindrone is a suggested drug.

d. *Ginseng extract* and *Vitamin E* work for some women and certainly hold little risk in *moderate* doses.

29. Other side effects of estrogen-replacement therapy

a. Breast tenderness is a frequent side effect, most pronounced in women with a tendency toward cystic mastitis. (See p. 359) If this happens, lower the dose, or take the pills every other day, and take progesterone two weeks during the month.

b. Edema and weight gain may also appear as side effects. If these side effects are excessive, either go off the drugs, lower the dosage, or switch to another brand of estrogen.

30. Bleeding during estrogen-replacement therapy

If women are still menstruating when estrogen therapy is begun, the usual menstrual pattern should continue. Sometimes women on combined estrogen and progesterone replacement have continued to menstruate into their sixties; an undesirable result for many women. Women who have stopped menstruating before estrogen administration will usually experience no return of bleeding as a rule.

Bleeding in the middle of the cycle, prolonged bleeding, or bleeding after the menses have once stopped are all abnormal patterns (see ⚔18 above) and must be evaluated by endometrial biopsy, endometrial washing, or D & C.

31. Testing for changes in the breasts and endometrium should be routine during estrogen-replacement therapy

Many physicians are now performing routine endometrial biopsies or washings before starting women on estrogen if they are at 'high risk for endometrial cancer. (See pp. 364–65) Others recommend these studies yearly for all women on estrogen-replacement therapy. Mammography every one to two years may also soon become a recommended procedure for women on estrogen.

WARNING: Never take estrogen without checking routinely for possible side effects!

32. Who should avoid oral estrogen-replacement therapy

Women with:

a. Breast cancer or severe cystic disease of the breasts

b. Endometrial cancer or hyperplasia

c. Ovarian cancer

d. Large fibroid tumors of the uterus

e. History of phlebitis, severe varicose veins, or other clotting disorders

f. Severe heart disease, kidney disease, diabetes, or hypertension

33. Estrogen-replacement dosages are not sufficient to protect against pregnancy

Other birth-control methods should be continued if a woman is still menstruating. Birth-control pills should not be used by women over age forty. (See p. 47)

34. Estrogen-replacement therapy does not protect against cardiovascular disease

The incidence of heart attack, stroke, or hardening of the arteries is lower in women under fifty than in men. After that age women apparently catch up with the men in the incidences of these diseases. For this reason it has long been thought that estrogen, present before menopause, had a protective effect against these diseases. Estrogen replacement was believed to be effective in guarding against these diseases after menopause.

This theory is generally discredited.

Cardiovascular disease has now been related to other factors, like overwork, smoking, high-serum cholesterol, and triglycerides, any one of which complicates your chances of a heart attack more than estrogen. In addition, now that extensive autopsy data is in for men and women older and younger than fifty years, the rates of coronary artery disease appear to be identical. (Ref. 1) Most important, there is new evidence that women over thirty-five taking high-estrogen birth-control pills are *more* prone to heart attacks. (See p. 47) Men who receive estrogen as a treatment of prostate cancer have a higher incidence of heart attacks. *It is plain common sense to conclude that estrogen-replacement therapy likewise may carry a slight danger of, if anything, increasing the tendency to cardiovascular complication.* In fact, a recent study documented that replacement hormones double this risk. (Ref. 17)

35. Osteoporosis—the role of estrogen is unclear

Osteoporosis (oss-tee-oh-por-OH-sis) is a thinning of the bones and actual loss of bone matter which occurs in postmenopausal women more frequently than in premenopausal women or in men at any age. It is usually not a problem for women at change of life, but seems to start then and grow serious in elderly women. It can lead to hump back; to a softness in the hip bones and in the vertebrae (the connected sections of the spine) so that these may break very easily in old age. It is estimated that osteoporosis causes a million American hip fractures every year, 85 per cent of these in women.

36. Causes of osteoporosis

There is considerable debate over the role of estrogen in the prevention and treatment of osteoporosis. Some studies show that bone density is considerably higher in women who have been on replacement estrogen and that bone thinning can be prevented by giving estrogen after menopause. (Ref. 7, 18) These are very promising studies but so far do not tell us whether there are some women who will benefit and others who will not, from estrogen therapy. Since only one in four women suffer from osteoporosis, this means that a lot of women would be exposed to the dangers of estrogen to prevent fractures in a small group.

On the other hand, there is no proof that osteoporosis is *caused* by estrogen deficit. It results from an alteration in the body's ability to metabolize calcium (the major bone mineral) and phosphorus, which comes with age. Men and women seem to metabolize these minerals differently; in women, the metabolism which supports bone formation tends to fall off more greatly as the years pass. This may be caused by a change in kidney function; a change in the ability of the intestinal tract to absorb these minerals; or from a hormonal imbalance (having nothing to do with sex hormones) from the adrenal gland that affects the metabolism of bone. (Ref. 19) Even more simple, it may be that women need to supplement their diets with calcium more than men do, just as younger women have to supplement their diets with iron on occasion.

Other factors which *increase* the risk of osteoporosis are heavy smoking, thinness, inactivity, and heredity. Women whose ancestors came from northern Europe have a higher risk for osteoporosis. Excess consumption of antacids containing aluminum hydroxide may contribute to bone thinning by interfering with calcium and phosphorus metabolism. (Ref. 20)

37. Diagnosis of osteoporosis

Ordinary X rays will not detect a thinning of the bones until osteoporosis is relatively far advanced. Special X-ray density studies can detect this condition at an earlier stage. LOOK AHEAD: In the future, testing to determine the density of your bones as change of life nears may become routine to treat early stages of osteoporosis. (Ref. 7, 18)

38. Good diet and exercise can prevent and control osteoporosis in most women

Starting at age thirty, make sure you are getting at least 800–1,200 mg of calcium per day: it is available in milk, cheese, and other dairy products. Exercise daily; that increases your body's ability to metabolize calcium and phosphorous, and most important, good muscles can shore up weakening bones considerably. Take the minimum daily requirement of Vitamin D but *be careful not to take more: excess Vitamin D can actually aggravate osteoporosis.*

Fluoride in the water supply may help to delay osteoporosis. If your community's water supply is not fluoridated, take supplemental tablets. (See p. 248)

39. Routine estrogen-replacement therapy is not recommended treatment to prevent osteoporosis

At the present time, the risks of estrogen therapy are too great to warrant its routine use to prevent osteoporosis in all women. The FDA has recently approved the use of estrogen in *treating* osteoporosis, but it seems advisable to wait and see if 'high-risk women can be more accurately identified before the drug is used routinely as a *preventive* measure. If you are at high risk (see ⚹36 above) discuss this with your physician.

The important exception to this is young women with premature menopause (either surgical or spontaneous) in whom estrogen has a definite effect in preventing osteoporosis. (Ref. 1)

EMOTIONAL CHANGES

---

40. Emotional and psychological aspects of change of life

An elaborate mythology in many cultures suggests that women go crazy at change of life. This has been the rationale for denying mature women, at the peak of their judgmental powers, real power in politics, for example. It has been the cause of thousands of unnecessary hysterectomies and millions of unnecessary estrogen prescriptions. It has its impact on family life, giving teen-agers an excuse to disregard their mothers and men a sorry tale to tell to younger women. It is a kind of madness of its own—because women do *not* go crazy at change of life. Some go through, at worst, a difficult time.

a. *Endocrine changes may cause emotional problems*. The change in hormonal cycles, the switchover from an endocrine machinery whose center is the ovaries to an endocrine machinery whose center is the adrenal glands, often affects the hypothalamus, the endocrine center in the brain which controls a number of chemical reactions in the body, including some emotional reactions. This means that a woman at change of life may feel more tense; may be moved to tears more easily; may experience sensations of great well-being. How strong these impulses are depends to a great degree on *the other emotional strains* that operate in a woman's life at this time. (See ⚥b below) If her life is calm and she is feeling happy, the endocrine changes will not be much of a problem.

Avoid long-term drug therapy for the emotional crises of change of life.

Just because you find yourself weeping easily does not mean that you must be treated with tranquilizers. Dangerous drug habits are often formed at this time because of the tendency to overmedicate symptoms that are normal and will surely pass. Try tennis instead; millions have. Try a new job, a long vacation, going to school, painting watercolors, running for office; anything that diverts and refocuses your energy. Your children may laugh at you, but at *their* age, they should be laughing at themselves.

b. *Outside pressures deepen the tensions of change of life*. Between the ages of forty-three and fifty-five, a number of events may be complicating a woman's emotional environment. Her parents may be old and sick; their imminent death is a forewarning of hers; frightening and draining. Her children may be leaving home, creating a great empty space around her. Careers, in which so much time and money have been invested, have a tendency not to be so satisfying now that you have been working at them for twenty years. Likewise for relationships. It is not estrogen that must be replaced now, but the splintering pieces of a lifelong environment.

The worse these outside pressures are, the more likely a woman is to suffer emotionally at change of life. The feminist movement has been a great help in giving women a sense of their possibilities for *renewal*, and even if you have never read feminist literature before, you should take a look at it now; it suggests plans of action that can help a woman change her environment, rework her attitudes toward herself; it is preventive medicine for the awful feeling that you are suddenly in the denouement before the end of the play; you are not in any such thing; on the average you have thirty to forty years to go, and there are millions of women in this country who can by their example suggest the ways you may go with it.

c. *Change of life happens to men too—and that is part of a woman's problem.* Obviously there is no male menopause, because menopause refers specifically to the cessation of menstrual flow. But men do experience the crises of change of life and often actually have fewer resources to deal with them. If there were such a thing as testosterone-replacement therapy, they would probably be taking it with abandon (and quite uselessly)—to thicken their thinning hair, quicken their slowing sex drives (some do use testosterone for this), smooth out their wrinkles, shore up their overworked hearts and stiffening bones. Change of life is a bad time for everybody, but it is in *itself not a disease, merely a natural phase of life.*

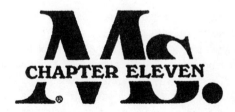

CHAPTER ELEVEN

DISEASES OF WOMEN

A number of diseases afflict women specifically; some relate to age and stage of life; some stem from pregnancy and childbearing; some relate to sexual activity; some, arthritis, for example, are apparently unrelated to sexual and reproductive character, but select women as their primary targets anyway. The best way to avoid a disease is to know about it before it happens, or to know what it looks like at the earliest stages, so that if it happens to you, you can get to work right away on a cure. Knowing about a disease means talking about it, even it if is a disease that society would prefer not to discuss.

The taboo on talking about breast cancer, for example, was broken by wives of political leaders, who openly discussed their surgery. As a result, millions of American women who might not have dealt with breast cancer until it was far advanced, went to early detection clinics. These women practice *preventive* medicine against a disease which had previously been so hushed up that few people understood that it could be detected at a curable stage.

Younger women are fortunate to be growing up in a society where public discussion about women's health is the rule, not the exception, and *they should never for a moment allow the quiet to set in again.* Shyness and secrecy are the twin demons that, for centuries, kept women sick or thinking they were sick when they really weren't. What is true for public communication is true for communication between mother and daughter, between friends, between doctor and patient as well. Talk to the women around you; talk to your doctor; talk to the *men* around you. The more people talk to each other about their health, the more they can do to keep each other healthy.

VAGINITIS AND VENEREAL DISEASE

---

1. Types of vaginitis

Vaginitis (va-gin-EYE-tis) refers to all inflammations, irritations, and infections of the vagina. Some of its non-specific symptoms include discharge, itching, burning, and odor. These same symptoms may be caused by infectious agents such as trichomonas (trick-a-MOH-nas), monilia, bacteria, or by allergies to sprays, douches, or tampons. (See p. 230)

Vulvitis (vul-VYE-tis)—redness and itching of the labia—often accompanies vaginitis.

2. Vaginal discharge is not always a sign of vaginitis or any illness at all

The vagina is a moist and constantly changing environment, responsive to every step in the menstrual cycle, and to sexual arousal. Most women experience a certain amount of vaginal discharge at all times. You can tell that the discharge is normal if it is not foul-smelling, if it does not cause itching or burning, if it is not accompanied by any other symptoms of illness like fever, headache, extreme fatigue. *A feeling of wetness or a light yellow to white smear on your underwear is in itself nothing to worry about. In fact, it signifies that you are functioning normally.*

3. Vaginal odor is not always a sign of vaginitis

Some drug and cosmetic companies, always in search of a new "problem" that requires a new product to conquer it, have attempted through national advertising to make vaginal odor much more of a problem than it really is. Because the power of suggestion is so great, a woman who never thought she smelled bad can watch television and conclude that she must have smelled bad all along, and run out to her drugstore to purchase a douche or spray that will make her and her underwear smell like a field of flowers. (See pp. 228–29)

Don't be fooled!

Of course, vaginal secretions and sweat glands in the pubic area cause odor. But it is almost always not very unpleasant and it is almost always undetectable to anyone except you. If you are concerned about offending a sexual partner, then wash with soap and water.

Excessive douching to eliminate all odor is not only pointless but may even be risky—it may cause an irritation of the vaginal wall that makes you more susceptible to a *real* vaginitis. Only if vaginal odor is very strong should you worry about it and be checked for vaginitis.

4. What to do if you think you have vaginitis

If the normal vaginal discharge increases and you think you are developing vaginitis, try several things before going to a doctor:

a. If you have been wearing underpants made of synthetics, switch to cotton. It is more porous, allows greater circulation of air in the vaginal area, and absorbs moisture. Synthetic materials tend to trap moisture so that it persists and causes irritation.

b. If you have been using bubble bath or a perfumed douche, stop—and use plain soap and water. Maybe your body is just reacting adversely to the application of strong chemicals.

c. If you have been using harsh, perfumed soaps around the vulva, switch to a milder soap.

d. If you have been using harsh laundry detergent, try a milder laundry product or try rinsing out your underwear by hand with a mild soap.

e. Take frequent tub baths and try douching with two tablespoons of white vinegar mixed in one pint of warm water.

If symptoms persist for three to four days, get worse, or are accompanied by fever, abnormal bleeding, or severe pain, *see a doctor*.

f. If you have a vaginal infection, or the symptoms of one, you can expect the following from your doctor. She or he will:

—take a complete history.

—do a complete pelvic examination (see p. 407), including a culture for gonorrhea if appropriate.

—take a Pap smear, if this was not recently done. (Sometimes infections can be diagnosed from a Pap smear which cannot be seen on smears made in the doctor's office.)

—do cultures for monila and trich sometimes, if the organisms cannot be identified on the wet smears. The wet smears *must* be done. The cultures are optional.

—take a smear of the suspicious vaginal discharge, to be analyzed in the office.

INSIST THAT ALL THESE SMEARS BE DONE! Discharges from the various vaginal infections mimic each other, so that it is very frequently hard to diagnose them just from observation. You will augment your chances of a cure if you insist that your doctor does the smears.

5. Moniliasis

Moniliasis (mow-NILL-eye-a-sis) is the most common form of vaginitis. Sometimes called a "yeast" infection, it is actually caused by a fungus called Candida albicans (in Latin, Candida means dazzling white, *albicans* means white). Under a microscope the monilia fungus looks like a scattering of white necklaces (*monile* means necklace in Latin).

6. What are the symptoms of moniliasis?

a. A thick, white discharge that often has the consistency of cottage cheese;

b. Severe itching in the vaginal area;

c. Irritation and redness around the vulva and sometimes around the anus

7. Who is likely to get moniliasis?

Women in the menstruation-age group are most likely to get monil-iasis. Premenarchal girls and postmenopausal women rarely find it a worry. However, several factors predispose women to monilia beyond general chronological factors.

a. If a woman is taking steroids like cortisone to counteract another illness, that may upset the bacterial balance in the vagina and favor the growth of monilia.

b. The same is true of antibiotics. For example a premenarchal girl or older woman may contract monilia while taking antibiotics to cure a strep throat or urinary infection. The antibiotics kill off the bacteria which usually keep the fungus in check.

c. Women with diabetes are prone to moniliasis. When the diabetes is under control, the moniliasis is usually under control. It tends to become a problem when blood sugar gets high or when sugar builds up in urine.

d. Any state which produces high levels of progesterone favors moniliasis. Therefore, the premenstrual phase of the cycle is the time when many women get it. Women taking high-progestogen birth-control pills (see p. 45) and pregnant women may be bothered by it. If the moniliasis is caused by high progesterone premenstrually, then it may go away by itself a day or so after the period, as the body chemistry alters naturally.

8. The treatment of moniliasis

WARNING: Whatever you do to treat moniliasis, *don't scratch!* The itch may be driving you crazy, but scratching will only make it worse. Literally dozens of prescribed medications can give almost instant relief —gels, creams, vaginal tablets which can be applied directly to the vagina once or twice a day.

For a new case of moniliasis, therapy should last seven to fourteen days. Keep using the medication even after the symptoms are gone, as long as your physician or clinic has told you to use it; that will increase the chances that the monilia will not return. When itching is very severe, a low-dose steroid cream or lotion can be applied directly to the vulva to relieve the discomfort.

Most moniliasis medications are available only by prescription. RECOMMENDATION: *Over-the-counter drugs that claim to relieve vaginal itching are not ideal for this condition.* They will not eliminate the fungus. There are two treatments you can buy yourself in the supermarket: yogurt and plain white vinegar. Yogurt—the plain kind (without fruit)—appears very effective for mild cases. Put the yogurt into a plastic squeeze bottle or a pastry tube and apply it directly to the vagina. It contains a *lactobacillus* (lac-toe-ba-SILL-us), a bacteria derived from milk, which is similar to that normally found in the vagina. This bacteria blocks monilia naturally. Some women prefer to use the yogurt starter material (which also contains lactobacillus)—available in health food stores—as a douche ingredient. Two tablespoons of white vinegar to a pint of water is also a helpful douche; although it may not cure the moniliasis by itself, it is very helpful as a companion treatment with medical therapy. Like the lactobacillus in yogurt, the acid in vinegar helps to make the vagina inhospitable to moniliasis (and to other infections).

9. What to do if moniliasis is chronic

Some women get moniliasis so frequently that they begin to feel it has never gone away. Usually, some environmental factor is to blame. If you can isolate it and excise it from your life, you can probably control the moniliasis.

If you are taking the pill, switch to a brand with lower progestogen or find another form of birth control. If you have a family history of diabetes, suspect diabetes as the cause and get a blood sugar test. If you have contracted moniliasis as a result of antibiotic therapy in the past, get some moniliasis medication and use it as *preventive* medicine *every time* you must take antibiotics. Sexual partners, male and female, should be treated if the disease persists. Ask your physician what medicine they should use.

Many women with recurrent moniliasis harbor the fungus in the bowel; reinfection occurs chronically from the anus. Nystatin, a prescription medication taken orally, can clear the bowel of the disease. Sometimes, diaphragms are contaminated with monilia: if you think this is the case, replace the diaphragm or soak it in antiseptic solution.

Another way to treat chronic moniliasis is to anticipate it. If you often develop the infection in the last phase of your cycle, treat yourself prophylactically with antimoniliasis medication several months in a row.

10. How moniliasis is diagnosed

Most women get to know the symptoms of moniliasis and are quite sure when they have it. If you have had the infection verified *at least once* by a physician, if predisposing illnesses have been ruled out, and if you can learn to make the infection go away on your own (see ※8 above), you certainly do not have to visit a doctor each time.

The initial diagnosis is usually made in the office. A sample of the discharge is placed on a microscopic slide with some 10 per cent potassium hydroxide. This solution kills off the other cells present and allows the monilia to stand out. A culture can be performed to further verify the diagnosis.

Sometimes a routine Pap smear will turn up evidence of moniliasis that has given no symptoms. If you have no discomfort, these cases do not have to be treated.

11. Side effects of moniliasis medications

If the problem seems to be getting worse, it may be that you are having sensitivity reactions (itching, swelling) to the monilia *medications*. Relief from the symptoms of moniliasis should be expected within two to three days. If you don't get it, suspect the medication and switch to one of the many alternatives.

12. Trichomoniasis

This form of vaginitis is caused by a one-celled organism called *Trichomonas vaginalis,* which lives in the vagina, cervix, urethra, and bladder of women and the urethra and prostate of men. This organism can cause an inflammatory reaction that is very uncomfortable.

13. What are the symptoms of trichomoniasis?

a. A thin, frothy, yellow-green discharge with a foul odor;

b. Itching or vaginal irritation, usually worse just after the menstrual period;

c. Burning and frequency of urination. The "trich" organism can be seen in a wet smear of the discharge mixed with saline solution—it is alive, swimming around on the slide. It will also be detected on the Pap smear. If the Pap smear is class I (normal) and there are no symptoms, treatment is not necessary. The only medication which kills the organism has several side effects—so if you don't *need* to take it, don't take it. (See ⚜16 below)

14. Who is likely to get trichomoniasis?

With very few exceptions, only sexually active women get "trich." For this reason it is considered a form of venereal disease. (All sexually transmitted diseases are classified as "venereal"—pertaining to Venus.) Men do not usually have symptoms when they harbor trich, but they may have a slight discharge from their penis and some burning on urination. They usually think they have gonorrhea, and unfortunately some doctors will treat them for gonorrhea without checking for trichomonas. Since 90 per cent of the sexual partners (male or female) of infected women harbor trichomonas, they *must* be treated to keep from reinfecting the women.

15. Trichomonas can cause cystitis

These organisms can invade the urinary bladder and urethra and cause a full-blown cystitis which does not resolve until the trichomonas is treated. (See ✂54 below)

16. Treatment of trichomoniasis

Metronidazole (Flagyl) is the only drug currently on the market which kills the trichomonas protozoan. Both partners usually take one 250 mg tablet three times a day for 7 days. More recently, studies have shown that one dose of 8 tablets for each partner also gives a good cure. (Ref. 1) This may be preferable because of the side effects of Flagyl. (See below) A variety of creams, suppositories, and douche products such as triple-sulfa cream, clotrimazole suppositories, and Trichotine douche preparation may also help, but if the partners are not treated with Flagyl the problem of reinfection remains.

17. Watch out for the side effects of Flagyl

Flagyl is currently under investigation by the FDA. It can irritate the throat or stomach, and should, therefore, always be taken *with meals*. During Flagyl therapy, avoid alcoholic beverages; the combination causes abdominal pains. Some women find that the drug leaves them with a strange taste in their mouths, a feeling of furriness on the tongue. Urine sometimes turns dark. WARNING: *During pregnancy, when it is quite possible to contract trichomoniasis, Flagyl should not be used at all.*

In very rare cases, Flagyl suppresses production of blood cells in the bone marrow, leading to severe anemia. OPINION: *For this reason, Flagyl should never be taken for more than a week.* If a dose must be repeated, a white blood cell count should be taken.

The major worry about Flagyl are the reports that it causes cancer in animals. There have never been any reports of Flagyl-caused cancer in humans. In fact, a recent study showed no increase in cancer rates in people who had taken Flagyl—a reassuring but not completely conclusive report. (Ref. 2) Therefore, the FDA has approved the drug for continued, short-term use only. Drug companies are experimenting to find a safer alternative. However, at this time, the complete banning of Flagyl would cause a lot of women a lot of chronic problems with trichomoniasis. *Watch the news.* Be aware when a less risky drug appears, so that you can insist on it.

18. Non-specific vaginitis

This name refers to a category of vaginitis caused by a number of bacteria, 90 per cent of the time by *Hemophilus vaginalis*. (Hemophilus derives from *haima,* Greek for blood, and *philo,* Greek for love, indicating that the bacteria grows in places where blood is present.)

19. What are the symptoms of non-specific vaginitis?
a. Very foul odor
b. Grayish, watery discharge and itching
c. Coexistence with trichomoniasis infection in 25 per cent of cases

20. Who is likely to get non-specific vaginitis?
The infection usually occurs in adult women and the vast majority of cases are sexually transmitted (along with the regular companion infection, trichomoniasis). Unlike monilia, the disease is associated with excess *estrogen* production. Therefore, pregnant women and women taking estrogen-heavy medications are more prone to it, and it tends to occur in the *first* part of the menstrual cycle.

21. How non-specific vaginitis is diagnosed
It can only be diagnosed by lab test. A wet smear will show no monilia, sometimes trichomonas, but will also show large cells from the lining of the vagina with bacteria stuck to them. These are the "clue cells." Even if they are not present, and no trichomonas or monilia show up on the slide either, but the woman has a very evil-smelling discharge, then the diagnosis will usually be non-specific vaginitis. Exceptions are the possibilities of infection from an IUD or gonorrhea. If there is still doubt, or the disease is recurrent, repeat wet smears should be taken and cultures too, if the laboratory is adequate for the task. (It is very difficult to culture Hemophilus; special media and incubators are needed, and some labs don't have them.)

22. Treatment of non-specific vaginitis
The ideal treatment is ampicillin, 500 mg four times daily for seven to ten days for partners. If you are allergic to penicillin, use tetracycline. Some reports show Flagyl to be effective for this condition (Ref. 3), but the side effects of the drug must be considered. (See ⚹17 above) Other methods of treatment include vaginal creams and suppositories of tetracycline or sulfa, used twice daily for ten days. If both partners are not treated, the infection may recur (like trich).

23. Side effects of the drugs used to treat non-specific vaginitis
Some women taking ampicillin may develop moniliasis, but this usually clears when the antibiotic is stopped. The only other side effects would be allergic reactions to the antibiotics.

24. Gonorrhea as a cause of vaginal discharge

All sexually active women with vaginal discharge should be tested for gonorrhea, which frequently causes infection in the cervix. (See ⚹41 below)

25. Other causes of infectious vaginitis

Several other organisms have been reported to be increasingly prevalent causes of vaginitis, cervicitis, and pelvic inflammatory disease.

a. *Chlamydia* (klam-ih-DEE-ah) are organisms between bacteria and viruses, which have been cultured from the vaginas and cervices of women with vaginitis symptoms. It is believed that these organisms are transmitted sexually, that they cause most "non-specific" urethritis (inflammation of the urethra in men), and also Salpingitis. (See ⚹42b below) The treatment is tetracycline, 500 mg 4 times daily for seven to twenty-one days, for both partners. (Ref. 4)

b. *Mycoplasma* (mike-o-PLAS-ma) are organisms similar to chlamydia and are believed to cause similar symptoms. In addition, mycoplasma may cause recurrent abortions and thus infertility. (See p. 98) This disease is also transmitted sexually and both partners should be treated with tetracycline. (Ref. 5)

Watch the news for results of the ongoing research on these organisms.

c. In rare instances, other bacteria such as streptococcus, staphylococcus, Escherichia (esh-er-ICK-ia) coli (a bacteria named for the German physician who discovered it) can cause vaginitis symptoms. Usually these bacteria cause worse trouble elsewhere in the body and the vaginitis is a secondary problem.

26. Venereal warts (condylomata acuminata)

From the Greek work *kondyloma* (a knob) and the Latin *acumino* (to sharpen) condylomata (con-dill-OH-mat-a) acuminata (ak-KU-mi-na-ta) are increasing in frequency among women and men. Small warts grow on the vulva and vagina, sometimes on the cervix. The disease is caused by a virus similar to that which produces such warts on other parts of the body, usually spreads through sexual contact and may be associated with other vaginal infections.

27. Treatment for venereal warts: Podophyllin

For men and for women, the treatment is the same. Small areas of warts are touched with Podophyllin (po-DOF-fill-in) which kills the virus that caused them. Podophyllin is a very caustic substance; a touch will do; rinse the treated area with *lots* of water within two hours after the application. Repeat the treatment weekly until the warts disappear. Any concurrent vaginal infection should be treated simultaneously.

28. When not to use Podophyllin

Women who suffer from warts inside the vagina cannot have the Podophyllin treatment—it is too harsh. WARNING: *Pregnant women must not use it either because the medication may hurt the fetus.*

29. Treatment for venereal warts: cryosurgery

Good news: Cryosurgery (from the Greek *kryos,* meaning cold) is a new process with enormous potential. Small areas of affected tissue are killed by application of a solution that freezes them and removes them for good. Although the treatment sounds cold and uncomfortable, it is in fact almost painless. It can be used on *warts inside* the vagina, and has the added advantage of being fast and can be done in a doctor's office. Cryosurgery is also being used extensively to treat cervicitis (see ✕37 below) and chronic severe hemorrhoids.

30. Folliculitis

Folliculitis (fol-lick-you-LIE-tis) is a very common disorder, in which the pubic hair roots become inflamed, starting as small red bumps that can grow large and painful like a boil. Hot soaks and frequent scrubbing are the recommended treatment. Folliculitis can happen to anyone and commonly recurs premenstrually. Cloxacillin is the preferable drug for women who get recurrent large boils. These are usually due to a staph infection.

31. Herpes simplex and herpes progenitalis

Herpes simplex is a commonly occurring virus of which there are two types. The first type usually infects the mouth and lip but can be transmitted to the genitals by oral sex. So if you or your partner have a cold sore or other mouth infection, avoid oral sex until it is completely healed. Also avoid sex with anyone with genital sores. The second type of herpes simplex virus affects the vulva, the vagina and the cervix and causes herpes progenitalis. Women who have had the first variety seem to develop some resistance to the second.

Herpes progenitalis comes in varying degrees of severity, but can be extremely painful and incapacitating, especially during the first bout. It is transmitted primarily through sexual contact, and has been on the rise like other forms of venereal infection. *Most serious, this virus may have a role in causing cervical cancer.*

32. Symptoms of herpes progenitalis

After a three-to-seven-day incubation period, a woman will note many small blisters in the genital region. The blisters pop rapidly and leave a multitude of small but extremely painful ulcers with red edges. The first episode of herpes progenitalis may last up to three to six weeks, accompanied by fever and swelling of large lymph nodes in the groin. Urination is extremely painful, for the burning caused by the ulcers is irritated by the passage of the urine over them. Sometimes the disease does not come back. Sometimes it recurs, every six to eight weeks, usually with a decline in severity and the number of ulcers each time.

33. Treatment of herpes progenitalis

Viruses, in general, have eluded cures by medical science, so, at this time only *the symptoms,* not the source, of herpes can be treated. See a physician for diagnosis. This can be made by culture or Pap smear of the lesions.

a. Try antiseptic creams such as Betadine.

b. Apply ether or chloroform to the lesions to relieve the stinging and pain.

c. Bathe in cool water several times a day.

d. Relieve the pain of urination by pouring cool water over the area while you are voiding, or void in the shower.

e. Sex is taboo if either partner has active herpes; it will probably be too painful to be pleasurable anyway.

f. Some vaginal contraceptive creams, applied to the sores may relieve the symptoms.

WARNING: In past years, various dyes—Congo Red, Acridine Orange—were applied to the herpes lesions and then subjected to ultraviolet light. This treatment is now discredited. It seems to have had no therapeutic effect; *in fact, recent evidence shows it may increase the danger of cancer later on.*

LOOK AHEAD: Watch for a breakthrough with promising antiviral agents now being tested. These include 2-deoxyglucose, adenosine arabinoside, and 5-iodo-2-deoxyuridine (Stoxil ointment—on the market for eye infections).

34. Relationship of herpes progenitalis and cervical cancer

In several large studies of women with cervical cancer, blood testing showed that a much larger number of them had had herpes type II than a group of women with no evidence of cervical cancer. (Ref. 6 and 7) This is by no means an all-or-nothing effect; all women with herpes do not get cancer. *It does mean that all women who have had herpes progenitalis must be absolutely religious about getting a Pap smear every six months,* for only in this way will cervical cancer be detected at an early, curable stage. (See ⚹180 below)

35. Regional centers for gynecologic cancer are interested in following and treating women with herpes

Most research into the possible relationship to cervical cancer goes on at centers which treat cancer of the female genitals. If you have recurrent herpes, these centers would offer the most up-to-date treatments.

36. Vaginitis and vulvitis not caused by infection

a. Menopausal women (see p. 283) may suffer from *atrophic vaginitis* —a discharge and itching caused simply by the decrease in estrogen.

b. Allergy can cause vaginitis-vulvitis symptoms. For example, you may be allergic to clothing material, soap, detergents, vaginal sprays, contraceptive jellies, anything that, when applied to the area, creates a "contact dermatitis," an itching and skin reaction. If examination and lab tests indicate no infection, look for an allergy, eliminate the offending material and you will feel fine again.

c. Overuse of douching or vaginal medications can create the symptoms of vaginitis. *Do not use prescribed vaginitis creams after the condition is cured:* the treatment itself may become counterproductive.

d. Oral sex may cause vaginal burning and redness in some women, probably because of allergic reaction to substances in saliva. If this occurs, try alternative sexual techniques.

e. Forgotten tampons, pessaries, and infections from IUDs can cause symptoms similar to those of vaginitis.

37. Cervicitis

This is an inflammation of the cervical glands, frequently accompanied by vaginitis. The cervical mucus becomes profuse, creating an annoying discharge. Sometimes, treatment for vaginitis will not eliminate the cervicitis and a whitish discharge—leukorrhea—will continue. Sometimes, small, mucus-filled cysts (called Nabothean cysts) occur in the cervix.

Generally, if the cervicitis is not severe, and the Pap smear is normal, treatment is unnecessary. The inflammation will clear by itself.

If the discharge becomes chronic, then the cervix can be cauterized in one of several *painless* office procedures. Either by cryosurgery (freezing) or silver-nitrate application, the superficial layers of the cervix are destroyed, along with the glandular areas. The cervix heals, becomes smoother and less irritated. Severe cases may also be associated with cystitis, and must be treated with antibiotics. (See ⅍63 below)

38. Cervicitis after childbirth is normal

A woman who has just had a child may experience minor inflammation of the cervix, which usually repairs itself.

39. Cervical erosion

This term has two meanings:

a. It may refer to *advanced cervicitis,* in which real inroads have been made into the cervical tissue, or to

b. *cervical eversion,* in which the lining of the cervical canal is turned outward, becoming visible in the center of the cervix and making the cervix more susceptible to infection and irritation. Sometimes there is an excess mucus discharge that cannot be controlled except by cautery. (See ✗37 above) This is also called a cervical *ectropion.*

40. Psychosomatic vaginitis: Is there such a thing?

In very rare instances, a woman may have all the symptoms of vaginitis with no infection or irritation to cause it. After careful evaluation and discussion, her physician may conclude that some psychological problem is expressing itself this way. It is possible. If other diseases such as ulcer, colitis, and migraine headaches can have a psychosomatic etiology, so can vaginal discharges. *The problem with this diagnosis is that it is used too often as an excuse for not evaluating a discharge completely.* Make sure that wet smears and cultures are done before accepting the conclusion, and verify it with a second medical opinion.

VENEREAL DISEASE

41. Gonorrhea (gon-nor-REE-a) ("clap," "drip")

More people get gonorrhea from each other than any other disease except the common cold. Public health officials say gonorrhea is an epidemic, complicated by the penicillin-resistant strains brought back by soldiers returning from Vietnam. The disease is most common among people under twenty-five, and people who have many sexual partners. Recently, the epidemic seems to be lessening, perhaps because of growing dissatisfaction with the pill (which may encourage transmission of the disease), and renewed interest in VD-preventing condoms and foams. (See p. 73) Also there has been vigorous anti-VD propaganda, involving everything from signs on buses to television specials with the late Zero Mostel playing a gonorrhea bacillus.

Gonorrhea is caused by a bacteria. *Neisseria gonorrhea,* named for the scientist, Albert L. S. Breslau Neisser, who discovered it in Germany in the late nineteenth century. It can infect the mucus membrane of the vagina, the cervix, the urethra, Bartholin's glands (see ✗133 below), rectum, and throat. The gonorrhea organism dies very quickly if it does not lodge in these places—therefore, it is next to impossible for it to be transmitted by any means except sexual contact. You cannot, for example, get it from a toilet seat.

42. The vast majority of women with gonorrhea (85 per cent) have no symptoms at all

They may have the disease, may be transmitting it to others who are transmitting it to others. It may be infecting the tubes and ovaries, without the woman herself ever knowing it.

a. RECOMMENDATION: For this reason, sexually active women *must* have tests for gonorrhea once or twice a year if appropriate. *Only the lab* can tell for sure. A culture is taken from the cervix, and sent to the lab for verification, as part of the regular gynecological examination. *Do not let a physician or other examining practitioner tell you that you have gonorrhea without verifying the diagnosis with a culture.* This takes about forty-eight hours and *must* be done because other organisms in the vagina are very similar to the gonorrhea bacteria and may be confused with it. The culture misses the disease in 15 per cent of cases because the bacteria is so difficult to grow.

b. Another way to be quite sure that you have gonorrhea is when your sexual partner develops it. In this case, seek *treatment* (not just testing) immediately.

c. If a woman has symptoms of tubal infection—fever, severe abdominal pains, heavy vaginal discharge—gonorrhea may be the cause. She should be started on therapy at the same time that she gets the gonorrhea test. (See ※45 below)

Other possible symptoms of gonorrhea include: a discharge from the urethra; burning on urination (this symptom, shared by men and women, accounts for the common reference to the disease as "getting burned"); irritation of the vulva; vaginal discharge; proctitis (prock-TIE-tis)—pain on defecation, a foul-smelling discharge from the anus. These things may not always indicate gonorrhea but they are all signs of ill health and require medical attention.

43. Symptoms of gonorrhea in men

Frequently a man will experience a discharge from his penis, a sign that the urethra is infected. Another symptom is a feeling of burning during urination. However, up to 40–50 per cent of men have no symptoms at all, contrary to the once popular view that men *always* have symptoms. (Ref. 8)

If your partner has a discharge from the penis, don't let him delay in being checked by a physician. Also, don't believe him if he says that the discharge is due to "straining," (a common rationalization). He may be kidding himself; don't let him kid you. Make him use a condom if you have intercourse.

44. Effects of gonorrhea in women

The Bartholin's glands may be affected; the ovaries and Fallopian tubes may be infected, causing infertility. In both sexes, generalized gonorrhea can cause serious skin rashes, hepatitis (liver infection—Fitz-Hugh-Curtis Syndrome), and arthritis. (See ※243 below)

If a baby is born to a mother with gonorrhea and silver nitrate or penicillin drops are not placed in the eyes, blindness may result. Thus the silver nitrate or penicillin treatment has become standardized medical care. WARNING: *Women having their babies outside of hospitals should take care not to overlook this treatment.*

45. Treatment of gonorrhea

When the disease has no symptoms, there are several alternative treatments.

a. Procaine penicillin injection, one dose of 4.8 million units, can be given along with Probenecid, a drug which heightens the level of penicillin in the blood.

b. Or ampicillin (3.5 grams) along with Probenecid can be given orally.

c. For people allergic to penicillin, 1.5 grams of tetracycline can be given orally followed by 500 mg., 4 times each day for 4 days, or spectinomycin (4 grams) by injection.

d. When gonorrhea has caused *severe pelvic inflammatory disease* (PID) (tubal infection), a woman must be treated with doses of penicillin given intravenously in a hospital. (Intravenous medication is given by inserting a needle into a vein, usually, on the back of the hand.)

Since some strains of gonorrhea resist penicillin, cultures must be done at one to two weeks and at six weeks to make sure that the drug has worked. This also tests that a woman has not become reinfected. (Other bacteria cause pelvic infections as well—chlamydia, mycoplasma, TB, strep.)

e. *Sexual partners must always be treated.* If you find that you have gonorrhea, don't be embarrassed to tell the people you've been sleeping with: you are endangering them and their sexual partners if you don't.

46. How to prevent gonorrhea

Know your sexual partners as well as you possibly can. Not knowing a man is reason enough to suspect that he may be carrying gonorrhea, so insist that he use a condom. Vaginal foams and jellies have been shown to have a preventive effect, so use them. (Ref. 9) If the man has any discharge from his penis or any sores in the genital area, don't have intercourse; these are very likely symptoms of VD.

Have regular checkups and gonorrhea cultures at least every six months, more often if you have had possible contact.

47. Syphilis

Syphilis, less common but much more serious than gonorrhea, spreads in exactly the same way—by sexual contact. If left unchecked, it can affect the brain, the heart; it will destroy the sufferer long before it kills, and the children of syphilitic parents will be grievously affected if they survive. Like gonorrhea, syphilis—virtually wiped out as an epidemic disease in the forties and fifties—has been on the rise again, a price we are paying for the sexual revolution and the decline in the use of condoms.

48. The four stages of syphilis

a. Stage One: Primary syphilis occurs ten to ninety days after sexual contact in the form of a chancre, a *painless* ulcer with an elevated edge usually around the genitals. If the man you are with has an ulcer on his penis, be suspicious. Send him to a doctor and avoid sexual contact. Frequently, a woman does not notice this stage in herself because the ulcer may be inside the vagina. The chancre may also occur on the labia, the tongue, lips, or nipples and lasts from three to nine weeks.

If you have any sore that does not heal after a matter of days, get it checked. Even if it isn't syphilis, it may signify another disorder.

A blood test will verify the first stage of syphilis about three to four weeks after it has been contracted. However, it can be detected earlier if the chancre is found; a scraping from it is taken and tested for the presence of the syphilis organism, a long, thin bacteria called *Treponema pallidum.*

b. Stage Two: About three months after contact, warty growths may appear around the vagina. Called *condyloma lata,* these are flatter than condyloma acuminata (venereal warts) (see ✳26 above). A spotty rash may show on the palms and soles, and sometimes all over the body.

A blood test during this phase will always be positive. The disease may have no obvious secondary stage but may pass directly into the latent phase.

c. The *latent phase* of syphilis has no symptoms and may last from two to twenty years. During this phase the blood test is always positive.

This stage may not occur at all and the disease may pass directly to the tertiary stage.

d. It is during the *tertiary stage* of syphilis that the heart and brain may be affected. It may start any time after Stage Two, so that early detection of the disease is vitally important.

49. How syphilis is detected

Routine screening blood tests are very accurate in detecting syphilis. This blood test is required throughout the United States for most people who are about to get married. It should be obtained every year without fail by women who have had more than one partner.

If the screening test (RPR or VDRL) is positive, the blood is sent for a more exact test. This is because the first test can sometimes be falsely positive: some viral illnesses and other medical problems such as Lupus (see ✻236 below) can cause the same blood results as syphilis.

Once the specific test shows positive, treatment should begin immediately for *all* the sexual partners of the person on whom the test was done as well. The law requires labs to report all cases of syphilis. In most localities investigation of sexual contacts is undertaken immediately. There is no legal way to conceal the fact that you have had syphilis. A case becomes part of the permanent medical records of the locality and the person affected. For example, if you have had syphilis in the past and apply for a marriage license, verification that you were treated and cured will be required before the license is authorized.

50. Blood tests for syphilis are required during pregnancy

Blood tests for syphilis should be given in early and mid-pregnancy, for untreated syphilis can cause serious congenital deformities if not the death of the fetus.

51. Treatment of syphilis

Bicillin, a long-acting penicillin, is given by injection.

a. For cases under two years duration, one shot of 2.4 million units is adequate.

b. If the disease has been present longer than two years, several doses will be required.

c. If a person is allergic to penicillin, Erythromycin or tetracycline can be used for fifteen days.

Generally, the test for syphilis remains positive after treatment but the titer (or concentration of antibody) in the blood decreases. It is important that routine blood tests continue because a person can catch syphilis again, and if so, the titer in the screening test will rise again.

52. Other venereal diseases

Some other venereal diseases—chancroid, granuloma inguinale and lymphogranuloma venereum—occur rarely in the United States. They strike mainly in tropical countries and are all characterized by sores or lesions on the vulva and swollen lymph nodes in the groin. If you have any of these symptoms, seek medical treatment immediately, for these can be chronic debilitating diseases if allowed to continue for any length of time.

WARNING: Other non-venereal diseases, such as hepatitis, can be transmitted by sexual contact. If your partner develops hepatitis, consult a physician about this possibility.

53. Pubic lice and scabies

Pubic lice, tiny bugs which burrow into the roots of the pubic hair and cause intense itching, can be transmitted from a sexual partner and also from bedclothes, towels, toilets. Treatment is a shampoo (Kwell or Eurax), which is washed into the pubic hair, left in for about twenty minutes, then showered off. This treatment may be repeated in twenty-four hours. Reinfection is a danger unless sexual partners, all linens, bathrooms are disinfected as well. If the disease recurs and doesn't go away, pubic hair may have to be shaved.

This has long been thought of as a disease of poverty. But it has been known to strike the unwary traveler, even in not-so-impoverished hotels, particularly overseas.

Scabies is also caused by a small bug, which typically burrows into the skin around the elbows, wrists, buttocks, and genitals, causing a track of red dots and intense itching. It is passed sexually, as well as by any close contact, and has been on a dramatic upswing over the past few years. The treatment is the same as for pubic lice—except that the sufferer uses a lotion, not a shampoo.

CYSTITIS AND URINARY TRACT PROBLEMS

54. Cystitis

Cystitis (siss-TIE-tis) is a general term for *inflammations* of the urinary bladder. It is much more common in women than in men, because women have a very short urethra—the tube leading from the bladder to the vagina. Most cystitis infections are caused by introduction of organisms from the outside, from the vagina or anus; these then spread up through the urethra and into the lining of the bladder. In some cases, the symptoms of cystitis can occur without any disease process—for example, through an allergic reaction. This is cystitis at its best—a temporary annoyance, not threatening to general good health. At its worst, cystitis is caused by an infection of the bladder which can spread to the kidneys and cause pyelonephritis, which seriously impairs kidney function. Thus, the symptoms of cystitis, if they persist for two or more days, must always be evaluated by a physician.

55. Symptoms of cystitis
These include:
a. Frequent need to urinate
b. Pain on urination
c. Having to get up at night to urinate
d. (Occasionally) blood in the urine (if present see a physician as soon as possible)

56. Major causes of cystitis
These are:
a. Improper toilet habits
b. Sudden increase in intercourse (this is the usual case of "honeymoon cystitis")
c. Catheter placement
d. Infection of the upper respiratory tract
e. Chronic cervicitis or vaginitis
f. A large cystocele (see ✕70 below)

57. Causes of cystitis other than infection
These include:
a. Allergic reactions
b. Irritation from soaps, bubble bath, other toiletries
c. Anxiety
d. Excessive fluid intake
e. Pelvic congestion
f. Estrogen deficiency after menopause
g. Coffee, tea in excess
h. Irritation from an improperly fitted diaphragm

58. Improper toilet habits as a cause of cystitis
Fecal contamination can cause cystitis when a woman who has moved her bowels wipes from the back to the front. Always wipe the anal area separately from the vaginal area. Teach your daughters to do so at the beginning of toilet training.

59. Diarrhea as a cause of cystitis

A woman who is suffering from diarrhea may contract cystitis because of contamination of the urethra from the frequent bowel movements. So, if you have diarrhea, take extra care in cleansing the genital area.

60. "Honeymoon cystitis"

This cystitis, usually associated with a sudden increase in the frequency of coitus, probably comes from irritation at the base of the bladder during repeated penile thrusting and from the deposit of organisms at the opening of the urethra during intercourse.

Women who find they contract cystitis after times of intense sexual activity should

a. urinate *before and after* intercourse, since the urine may wash away the organisms that have been deposited in the urethra;

b. use a vaginal lubricating jelly, which may minimize irritation at the base of the bladder.

Some practitioners suggest that, when the condition is recurrent, antibiotics be taken for short periods of time before and after intercourse.

61. Catheter placement as a cause of cystitis

After surgery or childbirth, if a woman is unable to empty her bladder naturally, a catheter (KATH-eh-ter)—a long plastic tube—may be placed in the urethra to help urination. The simple presence of the catheter may cause cystitis by allowing bacteria to get into the urethra.

OPINION: *Catheterization, therefore, should never be a routine procedure.* It should only be done when a clean urine specimen is otherwise unobtainable, or in urological and gynecological tests that absolutely require the procedure. Some physicians routinely collect urine specimens by catheterization: *Do not allow this if you can void normally.*

62. A respiratory infection may cause a cystitis side effect

A viral or bacterial infection of the throat may also lead to cystitis—inflammation of the urinary tract by the same organisms—especially in children.

63. Chronic cervicitis as a cause of cystitis

Some practitioners believe that when a cervix is chronically infected, bacteria that are causing the cervicitis (see ⚹37 above) can pass through the lymph channels into the bladder, causing cystitis as well. A woman with cervicitis who has recurrent episodes of cystitis should have both treated. Trichomonas organisms can infect the bladder. (See ⌗15 above)

64. A large cystocele can lead to cystitis

A cystocele (SIS-toe-seal) or hernia in the bladder wall can prevent complete voiding and lead to stagnation of the remaining urine in the bladder. This in turn can create an infection and cystitis. The cystitis can be relieved through medication until the cystocele is corrected. (See ⌗70 below)

65. Factors other than infection which can cause cystitis symptoms

Some women are allergic to foods (lobster, for example) and get cystitis symptoms as a result. Others get these symptoms because of irritation from soaps, bubble baths, detergents, sprays, and douches. Pelvic congestion before menstruation (see ⌗96 below) can sometimes have the cystitis side effect. Anxiety leading to frequent urination produces at least this one effect of cystitis, as does excess intake of coffee, tea, or other liquids.

If you use a diaphragm, have the size checked.

66. Cystitis is more common in pregnancy

Because of pressure of the growing fetus on the bladder, pregnant women are susceptible to relative stagnation in the urinary system. Therefore, the incidence of cystitis is somewhat higher. Some symptoms, such as frequency of urination in early pregnancy, are just due to pressure.

67. Kidney disease (pyelonephritis) and cystitis

Pyelonephritis (pie-low-ne-FRY-tis), an infection of the kidneys, can result if cystitis infection spreads from the bladder to the kidneys. *This may be a serious, debilitating disease and should never be allowed to develop from cystitis, which can be stopped at a much earlier stage.* The symptoms of pyelonephritis are fever, back pain high under the ribs, and the symptoms of cystitis. A woman can frequently be very sick with abdominal pain and vomiting as well.

68. How cystitis is diagnosed

If the symptoms of urinary infection last three days or if they are severe, you *must* seek medical evaluation.

For a first attack of cystitis, a urine culture is usually not necessary, but a pelvic examination is recommended to rule out trichomoniasis or gonorrhea, both of which can give symptoms of cystitis.

If the infection is in the bladder, the first line of treatment is usually sulfa drug therapy. Some physicians insist on doing a urine culture right away; it can cost up to $35.00. OPINION: A more moderate course of action is as follows:

a. A simple urinalysis to see if white blood cells and bacteria, the signs of infection, are present; and if present:

b. Therapy with sulfa drugs for ten days; (80–90 per cent of the cases are cured by this therapy);

c. At the end of this time, a repeat urinalysis to see if the infection has cleared.

Fluids should be taken in increased amounts during treatment.

If the symptoms don't clear up with the first few days of sulfa therapy, the woman should go off the drugs for forty-eight hours and then get a culture of the urine to tell exactly which organism is causing the problem and what the proper antibiotic would be to cure it. Ampicillin or macrodantin can be used if a woman is allergic to sulfa.

Women with recurrent, infectious cystitis need careful follow-up and repeat cultures.

PELVIC RELAXATION

69. "Pelvic relaxation": tissue injury in the pelvic area

Pelvic relaxation is a general term referring to disorders of women caused by the tearing, stretching, or loss of tone in the pelvic muscles and fibrous tissue. Often called hernias, these disorders usually occur after a number of pregnancies, and tend to be aggravated post-menopausally. Obese women and women engaged in hard labor that puts a great strain on the stomach muscles are also susceptible to pelvic relaxation. Sexual activity, no matter how strenuous, can almost never cause this problem.

70. Cystocele

A cystocele (SISS-toe-seal) is a bulging of the bladder which amounts to a hernia in the upper wall of the vagina. The size can vary depending on how badly the tissue is damaged. A large cystocele can put painful pressure on the vagina or actually protrude through it. Women with large cystoceles have a predisposition to urinary tract infections.

Another frequent association with cystocele is *urethrocele,* (yur-EETH-roh-seal) in which the urethra bulges down below the pubic bone. Sometimes, the ligaments which normally hold the uterus in place are so stretched that the uterus descends into the vagina and sometimes even to the opening of the vagina. This is called *uterine decensus* (dee-SEN-suss) (fallen womb) or prolapse.

71. Rectocele

A rectocele is a weakening in the muscular support of the rectal wall so that the wall bulges into the vagina. When a woman is moving her bowels, the pressure will be most uncomfortable; she may be unable to defecate without placing a finger into the vagina to give support to the wall.

72. Enterocele

This is a hernia where the top of the vagina bulges into the lower part. In effect, the vagina is doubling over into itself.

73. Symptoms of pelvic relaxation

a. A woman may feel unusual pressure in the vaginal area, or just general discomfort in the pelvic area often accompanied by backache.

b. She will feel tired; will find that she wants to put her feet up, or that she is more comfortable wearing a girdle.

c. *Sexual dysfunction* is a symptom of pelvic relaxation, for the vagina may become so enlarged that the woman (or man) may have difficulty reaching orgasm due to lack of friction. In addition, the simple pressure of the descending organs may make sexual relations uncomfortable.

d. Because of pressure in the pelvic area, a woman may urinate uncontrollably, especially when she coughs or sneezes or does anything else to increase the pressure, even momentarily. This is called *stress incontinence*.

Most women experience incontinence—the inability to control urination—at one time or another. Usually, this is only a matter of a few drops. But stress incontinence involves a heavier flow of urine. It is different as well from "urgency incontinence," where urine leakage is caused by pressure of an overfull bladder. Women who have stress incontinence can live with the condition for a time—but as it grows more serious and interferes more profoundly with normal, everyday living, they should have it evaluated.

74. What causes pelvic relaxation?

a. Too rapid delivery may be a cause. For example, a woman may bear down to expel an infant before the cervix is sufficiently dilated.

b. Forceps delivery when the head of the infant is still too high in the vagina may lead to pelvic relaxation.

c. If a baby has a very large head and a mother a very small pelvis, and the second stage is prolonged, damage may occur.

d. Extraordinary muscular injury outside of childbirth may lead to pelvic relaxation. This is usually prolonged hard labor or strenuous athletic activity. In short, the same conditions that produce hernia in men can produce it in women. The rigors of childbirth are the critical additional cause among women.

e. Obesity and chronic cough aggravate the condition.

75. Episiotomy cannot prevent pelvic relaxation

Episiotomy (eh-PEEZ-ee-ot-omy)—a surgical procedure by which an incision is made to widen the birth canal during delivery (see p. 45) may prevent tearing of the perineum and the urethra as well. It is *not* effective in preventing cystocele, rectocele, or enterocele, the tearing of the muscles that support the upper vagina, which is the most common form of pelvic relaxation.

76. Pessaries can relieve the symptoms of pelvic relaxation in some cases

These hard rubber rings are placed in the vagina and when properly fitted can reduce the symptoms of incontinence and vaginal relaxation. They are particularly good for older women, for whom surgery is too risky. They must be periodically removed and washed.

77. Opinion: Before you decide on surgery for pelvic relaxation, do the following:

a. Try Kegel's exercises. (See p. 157)

b. If you are postmenopausal, try low doses of estrogen cream for several months.

c. Stop all strenuous activity, if possible;

d. If you are fat, lose weight.

e. If you have chronic bronchitis from smoking, stop smoking.

In addition, these tests are usually done before surgery:

f. A urine culture to rule out infection;

g. An X ray of the bladder (dye is inserted into the bladder through a catheter and an X ray taken to see if the bladder and urethra are misshapen and causing the symptoms of pelvic relaxation);

h. A cystometrogram, a test to determine the capacity of the bladder and the amount of pressure inside it, to rule out other disorders which might be causing incontinence;

i. X ray of the kidneys and ureters (IVP).

When stress incontinence is chronic, and all possible other causes have been ruled out, surgery is appropriate.

78. Vaginal hysterectomy with repair of bladder or rectum is the usual surgery to correct pelvic relaxation

The uterus is removed and the torn tissue repaired. Sometimes the bladder can be repaired without removing the uterus, but a woman must understand that this may only be a temporizing procedure. If the uterus descends into the vagina to a significant degree, it may have to be removed in another later operation. Sometimes, the results of the tests in ✕77 show that a Marshall-Marchetti procedure, an abdominal operation, would have better success for correction of stress incontinence. Discuss this with your gynecologist.

If a woman who has only had a bladder repair becomes pregnant, she should deliver by Caesarean section: a vaginal delivery would tear down the repair.

DYSMENORRHEA AND PREMENSTRUAL TENSION

---

79. What is dysmenorrhea?

Until endocrinology (the study of hormones and body chemistry) developed as a sophisticated medical science, little was known about dysmenorrhea (or painful menstruation) except that an enormous number of women suffered from it.

An aura of mystery surrounded dysmenorrhea (diss-men-o-REE-a). Often it was dismissed as untreatable or psychosomatic. Your mother's home remedies hardly ever alleviated your discomfort. Your physician often had no remedy at all and sometimes produced a complex-sounding explanation for why these menstrual miseries were "all in your head." This left you not only with stomach cramps but with ego cramps as well.

Fortunately, the mystery of dysmenorrhea is coming to an end, although the total cure is not yet at hand.

We can now broadly classify two major types of painful menstruation:

a. Primary or spasmodic dysmenorrhea

b. Secondary or congestive dysmenorrhea (frequently associated with premenstrual syndrome)

80. Primary dysmenorrhea affects young women

Primary dysmenorrhea usually begins in the early years of the menstrual cycle and rarely continues after first pregnancy, or, if there is no pregnancy, after age twenty-five. It is most common among teen-agers and is characterized by pain resulting from spasms of the uterine muscles.

81. Secondary dysmenorrhea affects older women

This type of dysmenorrhea usually occurs in women over thirty. It is more likely to be associated with some other menstrual problem, such as premenstrual syndrome and pelvic congestion syndrome, or with other pelvic problems such as fibroid tumors of the uterus, endometriosis, or pelvic infections. (See below) The two types of dysmenorrhea are sometimes not easy to distinguish, nor are the symptoms so different.

82. Diagnosis and treatment of dysmenorrhea

You don't need a physician to diagnose dysmenorrhea. Your own body, your own menstrual cycle will tell you what you are suffering from. Fortunately for most women, the discomforts of primary dysmenorrhea usually pass quickly, occur in mild forms, and can be lived through without special care or medication or interruption of normal activity. The whole condition is certainly made much more tolerable by the foreknowledge that it will end within a few days.

When you are so uncomfortable that you cannot continue normal activity, treatment is in order. Just as your menstrual cycle quickly establishes a routine pattern, you should quickly ascertain a routine treatment for the symptoms of your particular dysmenorrhea.

For years physicians who simply didn't know better gave women psychological diagnoses for dysmenorrhea. How often has a doctor told a young woman that she is getting these terrible menstrual cramps because she hasn't "resolved her sexual identity" or because she "wants an excuse to cop out from the pressures of life"? *Watch out:* If you believe this stuff, it may come true.

On the other hand, when a girl complaining of dysmenorrhea is encouraged to stay home from school or sit out her gym class, she is being *rewarded* for her pain—not relieved of it. If she receives lavish parental attention during her period, she is encouraged to think that it makes her a queen for a couple of days—special, exotic, unapproachable; Camille wearing her red camellia.

The sooner it is understood by everyone that menstruation is a routine physical occurrence and dysmenorrhea an unpleasant side effect that can usually be controlled, the sooner women will be able to find relief and get on with their lives.

83. Primary dysmenorrhea is rare without ovulation

At the onset of menstruation, when a girl's periods are still irregular and she has not begun ovulating, dysmenorrhea is rare. Classically, the teen-ager develops the pain over the next few years. (This absence of pain is also common among older women who have ceased ovulating and whose menstrual periods are coming to an end.)

84. What causes dysmenorrhea?

No one knows for sure, but there are several theories.

a. The relation of *prostaglandins* to dysmenorrhea is only now being understood. A large class of physiologically active compounds, prostaglandins stimulate the smooth muscles of the intestine and stomach and the muscles of the uterus. Because of their effect on the uterus, they are sometimes used to stimulate abortions. (See p. 197) This usually involves side effects of nausea, vomiting, and diarrhea caused by simultaneous prostaglandin effect on the gastrointestinal tract muscles.

The same process is at work in dysmenorrhea; prostaglandin effect is now thought to cause cramps, nausea, diarrhea, and vomiting. *Encouraging experiments* show that drugs to control prostaglandin effect greatly reduce the pain of dysmenorrhea. (See #86 below)

Menstrual blood has very high levels of prostaglandins. Any factors (still unknown) which elevate prostaglandins probably increase menstrual cramps.

b. *High levels of estrogen and progesterone late in the cycle* may cause the body to retain sodium (salt) and therefore, in turn, fluid, causing increased blood flow to the pelvic area and an uncomfortable, bloated feeling. This would be especially pertinent to the pelvic congestion syndrome (#96) and dysmenorrhea associated with premenstrual syndrome.

c. Don't pay too much attention to the theory that cramps are caused by narrowing or stenosis of the cervix which prevents menstrual blood from escaping. Except in very rare cases, this theory remains unproven.

85. How to relieve menstrual cramps

Cramps both in the stomach and the rectum usually can be relieved by mild pain-killers or muscle relaxants. Aspirin works well because it blocks the prostaglandins somewhat. If mild products which can be bought over the counter do not work, a physician may have to prescribe something stronger. A very few women may have to take low doses of narcotics during the first day of the period if they are severely disabled by pain. Calcium supplements help some women.

86. Recommendation: Prostaglandin inhibitors are very effective in relieving spastic dysmenorrhea

Theoretically, drugs which inhibit prostaglandin production should alleviate most of the pain, vomiting, and diarrhea associated with menstruation. In fact, several medications used widely for arthritis have an antiprostaglandin effect and are excellent in treatment of dysmenorrhea.

First try simple analgesics—aspirin or acetaminophen. If they don't work, *insist on* antiprostaglandin drugs. These include naproxen (Naprosyn), mefamic acid (Ponstel) and ibuprofen (Motrin). (Ref. 10, 11)

87. To prevent cramps, avoid constipation before menstruation

The constipation many women experience before their periods probably stems from the effect of high hormone levels on the smooth muscle of the bowel. The hormones cause the muscles to relax: constipation results.

Constipation aggravates menstrual cramps by distending the bowel, producing gas. If you take steps before and during your period to avoid constipation, you may be able to avoid cramping pain completely. Eat plenty of fresh fruit; try bran cereal. A mild non-prescription stool softener may help too. (See p. 240)

88. Diarrhea and vomiting with menstruation

These symptoms are probably caused by high levels of prostaglandins in the body. Some women may have to take antivomiting drugs during the first day of bleeding; the antiprostaglandins (see above) may help as well.

89. Exercise may help dysmenorrhea

Rather than believing the female hygiene advertisements, which suggest you *may* exercise during menstruation, experiment with the idea that you *should* exercise at these times. Many women report that exercise, with all that it means in terms of increased blood circulation and relaxation of muscles, is a way both to avoid and alleviate dysmenorrhea.

It may be necessary to put your feet up for an hour or so during menstrual pain, as a kind of brief interlude between the time you take your muscle relaxant or analgesic and the time you've begun to feel better.

Try and continue the exercise pattern that you're used to. Even women athletes who are in competitions find that they can continue, and win, while they are menstruating. (Contrary to what many people seem to believe, bleeding does not stop during swimming or other athletic activities; but that shouldn't stop you from swimming.)

90. Orgasm may help

Orgasm during sexual relations or by masturbation decreases the amount of pain felt by many women. This is more true of congestive symptoms common in older women than the spastic symptoms affecting young girls. Orgasm during menstruation actually increases the flow of blood and relieves the pressure of pelvic congestion.

91. Drinking may help

Alcoholic beverages act to decrease uterine contractions and therefore may help menstrual cramps. (See p. 171)

92. Tampons may increase cramping

Use of tampons increases cramping in some women, especially during the first few days of bleeding. One theory has it that the tampon may increase blood flow, by a sort of suction effect.

Another has it that the tampon expands, presses against the cervix and causes pain by stretching some of the pelvic ligaments. The tampons which expand laterally rather than in length may be more comfortable for some women. You are the best judge. If you have more discomfort wearing tampons, try wearing pads again.

93. Opinion: Don't use oral contraceptives as a remedy for dysmenorrhea except as a last resort, and then only briefly

Birth-control pills work very well to eliminate cramps and other symptoms of dysmenorrhea. The exact mechanism is unknown, but since they eliminate ovulation, they eliminate whatever there is about ovulation which causes cramps in the first place (probably the prostaglandin effect).

However, the multiple major side effects of the pill (see Chapter Four) do not warrant its use except for short periods of time and only in women with very severe discomfort.

94. Pain associated with ovulation: mittelschmerz

Many women, from time to time, note a twinge or sharp pain in one side of the abdomen about the time of ovulation. This pain is called mittelschmerz. Some women have the symptom every month, and a few experience severe pain for a day or two. The exact cause is unknown. It may be related to spasms in the Fallopian tube around the time of ovulation, or a small amount of fluid or blood may escape from the ovary at time of ovulation and irritate the lining of the abdomen. If you stop ovulation with the birth-control pills, the pain will go away—but WARNING! *this remedy should be used only in very severe cases.*

95. Premenstrual syndrome: progesterone as a treatment

Many women note that as they get into their thirties they develop one or more of the following symptoms in the latter part of their menstrual cycle:

a. Breast tenderness
b. Nervousness
c. Headache
d. Dysmenorrhea
e. Bloated feeling
f. Weight gain

All of these are part of the *premenstrual syndrome* so well described by Dr. Katrina Dalton in a book by the same name. (Ref. 12)

These symptoms probably result from imbalance of estrogen and progesterone in the late cycle, and are usually easily relieved by progesterone in low doses in the second fourteen days of the cycle. This treatment does not have the risks of estrogen therapy, but nevertheless, it should not be used unless absolutely necessary. (*Any* hormone-based drug should be taken with the greatest restraint.)

Try gentle diuretics or sedatives first. (Over-the-counter drugs with pamabrom or caffeine produce mild diuretic effects.) Only if these don't work and you are absolutely miserable with premenstrual syndrome should you ask for progesterone. It may be difficult to persuade your gynecologist to prescribe progesterone because Dalton's work and the efficacy of this treatment has been ignored by the medical profession. But if you are severely bothered, persist. Injections of pure progesterone or vaginal tablets may be used.

96. Pelvic congestion syndrome

This condition may actually be part of the premenstrual syndrome or may have other causes. Some symptoms resemble symptoms of pelvic relaxation: ache in the pelvic area, low backache, and an aching in the top of the thighs, but pelvic congestion syndrome is quite a different thing. Women often feel the symptoms most keenly seven to ten days before menstruation, that is, immediately after ovulation.

The syndrome usually begins to affect a woman when she is in her thirties (as does premenstrual syndrome—see ⊁95 above). The pelvic area can be very tender during examination or during intercourse; women suffering from pelvic congestion syndrome who undergo surgery are found to have a good deal of congestion in the pelvic organs and vessels, and muscle spasms throughout the area.

No one really knows the source of this problem.

It can be lived with and is lived with readily by many women who suffer from it, so serious investigation into its cause has been limited.

One *theory* is that it is caused by repeated sexual stimulation without orgasm. Masters and Johnson have found that pelvic congestion occurs immediately before orgasm; theoretically, therefore, pelvic congestion syndrome is a kind of chronic, preorgasmic state; some women do find that orgasm, either through sexual relations or masturbation, helps. (See p. 391)

Masters and Johnson showed that women with these complaints have an enlarged and tender uterus. After orgasm by masturbation (presumably after any orgasm) the uterus is its normal size again and the pelvic exam is painless as soon as ten minutes later. (Ref. 13)

SURGICAL PROCEDURES

DILATATION AND CURETTAGE (D & C)

D & C, dilatation and curettage, is one of the most commonly performed gynecological operations—frequently performed for diagnosis but often serving as a cure.

97. What is a D & C?

Under general or local anesthesia, the vulva, vagina and cervix are cleansed with antiseptic solution. A speculum is placed in the vagina; the cervix is grasped with a tenaculum. The uterus is then measured for length by a sound—a long metal device with distance markings on it, (a lot like the device used to check the oil level in a car). The cervix is widened gradually by insertion of increasingly wide dilators. When the cervix is sufficiently dilated to allow access to the uterus, the lining of the uterus is scraped off with a curette.

If a local anesthetic (usually a paracervical block) is used, it is injected just after the cervix is grasped with a tenaculum. Women who have the operation with local anesthetic may feel mild cramping during the scraping.

98. General usages of a D & C

a. A D & C is a cleaning of the interior of the uterus; this in itself is often a cure for various disorders. (See below)

b. A tissue scraping can be extracted during the D & C and sent for lab analysis. A report is usually available within twenty-four to forty-eight hours.

c. After the scraping, the physician can search the endometrial cavity with a special forceps, to detect polyps, for example.

d. The physician can also evaluate the shape of the endometrial cavity and detect any irregularities, such as fibroids, which might be causing excessive bleeding. These problems may be suspected as a result of office examination, but they can only be detected actually during the D & C, when the physician can feel into the uterus with a curette.

99. Normal postoperative course after D & C

There should be very little bleeding after a D & C; sometimes staining will last for a week; sometimes a woman will find that she passes small clots into the toilet. She may have cramps or backache for a day or two. Complications such as heavy bleeding are infrequent, for example. Avoid douching and tampons until bleeding stops. Condoms should be used during intercourse, for the first ten to fourteen days, for the cervix does not close right away. Resume bathing immediately, and anticipate returning to a normal work schedule a few days after the operation.

100. Complications are rare after a D & C

Relative to other operations on the uterus, a D & C poses few complications. Perforation of the uterus occurs occasionally. (See p. 201) Cervical stenosis (sten-OH-siss)—in which the cervix is scarred during the operation and fused shut by scar tissue—is a late but very rare complication. In the case of cervical stenosis, menstrual blood, mucus or pus (if the woman is postmenopausal) may accumulate behind the barrier that is closing the cervix and cause pain or swelling of the uterus. Unusual reactions to general anesthesia are a risk in any surgical procedure.

101. Irregular menstrual bleeding: the most common reason for D & C

A D & C is generally performed to diagnose the cause of irregular menstrual bleeding or postmenopausal bleeding, but *frequently it will cure the problem as well.* If no obvious cause for the irregular bleeding is found, then the diagnosis will be Dysfunctional Uterine Bleeding.

102. Some specific causes of irregular uterine bleeding

a. Endometrial polyps—small growths on the lining of the uterus—thought to be related to excess estrogen stimulation

b. Chronic inflammation of the endometrium (*endometritis*)

c. Fibroid tumors
d. Cancerous or precancerous growths
e. Simple hormone imbalance

103. Hormone therapy as an alternative treatment for irregular uterine bleeding in healthy women under thirty-five

When women under thirty-five are having irregular periods, with no reason to suspect serious disorder, hormone imbalance is a likely cause and hormone treatment to correct it may be suggested before a D & C is tried. This usually involves *no more than a few months* of hormone therapy to give the body time to retrieve its own balance, and in most cases is less dangerous than D & C and general anesthesia.

In women under thirty-five in whom hormone therapy fails, or in women over thirty-five, a D & C is the preferred treatment. For women bleeding after menopause, a D & C is the treatment of choice.

104. Recommendation: D & C is not for teen-agers

Menstrual irregularity is common among teen-agers and usually rights itself in time without treatment. If it is severe or disabling, it can be treated with hormones, and is more easily corrected than irregular bleeding in older women. (See p. 23) A D & C is more dangerous for a young woman who has had no pregnancies because the cervix is often very difficult to dilate, may tear, and the cervical lacerations affect future fertility. *Seek another opinion,* therefore, if your doctors recommend a D & C as the first line of treatment for a teen-ager.

105. D & C is frequently suggested at time of tubal ligation

With the woman's permission, a D & C is frequently performed at time of tubal ligation (sterilization) to eliminate the chance of a pre-existing pregnancy.

106. Other reasons—and non-reasons—for a D & C

D & Cs are often done in the treatment of Asherman's Syndrome (scarring in the uterus) and during infertility work-ups associated with laparoscopy and tubal lavage. (See p. 105)

WARNING: *It is a common fallacy that a D & C is "good" for a woman as a periodic "cleaning-out." This is nonsense.* If a woman exhibits no menstrual irregularity, then the inside of her uterus is probably in excellent shape and there is no reason in the world that she should undergo an operation to have it scraped off.

D & C is not in itself a treatment for infertility; it may serve as a necessary part of the diagnostic work-up for infertility but not before many other steps take place and other treatments have been tried. (See p. 106) WARNING: It is also *not* a treatment for cramps, no matter how severe these are (see Dysmenorrhea, p. 322) unless there is a need to make a diagnosis that only a lab test on the endometrial tissue can prove.

107. Opinion: If a doctor wants to do a D & C and can't give one of the above good reasons for it, check with another doctor

One of the most important ways to evaluate a physician is to judge whether he or she suggests unnecessary surgery. A great many doctors use the D & C as a diagnostic measure when less radical measures would suffice. *No surgery should ever be routine.* If you have the slightest doubt about the necessity for any operation, check with one or several other physicians and corroborate the first opinion before going ahead.

108. Laparoscopy as a diagnostic procedure

This is a method of looking directly at the pelvic organs and is discussed completely on p. 105

109. Hysteroscopy (hiss-ter-OSS-copy): a new diagnostic procedure

In this procedure, the inside of the uterus is visualized by a tube attached to a viewer, similar to a laparoscope, inserted through the cervix. This procedure may be used to remove lost IUDs or to see if there are any abnormalities in the endometrium, for instance, fibroids, as part of an infertility work-up. Some methods of blocking the Fallopian tubes for sterilization are performed with a hysteroscope. (See p. 86)

HYSTERECTOMY

110. What is a hysterectomy?

There are several types of hysterectomies, and the distinctions between them are vitally important.

a. *"Partial"* hysterectomy involves removal of the uterus and cervix. (Medically this equals a *hysterectomy. Subtotal* hysterectomy involves leaving the cervix but taking the uterus.)

b. When the tubes and the ovaries are removed as well, this is called *hysterectomy and bilateral salpingo-oophorectomy* (sal-ping-go-oo-for-ECK-tomy). It is also called *total hysterectomy.*

c. If only one tube and one ovary are removed, that is called *hysterectomy and unilateral salpingo-oophorectomy.*

d. *Radical hysterectomy* involves removal of tubes, ovaries, uterus, cervix, *and* pelvic lymph nodes. WARNING: *It should only be done in women with advanced cancer.*

A partial hysterectomy ("a" above) does not change a woman's hormonal status; she still has her ovaries, the source of most female hormones. She does not menstruate, however, and needs no contraception.

A hysterectomy in which only one ovary is removed ("c" above) also leaves a woman's hormone supply at normal levels.

Total hysterectomy (with removal of ovaries "b" above) and radical hysterectomy ("d" above) cause symptoms of menopause and climacteric. The hormone supply diminishes; physical and emotional changes are relatively severe in many cases. If a woman already past menopause has the operation, the changes will not affect her greatly: younger women may suffer much more and should take some hormone treatment to prevent the severe symptoms of climacteric too early in life. (See p. 289)

111. Opinion: Hysterectomy is a frequently performed unnecessary operation

Various estimates show that between 20 and 40 per cent of hysterectomies performed in the United States are unnecessary or highly questionable. A number of factors contribute to this alarming figure:

a. Many doctors dealing with women who have already completed their families use hysterectomy as a preventive measure against cancer and other degenerative diseases which increase in incidence as women grow older.

b. Many doctors perform hysterectomies when a woman wants to be sterilized; a simple and much less dangerous tubal ligation would do as well. The woman herself, ignorant of the safer alternatives, often urges the doctor to do this. *Both should know better.*

c. Some physicians perform hysterectomies for disorders in which a simple and much less dangerous D & C would serve.

d. The discretion that a physician has in deciding whether to perform a hysterectomy is narrowed or broadened depending on financial considerations. For example, women being treated by private physicians have more hysterectomies than women being treated under prepaid medical group plans, in which doctors get no extra money for doing extra surgery. In the same way, hysterectomy rates are much lower in countries where medicine is socialized (e.g., England). A recent study in Canada showed that when a committee watched over the indications for hysterectomy, this caused a drop of more than 30 per cent in the number performed. (Ref. 14)

112. Opinion: How to avoid having an unnecessary hysterectomy

A hysterectomy is a major operation, useful only to correct major disease, like cancer or fibroid tumors.

Therefore, anything less than major disease or injury should be disqualified as a reason for having the operation.

Never accept a hysterectomy as a treatment to achieve simple sterilization.

Never accept hysterectomy for menstrual irregularity, unless a D & C or hormones have been tried previously, or unless you have large fibroid tumors.

Always get at least one other opinion, preferably from doctors associated with different hospitals, if hysterectomy is recommended. Try to use insurance plans which cover second opinions.

Always know whether your physician is recommending a partial or a total hysterectomy. Know whether you are going to lose both ovaries or just one. These differences are *critical*—and they require a decision by the patient, not just her doctor. If there is not an *excellent* reason for the ovaries to be removed, opt for a partial hysterectomy, for this will leave you with an undisturbed hormonal cycle. If only one ovary is diseased, keep the other one, especially if you are under fifty; it will provide you with some if not all the hormones you need and make the change of life less troublesome. (See p. 287)

Talk to other women who have had hysterectomies. Their experience may serve as valuable counsel when you make your own decision.

Never accept hysterectomy as preventive medicine. It may be your doctor's view that the reproductive organs are unnecessary baggage for a woman who has completed her family, and is on her way to climacteric and possibly the degenerative diseases that afflict older people. This is a useless line of thinking; the odds are excellent that you will *not* get cancer of the uterus so the risk of the operation is greater than the risk of cancer if disease is not already present.

113. Abdominal hysterectomy—the most common form of this surgery

Abdominal hysterectomy involves general anesthesia. An incision is made in the lower abdomen either vertically or horizontally at the level of the top of the pubic hair (which is shaved before surgery). Some physicians pride themselves on making this horizontal incision as close to the pubic hair as possible, so that the resulting scar is all but invisible. It is called a Pfannenstiel incision, after the doctor who perfected it. *Request this incision.* Surgical values being equal, the Pfannenstiel incision is much more desirable cosmetically, and has better strength in healing. If large tumors are present, a Pfannenstiel incision is not possible.

The uterus is removed, as well as the cervix; the top of the vagina is closed. This wound just heals over, allowing intercourse as before. The bladder has to be moved a bit during the surgery: therefore, a woman will usually wake up with a catheter in her bladder to keep it empty; as the bladder relaxes into its natural position and the trauma to the surrounding muscles lessens, the catheter can be removed, usually the next day. The woman will probably receive intravenous fluids until her bowel starts working again and she can eat and drink normally. This should take two to four days.

In the few days immediately after the operation, a woman will experience considerable pain. Her physician can prescribe pain-killers to ease the discomfort.

She should get out of bed and walk around as soon as possible, preferably the first day after the operation. This prevents lung congestion that could lead to pneumonia; it makes leg muscles contract, helping to prevent phlebitis (clots in the veins, see p. 49); it encourages the circulation that promotes healing and helps the bowel to function normally again. When the hospital attendant suggests this first walk, you may with all your heart wish to resist. But the suggestion is a good one and should be followed, despite the pain.

The hospital stay for hysterectomy is usually five to ten days, depending on how quickly the individual recovers. Full recovery will need another three to six weeks' rest at home, and, in fact, a woman will probably not feel at full energy until some months after the surgery. Every prior arrangement must be made to allow the recuperation she needs. Women in good physical condition to start with will recover sooner.

114. Vaginal hysterectomy

Vaginal hysterectomy involves the same removal of organs, except that the incision is made through the top of the vagina. Recovery time is generally less than for an abdominal hysterectomy; there is less pain, because it is the vagina, not the belly, which must heal. Vaginal hysterectomy has some limitations. First, the uterus must be small enough to be drawn out through the vagina—this lets out women who suffer from large fibroid tumors of the uterus. It cannot usually be used in total hysterectomy, where diseased tubes and/or ovaries are being removed.

For stress incontinence and other forms of pelvic relaxation (see p. 322), vaginal hysterectomy is the preferred treatment, allowing repair of the bladder without a major abdominal incision.

115. Sexual response is not affected by hysterectomy

The physical aspects of sex should not be affected by hysterectomy—except that sex must be avoided until the woman is fully healed. Most women say that sex after hysterectomy is just as good or better than before, but attest that it does *feel* different—probably because there are contractions of the uterus during orgasm which a woman who has had her uterus removed no longer feels.

Sexual response of a woman should not be affected by partial hysterectomy. In the case of total hysterectomy, the removal of the ovaries and the interruption of the hormone supply may have an important effect in altering (not always lessening) physiological responses to sex (see p. 285). If vaginal dryness or severe hot flashes occur, discuss hormone therapy. (See p. 282)

116. Complications of hysterectomy

a. Urinary-tract infections sometimes occur because of the catheter in the bladder after surgery (※61 above).

b. Pelvic infection is a possibility. Blood may collect in the area where the uterus was, and then become infected. This is more common after vaginal than abdominal hysterectomy, because the vagina contains more bacteria that could infect the area than does the skin of the abdomen. Antibiotics are the common treatment; sometimes if pus has collected in the area where the uterus was, a drain must be placed through the top of the vagina to let it out. Antibiotics are frequently given before vaginal hysterectomy to prevent infection.

c. Wound infection in the abdomen is a possibility. This usually appears around the fourth or fifth day after surgery. The treatment is antibiotics and hot soaks. The rate of wound infection is much higher in obese women.

d. The bladder is the principal organ that must be moved to allow removal of the uterus. Therefore, *bladder damage* is relatively more common than other complications; it can usually be repaired on the spot, with no aftereffects. The greater difficulty comes when the damage to the bladder is not recognized during surgery and grows more severe after the surgery is over.

In less than one per cent of cases, and more frequently in complicated surgery, a *fistula* (FISS-tue-la) may form to complicate bladder function. A fistula is a small canal (the word comes from the Latin word meaning tube or pipe) which allows the contents of one hollow organ to drain into another. As a result of damage to the bladder or ureter during hysterectomy, a fistula forms and the urine may begin to leak out into the vagina. Treatment is usually to place a catheter in the bladder and allow it to drain for several months while the fistula seals itself. Further surgery is sometimes needed. A woman can be up and around during this waiting period, but the scope of her activity is limited.

117. Postoperative care for hysterectomy

Pelvic examinations should continue every six months after a partial hysterectomy, to check the condition of the pelvic cavity where the uterus was, and the ovaries and tubes. If a woman has had her ovaries and tubes removed as well, a checkup every one to two years is probably sufficient, with Pap smears to check for vaginal cancer. Breasts should be checked two times yearly by a physician.

118. Long-term complications of hysterectomy

a. *Hernia:* In overweight women or women who have suffered a postoperative infection in the wound, a hernia through the abdominal scar is a possible long-term complication. In this case the stomach muscle and fibrous tissue give way and a bulge appears under the skin. Some hernias are small and give no discomfort, others must be repaired surgically.

After hysterectomy, the top of the vagina can also herniate. Again, the treatment depends on the seriousness of the discomfort.

b. *Prolapse of the ovary:* After both abdominal and vaginal hysterectomies, there is a new empty cavity where the uterus used to be. In some women the ovaries may fall into this area behind the vagina and cause pain during intercourse. Rarely, surgery may be needed to pull the ovaries back into place.

119. Psychological complications of hysterectomy

Hysterectomy can have profound psychological effects that few women can anticipate. These stem from a feeling of having been cut off from one source of womanhood, from feelings of mutilation, or from the feeling (very common in major surgery) that one has actually seen death. If a woman has had a total hysterectomy and develops severe hot flashes the psychological problems may be aggravated by the physical. She should use estrogen replacement for *short periods of time.* (See p. 289) Mild depression following hysterectomy is common: if it is severe or prolonged, seek professional help.

If you know you are about to have a hysterectomy, and you are scared, do not be surprised if husband, children, and physicians are no comfort. They cannot be expected to understand what you are about to go through. Seek the counsel and comfort of other women who have been through it and know how bad it was and *how bad it was not.*

120. Fibroid tumors of the uterus: the most common reason for hysterectomy

Fibroid tumors of the uterus are benign tumors of the uterine muscle, which occur in 25–35 per cent of all women. Their cause is unknown, but they do seem to run in families. They tend to decrease in size after menopause (when estrogen supplies are low) and increase in size during pregnancy (when estrogen is high) and in women on high-dose birth-control pills.

If the fibroids are small, they may give no symptoms—and surgery to remove them is unjustified. Indeed, a woman may live comfortably and without any symptoms with small fibroids for years and years. (By "small," physicians usually mean that the tumor does not make the uterus bigger than it would be at three months of pregnancy.)

121. Symptoms of fibroid tumors of the uterus

a. The most common symptom is increasingly heavy menstrual bleeding, sometimes to the extent of hemorrhage. If untreated, this can leave a woman severely anemic. Bleeding is heaviest if the fibroid is on the *inside* of the uterus, right under the endometrial surface (submucous).

b. If the tumors are large, they can press on other pelvic organs, such as the bladder, rectum, and the ureters that lead from the kidney to the bladder, causing severe pain and sometimes kidney infections that only hysterectomy will assuage. For some women, severe backache may be a symptom of fibroid tumors.

Like all tissue, a tumor must have a blood supply to stay alive. If a fibroid loses its blood supply, dies, or twists on the uterus, severe pain will result.

Any or all of these symptoms—bleeding, severe abdominal pain, severe backache—should at once take you to a physician.

122. If fibroids are discovered on examination

A doctor who discovers small fibroids may do nothing about them.

OPINION: If they make the uterus larger than it would be at twelve weeks' pregnancy, have them removed. Beyond that size, they begin to cause pressure on the other organs. Since these tumors become cancerous in fewer than 1 in 200 women, their presence alone should not alarm you. However, if you have fibroids, have yourself examined at least twice yearly to assure that the tumors are not changing or growing fast.

123. Other reasons for hysterectomy

a. *Irregular bleeding* with no obvious cause that has not been stopped by D & Cs, or hormone treatments.

b. *Pelvic infection and pelvic inflammatory disease.* Women who have suffered from these disorders, often in the aftermath of gonorrhea or IUD infection (see pp. 60–61), may develop serious scarring of the tubes and ovaries. The scar tissue knits these organs together with the uterus, and may cause infertility, severe dysmenorrhea and severe pain during sexual intercourse. A diagnosis of pelvic inflammatory disease should be confirmed by laparoscopy (see p. 105) and antibiotics should be tried to dissolve the infection before surgery is attempted. Sometimes conservative surgery, such as lysis of adhesions, may work, and you should discuss this possibility. *However, in severe cases—and most heartbreakingly, among young women—the condition cannot be checked except by total hysterectomy.* Pelvic inflammatory disease that leads to total hysterectomy is on the rise with the increased incidence of gonorrhea and IUD use. So never imagine that venereal disease can be always cured quickly, without complication.

c. *Pelvic relaxation* (see ✂69 above)

d. *Cancer of the uterus, cervix, or ovary* (see below)

e. *Postpartum hemorrhage.* On rare occasions, a woman will hemorrhage so extensively after delivering her child that the only way to stop the bleeding and save her life is by removing the uterus. This is an emergency operation, usually conducted immediately after delivery.

124. Myomectomy: removal of the fibroid tumors alone

In a myomectomy fibroid tumors alone are removed; the uterus is left in place. It may only be a stopgap measure—that is, it can be done if small fibroids are rendering a woman infertile or causing heavy periods as a way of allowing her to conceive a child or keep her uterus. In about 20 per cent of cases, a hysterectomy is needed later on. But the myomectomy may have given the women those few years she needed to have the children she wanted. A woman who becomes pregnant after a myomectomy should expect to deliver by Caesarean section; vaginal delivery is usually impossible because of scar tissue on the uterus, resulting from the myomectomy.

OPINION: Some physicians don't like to do myomectomies. They feel the woman will just have to come back for a hysterectomy later on, so why not do the whole job in the first place? *This may make good sense to a doctor, but it is no answer for a woman who wants a child or who just does not want her uterus out.* While myomectomy is less radical than a hysterectomy, it may be more difficult technically, with greater blood loss. If fibroid tumors are unusually large, and the uterus very distorted, it is *not* the recommended treatment. However, if you really desire a myomectomy and your doctor refuses, get at least one additional opinion. A specialist in the treatment of infertility is a good choice.

125. Supracervical hysterectomy (subtotal)

This is a rare procedure, in which the uterus is removed *but not the cervix.* It is used for women who have widespread pelvic infection or very large fibroid tumors that make removal of the cervix impossible without damage to the ureters or bladder. A woman who has had a supracervical hysterectomy still must have Pap smears because she must continue to guard herself against cervical cancer.

OVARIAN CYSTS

126. Ovarian cysts

Ovarian cysts are very common, usually benign swellings, filled with fluid, that appear and sometimes disappear spontaneously. Most ovarian cysts are *functional*—that is, something goes slightly wrong in the normal menstrual cycle and excess fluid collects around the follicle or corpus luteum, then disperses by itself.

Sometimes, the cysts retain their fluid and actually collect more fluid, creating a cystic mass filled with the normal secretions of the ovaries. If this grows large, it must be removed surgically.

127. How ovarian cysts are detected

Frequently, ovarian cysts have no symptoms and are only detected by the examining physician. Sometimes they are indicated by pain on the affected side as well as by menstrual irregularity—usually *prolonged* bleeding.

If the cyst is less than 5 cm in diameter, in a woman under forty, another examination in three to six weeks is indicated. If the cyst has grown, *then* surgery is indicated. (In many cases, it will have disappeared.) In older women, ovarian enlargement is more serious and requires immediate evaluation by laparoscopy or laparotomy.

128. Birth-control pills may shrink functional cysts

When a woman takes birth-control pills, her ovaries do not go through the changes of complete follicle development and corpus luteum formation because she is not ovulating. *Thus, women on the pill almost never develop functional cysts of the ovary.* Sometimes the pill can be used to shrink functional cysts. This treatment should last for no more than two months: if the cyst has not disappeared, it is probably *not* a functional cyst. Further diagnosis is in order.

129. Other tumors of the ovary—benign or malignant

These include:
a. Dermoid cysts and other benign tumors
b. Polycystic ovaries
c. Cancer of the ovaries

130. Dermoid cysts (cystic teratomas)

These are common, benign tumors of the ovary in young women and fairly startling because they are believed to be embryologic remnants—frequently containing teeth, hair, brain and thyroid tissue. Usually they are detected during a routine gynecological examination and can be confirmed by X ray of the lower abdomen, that may reveal calcium in the embryologic content. Dermoid cysts do not usually cause menstrual irregularity.

Preferred treatment is surgical removal of the cyst, which can often be performed without removing the entire ovary.

131. Polycystic ovaries (the Stein-Leventhal Syndrome)

Polycystic ovarian syndrome is much misdiagnosed. It has another name—the Stein-Leventhal Syndrome (for Irving Stein and Michael Leventhal, the physicians at Michael Reese Hospital in Chicago who first described it in 1935). The syndrome describes a group of women suffering from hormone imbalance, with accompanying obesity, excess body hair, and chronic menstrual irregularities. In addition, they have enlarged ovaries with a great many follicle cysts. This part of the condition is called polycystic ovaries. These women frequently have difficulty conceiving.) (See p. 96)

WARNING: The reason it is so important for the Stein-Leventhal Syndrome to be correctly diagnosed is that women who have it run a somewhat increased risk of cancer of the endometrium and should have hormone treatments to prevent it. The *only way* to verify a diagnosis of Stein-Leventhal Syndrome is by examining the ovaries themselves by laparoscopy or laparotomy. Sometimes, this important step is skipped, and women who naturally tend to be hairy and are suffering from menstrual irregularities are diagnosed to be suffering from the syndrome incorrectly. *So take care. If polycystic ovarian syndrome has been diagnosed without laparoscopy, get another opinion, preferably from a gynecological endocrinologist.* Also, obtain blood tests for ovarian and adrenal hormones.

132. Polyps

Polyps are *benign* growths of glandular tissue which occasionally pop up in little lumps on the cervix or the endometrium. Cervical polyps are usually discovered during a regular pelvic exam or may cause bleeding after intercourse. Endometrial polyps almost always cause irregular vaginal bleeding, and if a D & C is done to relieve the symptom, the cause will be discovered at that time. A D & C is the best treatment for cervical or endometrial polyps and will usually get rid of them for good. Occasionally, a cervical polyp in a young woman can be removed in the office. If bleeding continues, a D & C is needed. Polyps are more common around menopause and are probably related to endocrine imbalance.

133. Bartholin's abscess

The Bartholin's glands are located at the lower part of the entrance to the vagina. Sometimes a minor irritation can inflame the gland, sometimes they can be infected by gonorrhea; in either case, the entrance to the gland is blocked and the gland fills with pus and fluid and swells up. If there is pus inside, an abscess is formed and a very painful, hot swelling can occur.

134. Treatment of Bartholin's abscess

If an abscess forms, and infection is clearly present, a woman should have herself checked for gonorrhea. Antibiotics will usually clear the abscess. Warm baths that help bring the infection up to the surface so that it can drain will relieve swelling and pain. If antibiotics and heat do not make the abscess drain, a doctor can incise it with a needle or small knife for immediate drainage. For women who suffer repeatedly from these abscesses, a permanent solution—marsupialization (mar-SOUP-ee-ill-ization)—is suggested. In this process, the gland is literally turned inside out so that fluid or pus cannot accumulate.

135. Bartholin's cysts

A Bartholin's cyst is just like a Bartholin's abscess except that the cyst is filled with fluid, the abscess is filled with pus. If small, a

Bartholin's cyst need not be treated. Small cysts sometimes occur after childbirth, if the episiotomy (see p. 145) cuts across the duct of the Bartholin's gland. If the cyst becomes annoyingly large, proper treatment is removal of the gland or marsupialization. This is a relatively simple operation. Compared with Bartholin's abscess, a Bartholin's cyst is not painful.

136. Cyst and abscess of Skene's glands

In exactly the same way as the Bartholin's glands, the Skene's glands —located just below the urethra—can become infected or cystic. Treatment is usually removal of the cyst or abscess by removal of the gland, again, a simple procedure.

137. Endometriosis (en-doe-mee-tree-OH-siss)

Endometriosis is a little-understood condition in which the lining of the uterus somehow appears outside the uterus—for example, in the pelvic cavity, behind the uterus, on the ovary and the tubes, in the cervix and vagina, and even sometimes on the skin of the vulva and the abdomen. The disease usually strikes women in their late twenties.

Common symptoms may be

a. Severe menstrual cramping in women who previously had little or no discomfort

b. Chronic pelvic pain

c. Pain during sexual intercourse

d. Infertility (because endometrial tissue may adhere to the Fallopian tubes, altering tube motility, causing scarring and preventing conception

e. Irregular menses

For endometriosis to be diagnosed, most or all of these symptoms must be present, and the diagnosis must be confirmed by laparoscopy.

138. Treatment of endometriosis

a. For many years, the main treatment method was hormones, given in the form of very high-dose birth-control pills. In many cases, this treatment made the patches of endometriosis shrink. Low-dose pills can often keep mild endometriosis under control. Obviously, pregnancy is impossible under these circumstances.

b. Some women have used progestogens (synthetic progesterone) such as medroxyprogesterone acetate (Provera) in high doses with great success.

c. *Good news—watch the papers:* A very promising new drug, danocrine or Danazol, seems to have had the best results yet. It may have other beneficial side effects, such as decreasing the severity of cystic disease of the breast. (Ref. 15) This drug's overwhelming drawback is that it costs an average of a hundred dollars a month, putting it way out of reach for many women. (Treatment is usually prescribed for six to nine months.) It is hoped that with increasing sales, the price will fall.

d. Surgery can work as well. The surgeon scrapes off all patches of endometriosis he or she can find and then reconstructs the tube, if necessary. Ideally, this should be done by an infertility surgeon.

CANCER

139. Cancer is a malignant (invasive) distortion of cell development which can affect any part of the body. Probably a group of diseases, rather than a single disease, it is the subject of intense research today, of two types:

a. *Basic research* to determine what causes cells to undergo the changes that eventually become a malignancy, and thereafter to multiply rapidly and spread throughout the body.

b. *Applied research* on how to detect the disease early and treat it. Applied research may *seem* more important, because of its assault on the concrete problem. But most of our great scientific breakthroughs required, somewhere along the line, research into the *basic* nature of the problem in its most abstract dimensions. For example, it is probable that Watson and Crick (and their unheralded colleague, Rosalind Franklin), in their Nobel Prize-winning work on the basic make-up of DNA, the genetic material in every cell, contributed greatly to applied cancer research. But they weren't *thinking* of cancer necessarily; they were just trying to find out more about cells and the genetic package they carry. Basic research can get nowhere for years and years until it finally hits paydirt. *The public and those appropriating public funds must understand how vital this basic contribution is to finding, for example, a cure for cancer.*

140. A carcinogen is a substance which starts the cancer process

A carcinogen (car-SIN-o-jen) alters a cell so that it becomes free of normal limitations on growth and can reproduce itself without control. It may be a virus (which causes breast tumors in mice) or a chemical (such as a hydrocarbon, present in air pollution, which causes tumors in animals and is implicated in lung cancer in humans), or a hormone (which is implicated in tumors of the breast and genital organs). Cancer may also be associated with failure of the body's immunologic responses, and the resultant inability to eliminate abnormal cells.

141. A promoter is a substance which speeds the cancer along once it has started

After the carcinogen has prompted the cell to change, certain *promoter* substances can hasten the process and contribute to the growth of the tumor. Hydrocarbons and hormones act as promoters in animals, and may do so in humans as well.

142. The "latent period" is the time it takes for cancer to express itself

The time from initiation of the cancer by the carcinogen to the time that the cancer invades and is expressed and observable in the body is called the "latent period." For cervical cancer, it is about two to ten years; for breast cancer, as long as ten to thirty years. The latent period may be shortened by promoter agents. *Thus, even a tumor that has started may not appear without a promoter to encourage it.* Thus control of promoter substances is *vital* to cancer control, a fact which should make us all dedicated environmentalists. It is during the latent period that cancer, if the cancer can be detected, is most easily arrested and cured. (See ✻184 below)

143. The risk of breast cancer

The chance that an American woman will get breast cancer is about 1 in 14—7 per cent of all women. About 100,000 new cases are detected each year; this number is increasing slightly all the time. Some women run a *higher* statistical risk than others. These include women who:
   a. Have a family history of breast cancer, especially at a young age
   b. Have had benign breast disease
   c. Have been exposed to high doses of radiation
   d. Have taken high doses of estrogen for long periods of time for menopausal symptoms (and possibly women who took DES during pregnancy)
   e. Have early menarche and late menopause
   f. Have their first child after age thirty or who have no children at all
   g. Ovulate irregularly
   h. Suffer from obesity, hypertension, and diabetes
   i. Have diets high in fat
   j. Have previously had cancer of the colon, or endometrium
   k. Take thyroid medications for a long period of time or who take

medications which increase the prolactin levels such as reserpine and tranquilizers. (These factors are debatable.)

Some women have a *lower* statistical risk of developing breast cancer. These include women who:

a. Have a pregnancy before age eighteen, and have many pregnancies

b. Have late menarche and early menopause

c. Breast-feed several children over long periods of time (not such an important factor as was once thought)

d. Have their ovaries removed at a young age (not to be encouraged as a prophylactic method) (Ref. 16, 17, 18, 19)

144. What causes breast cancer?

Several theories of causation seem relevant, including:

a. Environmental pollution

b. Viruses

c. Estrogen (and other sex hormones)

d. Prolactin

e. Immunologic breakdown

f. Excess radiation to the chest

145. Environmental pollution is probably the biggest cause of increase of cancers of all types

The pollutants in the air, water, and food supply are largely industrial wastes, the products of our advanced society. However, economic and industrial progress is being made at the cost of human health. Many researchers now believe that probably 75 per cent of human cancers are caused by environmental factors, and breast cancer is undoubtedly included here.

146. The viral theory of cancer causation

Certain viruses cause breast cancer in mice. Particles very similar to these viruses have been found in the breast milk and breast tumors of women. An enzyme has been isolated—reverse transcriptase—from human breast cancers which is known to occur only in viruses that cause cancer. (Ref. 20, 21)

In addition, some women with breast cancer have an antigen in their blood which causes the body to develop antibodies which in turn react *against* tumor tissue. This is the way the body normally reacts against a virus. The antigen seems to be identical in all breast cancers; sometimes blood serum from women who have the antigen and the antibodies it triggers can be given to women who aren't having the antigen-antibody reaction to help them fight their own cancers. This work is still highly experimental but very exciting. (Ref. 22, 23)

147. Estrogen as a carcinogen and as a promoter substance for cancer

During the last fifteen years, because of birth-control pills containing estrogens, estrogen-replacement therapy during menopause, and the addition of DES—Diethylstilbestrol—into feed for fattening livestock, women have been receiving more than their normal share of estrogen. Thus, the possible links of estrogen with cancer—both as an initiating carcinogen and as a promoter substance—have caused great and continuing controversy.

WARNING: *There is strong evidence that DES is a carcinogen.* (See ☀198 below)

It is associated with a tumor of the vagina which is virtually unknown except in the daughters of women who received DES during early pregnancy. The DES causes some changes in the cells of the vagina and cervix, so that after puberty, when hormones appear in large quantities, the cancer appears. In this case, estrogen may act as carcinogen *and* promoter. (Ref. 24, 25) Mothers who took the DES may have a higher risk for breast cancer, although this data is currently debatable. (See ☀199 below)

Estrogen replacement in menopause and the high-estrogen sequential birth-control pills have definitely been associated with endometrial cancer. (Ref. 26, 27, 28. Also see p. 290)

Some "purists" will say that this is not enough to prove that estrogenic compounds are carcinogenic. *However, this is one case where guilt by association is grounds for condemnation.* Estrogens have caused cancers in test animals; the DES daughters are the tragic guinea pigs in an inadvertent "test" on people. That should be proof enough that low-estrogen birth-control pills should be used instead of high-estrogen compounds; that estrogen-replacement therapy should be used only in the most severe circumstances of climacteric and then for a very short time; and that livestock should be fattened with something other than DES.

No matter what doubts many have about this theory of carcinogenesis, there is no doubt that estrogen is a promoter substance for breast cancer. In test animals, cancers initiated by viruses are promoted to maturity by estrogen. While studies show birth-control pills *decrease* the incidence of benign breast disease, they may *increase* the speed with which pre-existing tumors grow. (Ref. 29, 30, 31) This is a hotly debated issue at present. Watch for further studies.

Women who have irregular periods, obese women, women with early menarche and late menopause resemble each other in that they have higher body levels of estrogen, present over a longer period of time. These women all have a higher incidence of breast cancer.

Obviously, then, anyone who is at high risk for breast cancer (see ✕143 above) should not take estrogen! Everyone else should proceed with utmost caution, always using combined estrogen-progesterone therapy if these are absolutely necessary. (See p. 291)

148. The role of progesterone in cancer is debatable

In mice and dogs, progestogens (artificial progesterone compounds) can serve as promoters of breast tumors. However, in humans, evidence suggests that progesterone may have a protective effect. This is unclear at present.

149. The role of prolactin in causing or promoting breast cancer

Prolactin is the hormone which triggers lactation at the end of a pregnancy, allowing a woman to breast-feed her baby. (See p. 158) At all other times, it is blocked by the prolactin-inhibiting factor produced in the hypothalamus, responding to high levels of estrogen and progesterone in pregnancy and during the normal menstrual cycle.

Sometimes the prolactin-inhibiting factor is stopped, and prolactin released when it shouldn't be. At these times, many people believe prolactin works with estrogen in causing breast cancer; it is unknown which is the promoter, and which is the carcinogen, or whether both act as promoters. (Ref. 32, 33, 34)

Thus, drugs which elevate prolactin levels may be associated with rising incidences of breast cancer. They are:

a. *Reserpine,* commonly prescribed for hypertension, associated with elevated prolactin levels and increased breast cancer, (Ref. 35)

b. *Phenothiazines* (feen-o-THIGH-a-zeens), a group of tranquilizers,

c. *Tricyclic antidepressant drugs* (Aventyl, Elavil, Norpramin, Pertofrane, Tofranil, Sinequan, and others)

d. *Methyldopa,* also prescribed for hypertension.

If you take these medications, have yourself screened periodically for breast cancer and watch for further reports of the effects of these drugs.

150. Immunologic breakdown and the spread of cancer

One theory proposes that cancer is most common in childhood and in old age, when the immune system is not well developed or is deteriorating and cannot fight off invading cancer cells. That is why, it is believed, breast cancer occurs more frequently in older and post-menopausal women. The strong, healthy body does not necessarily give in to the onslaught of cancer: for example, an intense inflammatory reaction around a tumor means that the body's immune system is fighting it; the prognosis in these cases may be better, for the tumor so resisted may be less likely to metastasize (me-TASS-ta-size)—to spread. In addition, women who have the antigen/antibody reaction in their blood have good prospects for a cure. (See ⚥145 above)

151. Excess radiation to the chest causes breast cancer

Women who were exposed to radiation in Japan during World War II, and women who have received multiple doses of radiation during treatment of tuberculosis have higher incidence of breast cancer. (Radiation therapy of various benign diseases such as acne is to be condemned.) This is the reason that the use of mammography for routine screening of all women (see p. 182) is currently condemned. Although not yet proven, the risk appears to be greater than the benefit in young women. (Ref. 36, 37)

152. Mastectomy

Mastectomy is surgical removal of the breast. A "partial" mastectomy removes part of the breast tissue; a "total" mastectomy removes all of the breast; a "radical" mastectomy removes the breast, lymph nodes, and chest muscles; a "modified radical" mastectomy leaves the muscles.

Until about ten years ago, *radical mastectomy* was the only kind. It was presented as a surgical procedure by Dr. William S. Halstead to the Mayo Clinic Society originally in 1894. A radical mastectomy involves removal of the breast and the chest muscles and dissection and removal of all the lymph nodes in the armpit. At the time, the operation created wonderful improvement in the survival statistics for women with breast cancer. About forty years ago, the death rate for breast cancer began leveling off—at 25 per 100,000 women per year. Twenty years ago, researchers began looking at those statistics and wondering why there had been no further improvement. Perhaps the radical procedure was not necessary for everybody; perhaps greater selectivity was in order. Some physicians began performing *total mastectomy,* in which the chest muscles were left intact and the lymph nodes removed only in cases of large tumors. *The mortality rates have remained about the same.* Today, we are at the point with another twenty years of hindsight, where a variety of treatments other than radical mastectomy are being used for breast cancer, with greater and greater demand from patients and doctors that individuals be treated with different therapies suitable for *them.* (See ⚥158 below) This is a time of great confusion and experimentation in breast-cancer therapy. It's hoped that the next five to ten years will resolve some of the uncertainty for women.

153. Varieties of treatment for breast cancer

a. One group advocates *radical mastectomy* in all cases on the theory that this best guards against recurrence.

b. A steadily enlarging group advocates removing the breast and lymph nodes while leaving the chest muscles, on the theory that these additional excisions add nothing to a woman's chances of survival. This is a "modified radical" mastectomy.

c. A smaller group advocates removing only breast tissues—"total" mastectomy.

d. Another group advocates *lumpectomy* for small cancers, detected early—involving removal of the mass alone.

e. Sometimes either type of mastectomy or lumpectomy is coupled with chemotherapy or radiation or both.

The controversy will be much quieted only when hard statistics begin to come in on how women respond to these treatments fifteen to twenty years after they have had them—whether, in fact, recurrence rates are higher with the simple procedures or just the same. A nationwide study to gather these data is taking place now. *Watch your newspapers for the results.*

154. The concept of hormonal dependence of tumors and its use in treatment of breast cancer

Approximately 40–60 per cent of breast cancers which occur in premenopausal women are dependent upon estrogen for growth. This is known by the fact that the removal of the ovaries, which was previously routine in premenopausal women with breast cancer, causes regression of the tumor in 40–60 per cent of the women. If the tumors did not respond to removal of the ovaries, then removal of the adrenals and sometimes of the pituitary gland was helpful in some women.

It is now possible to predict which tumors will respond to the removal of these other endocrine glands. This is done by the analysis of the tumors for the presence of receptor proteins. If the breast tumor contains the receptor proteins for estrogen, progesterone, or androgen, it means that the tumor probably needs that particular hormone for growth. Women who do not have these receptor proteins are found to have little chance of benefit from further surgery, so they are spared the unnecessary removal of the organs.

Most tumors in postmenopausal women are found not to contain estrogen receptors, but some contain androgen receptors and respond well to the removal of the adrenals, the major source of androgen.

The converse use of receptor protein information is that, if the receptor proteins are absent, the tumor may respond well to administration of that hormone as a therapy.

This is an exciting new area of research. It is important that women with breast cancer have their treatment started at a center which is doing the analysis of the tumors for receptor proteins. (Ref. 38)

155. Chemotherapy

This involves the administration of powerful antitumor drugs either right after the original surgery or later if a recurrence is noted. Some drugs administered right after surgery to all patients have shown good results in decreasing the incidence of recurrence. (Ref. 39) Other centers administer these only to patients whose tumors are spreading to the lymph nodes. RECOMMENDATION: Try to initiate chemotherapy only at a regional cancer center. Watch for news about newer methods of chemotherapy.

156. Radiation therapy

Some people advocate radiation in addition to mastectomy; others use it instead of mastectomy and still others suggest its use only if there is evidence of spread of the tumor to the glands under the arm. The role of radiation therapy in the *initial* treatment of breast cancer is debatable at present. The national study currently in progress will determine whether there is any usefulness to this treatment. *Watch for further news.* However, radiation therapy is definitely useful in treating local recurrences and relieving pain from the spread of the tumor to bone.

157. Immunotherapy

WATCH FOR FURTHER NEWS: Some researchers working with the *immunologic response theory* (see ⚹150 above) are experimenting with ways to transfer immunity from women who have developed high levels of antibody to tumors to women who have not. The goal is to eliminate the tumor cells from the blood stream of the second woman. Other similar projects involve attempts to determine ways in which to stimulate a woman's own immune system to react more violently against the tumor cells. (Ref. 23) This is an interesting line of research but probably will not be used clinically for some time.

158. Opinion: The cautious approach to mastectomy

The controversy currently raging about which type of mastectomy is best was triggered by a rather all-or-nothing use of radical mastectomy by physicians and a feeling on the part of many women that they were being mutilated without sufficient cause. Until years of research and observation on mastectomy patients have been completed (see ⚹152–53 above) a woman must depend on the personal opinions of her physicians, and what she reads in the press.

The approach to treatment of breast cancer suggested here is an individualized one. A surgeon must evaluate each patient's breast lump and her personal desires, and then present the options to her.

Weigh the options carefully: vanity or fear may be your worst enemies now—they must not deter you from choosing the best option *for cure*. Ask for a second opinion and compare the two.

A biopsy is necessary to prove malignancy.

Often, the section of tissue will be removed for analysis and will be frozen and tested while the patient is anesthetized in the operating room. If the test shows malignancy, the mastectomy will be performed before she wakes up. *This is advisable only when there is absolutely no doubt that a lump is malignant.* Occasionally, a mistake is made in the reading and unnecessary surgery is performed.

Some surgeons now perform biopsies on an outpatient basis. The woman waits a few days for preparation and reading of the permanent slides. This delay of the mastectomy (if indeed it is necessary) does not alter long-term survival or complication rate. (Ref. 40)

Procedures for biopsy include:

a. *Needle or drill biopsy:* most reliable for large and/or superficial lesions, but unreliable for small and deep lesions. These methods have the advantage of not leaving a scar.

b. Deep or small lesions picked up on mammography usually require *open biopsy under general anesthesia.* Performing this procedure under general anesthesia prevents patient discomfort and also better enables the surgeon to remove the lesion completely, control bleeding, and restore the shape of the breast.

c. *Waiting for the permanent sections of tissue* gives a better guarantee that there will be no error in the biopsy reading. A second opinion on the pathology slides may be requested by the woman and the slides may be mailed or hand-delivered to a pathologist at a cancer center or university hospital. *Of great importance, this small delay gives a woman the chance to know what may be about to happen to her.* She can discuss with her doctor which surgery and combined therapy are best for her. She knows what to expect and has some chance to adjust, or if she has objection to surgery, she can stop it. She can also switch to a cancer-treatment center if she has any doubts about the facilities at her present hospital.

159. Remember, in 80 per cent of biopsies, no malignancy will be found, so no further treatment will be needed

160. Normal care after mastectomy

The usual hospital stay after a total or modified radical mastectomy is seven to ten days. A woman can expect pain in the incisional area and under the arm if the lymph nodes have been removed, but this is not severe and is readily controlled by pain medications. Small tubes are left beneath the skin and connected to a suction pump to drain blood and tissue fluid and help the skin adhere to the chest wall. They are removed within a few days.

Within the first five days, begin exercises to maintain the full range of motion in the shoulder and arm on the side where the surgery took place. This means that an already hurting area will hurt more—but it is absolutely imperative that the exercises be done. Not to do them is to risk having a frozen shoulder. (See ※161d below) Most of the exercises involve just lifting the arm from the shoulder, strengthening the grip, reaching a little higher every day as recovery progresses. (Hence, the name of the mastectomy patients' self-help group of the American Cancer Society—Reach for Recovery.)

After radical mastectomy, a woman may feel numb on the side of her chest which has been operated on or may find that the area is very sensitive to touch for up to a year afterward. Make adjustments in sexual relations to avoid this sensitivity. Partners should find a position that is comfortable for both without placing weight against the woman's chest.

161. Possible aftereffects of mastectomy

a. *Lymphedema, swelling of the arm,* is the most common long-term postoperative complication after radical or modified radical mastectomy occurring in about one-third of the women. It can occur immediately, or years later, because of the blockage in the small lymph vessels that ordinarily drain from the arm into the lymph nodes of the armpit. Women who have had postoperative infections or who receive radiation treatments to the underarm area are more likely to experience this complication.

Some methods of controlling lymphedema are

a. Diuretics (medications that cut down on the amount of water the body retains),

b. Low-salt diets which do likewise, and

c. Elastic sleeves. Physical-therapy machines are available which massage the arm, starting at the hand and gradually pushing all the accumulated fluid toward the shoulder. This treatment may have to be repeated frequently; an elastic sleeve is a must in conjunction with it.

Exercise of the arm and shoulder is the very best way to prevent lymphedema and to keep it under control after it occurs.

d. *Frozen shoulder, with pain whenever it is moved,* can be a problem if postoperative exercises are neglected. Heat treatments can help; some physicians suggest steroid injections into the shoulder joints, as though treating arthritis. Again, the best way to avoid this unnecessary complication is to do the suggested postoperative exercises no matter how much they hurt at the time.

162. Emotional aftereffects of mastectomy

Most women suffer depression and anxiety after this operation, partly because they have been sick with cancer and fear its recurrence, mostly because they feel mutilated, and anticipate rejection by friends and lover. Some people say that every woman who undergoes mastectomy needs psychotherapy. That may be extreme; psychotherapy is best kept for counseling *abnormal* emotional responses. Crying jags, depression after mastectomy is, if it is any comfort, a normal response. Seek counsel first from the volunteers at Reach for Recovery. They will come and see you in the hospital, or at home; they've been through it too; just meeting a woman who has recovered, who knows what the bad time is like, how important the exercises are, will be a source of strength for you.

Sexual partners adjust to mastectomy far more easily than many women expect them to. Discuss your feelings openly with the men and women in your life; resume sexual activity as soon as possible. (Medically, sex is fine as soon as you come home from the hospital.) A woman may find it more difficult to adjust if she does not have a loving relationship in her life, but *talk* to the people around you—*don't retreat* —you need them now, and they will rise to the occasion. (Ref. 41)

And remember: the most important thing about the millions of women who have had mastectomies in this country is not that they have come through harrowing and serious surgery but that they have, for the most part, been *cured* of cancer.

163. When do you know the cancer will not return?

It is certainly wise for women who have had a tumor removed from one breast to suspect that cancer might recur in the other breast, and to follow to the letter her instructions for postoperative care, to check herself frequently, and to have low-dose mammography (see ✕169 below) once a year.

Some cases recur as late as ten to fifteen years, but most physicians will estimate that after five years, a woman has a good chance at non-recurrence.

164. Prostheses—artificial breasts—after mastectomy

a. An exterior silicone prosthesis can be fitted and matched to the other breast before the woman leaves the hospital. It looks fine when you are dressed. It is not a good idea to wear it with your bra when you are making love—because of the possible discomfort and also because your partner needs to make his or her own adjustment to your surgery.

b. Reconstruction of the breast through plastic surgery, right after mastectomy or later on, is a growing medical project, and women should encourage research into its possibilities.

If the cancerous lesion has been small, and a total or modified radical mastectomy was performed, some surgeons now leave more skin than usual so that a silicone prosthesis can be placed under it. Initial reports show that when this is done in cases of cancer detected early, there is no additional risk of recurrence. (Ref. 42)

Check on the possibility of such an implant *before* you have your surgery—especially if you are not having a radical mastectomy. (*The possibility of prosthesis implanting is all the more reason to wake up between the biopsy and the surgery. (See ✕158 above)*

Many people believe that the worst psychological effect of mastectomy could be stopped if a fairly normal-looking prosthesis could be placed under the skin. (Ref. 43) This is one area of medical development in which women should be vitally concerned.

165. The earlier breast cancer is detected, the better chance for a cure

If all breast tumors could be detected before they were one centimeter in diameter, the cure rate by almost any therapy would be 80–90 per cent.

Like other cancers, breast cancer has a premalignant stage, a carcinoma-in-situ stage and an invasive stage. The earlier you find it, the better your chance of a cure *without* a radical mastectomy and the better your chance that mastectomy will not be followed by a recurrence.

166. How breast cancer is detected

There are five major ways in which breast cancer is detected:
a. Self-examination;
b. Examination by a physician;
c. Low-dose mammography, a new X-ray technique;
d. Thermography;
c. Newer experimental methods.

167. Self-examination

Women should learn to examine their breasts as soon as they have passed puberty. Do the examination every month on the last day of menstrual bleeding or immediately after the menstrual period ends. This timing will eliminate some of the unnecessary alarm that women feel when they examine their breasts during the week before menstruation, when swelling, tenderness, and prominence of the glandular tissue of the breast are quite normal. (After menopause any time will do.)

First. Look at your breasts in the mirror. Look for symmetry. Look to see if either breast has any bumps protruding or if there is any tightening of the skin, as though over a swelling or any puckering. If you press your hands on your hips, you will accentuate your breasts and be better able to observe them. Bend forward and look again.

Second. Still looking in the mirror, raise your hands over your head and watch to make sure that the nipples move upward with the rest of the breast. If either nipple seems stuck, if it doesn't move upward, and this is a change, see a doctor right away.

Third. Lie down on a firm surface. With your left hand, palpate all areas of your right breast; keep your right arm behind your head. Move your fingers in a rotary motion, pressing the tissue against the chest wall. Then switch sides. Put your left hand behind your head, examine your left breast with your right hand. Remember to gently squeeze both nipples to see if there is any discharge. A small amount of crusty discharge is normal. A bloody discharge is not, nor is a heavy discharge that seems continuous, not drying.

What you are feeling for and looking for is any swelling, or lump or any change in the texture under the skin of the breast. Breast tumors start out very small—the lump might feel like a pea or a marble under the skin, perhaps like a group of tiny pebbles. Remember, you are looking for something *under the skin:* an eruption, a pimple or sore perhaps from the chafing of a bra is almost surely not cancer. Compare the same areas in each breast. In addition, try not to confuse the breastbone, ribs, and the overlying muscles with a lump in the breast, or— and this is harder to differentiate—the breast glands that normally swell depending on what stage of the menstrual cycle you are in. *When in doubt, see a doctor.* It may be embarrassing to be told that the lump you thought you felt was really a rib—but it's also comforting.

168. Examination by a physician

When you have your annual or biannual gynecological examination, make sure your physician includes an examination of the breasts.

The doctor will feel the breasts with both hands, prodding, pushing, to make sure that no lump or thickening is present. You must undress for this procedure. *Examination through the clothes or inside the bra is inadequate.*

No woman should depend entirely on examination by a doctor in guarding herself against breast cancer. *You must do self-examination every month!*

169. Low-dose mammography

Mammography is a kind of breast X ray which is currently the most effective method of detecting incipient tumors *before they are large,* at a stage when they can be completely cured with surgery or other therapy.

The trouble is, X ray itself is a known carcinogen—and some feel that if breast X ray becomes a frequent, routine procedure, it will actually cause cancer in some women. This has not been proven, but only women in high-cancer-risk categories (see #143 above) should have their breasts X-rayed yearly, or every two or three years. Younger women with no reason to suspect their health, who are examining themselves monthly, having a doctor examine them yearly, should not use delmammography until they are fifty or older.

RECOMMENDATION: Choose low-dose mammography over regular mammography, because the radiation exposure is much less. The two differ only in the type of film on which the X rays are printed. One low-dose method is xeromammography, but other *lower*-dose methods are also available.

170. Who should have routine mammography?

Some women run a relatively high risk of breast cancer and they should have xeromammography every year, or every two or three years, depending on the severity of the predisposition. They are women

a. Over fifty;

b. Aged forty to forty-nine, with strong history of breast cancer in the family, or history of cancer in one breast;

c. Over thirty-five years old with a history of cancer in one breast.

Reports should be appearing in the next few years on the pros and cons of low-dose mammography, so *watch for them.*

In the meantime, younger women with an increased risk of breast cancer (see #143 above) should examine themselves routinely and have a physician check them every four to six months.

171. Opinion: Don't trust in thermography, a screening method for breast cancer which is not as reliable as delmammography

Thermography tests for hot spots on the breast with the idea that they may indicate incipient cancer. The great advantage of this method is that it is apparently without side effects. The disadvantage is that the method produces false results in many cases. At the present time it should not be relied upon as the sole screening method for women in the high-risk group. (See ⚹170 above) It is safe as a yearly check for women in low-risk groups, but should never replace self-examination and examination by physicians, and delmammography for high-risk women. (Ref. 44, 45) Other methods of screening, such as ultrasound and other heat methods are being tested. *Watch for news!*

172. What happens if a breast lump is detected?

If a breast lump is detected, or suspected, see a doctor *immediately.* Don't wait to see if the lump will go away; don't try not to think about it; have it checked. *Fewer than one-fifth of the breast lumps discovered by self-examination are cancerous.* A number of benign breast diseases can produce suspicious symptoms that are not cancer. *In 80 per cent of all cases,* lumps detected by any means will turn out to be benign.

The physician may attempt to aspirate the lump with a syringe in the office. If there is any fluid in it, that will be drawn off and usually sent for a Pap smear. Fluid generally indicates that the lump is a benign cyst. However, it is important that a woman who has had a cyst aspirated return for a checkup within a few weeks. *If the cyst reappears, it must be biopsied.*

Sometimes the lump is not a cyst but just a benign mass that has grown in the breast. It can be removed in hospital under local or general anesthesia.

173. Benign breast lumps that disappear sometimes occur in young women

Malignant tumors of the breast are very rare in women under twenty-five. Sometimes, as the breasts develop, lumps will appear that are no danger at all. These should be observed by a physician over time, and only if they don't go away is further treatment in order.

174. Pain is not usually a symptom of cancer

Generally, cancer is not accompanied by pain until it is far advanced. Pain is, however, a frequent sign of fibrocystic disease of the breast, as is premenstrual tenderness. (See ⚹176 below)

175. Nipple discharge is a possible symptom of cancer

A small amount of crusty discharge from the nipple is normal; only if it is continuous or heavy and *doesn't dry* is there something to worry about.

A watery or milky discharge sometimes results from vigorous manipulation of the breasts during sexual relations. Some tranquilizers, by their effect on the hypothalamus, can cause milky nipple discharge.

Similar discharge can occur when there is some misfunction of the hypothalamus after childbirth or after stopping the pill. (See p. 53) If the discharge persists or is heavy, consult a physician. The problem is not cancer in some cases, but an endocrine specialist will probably be needed.

If the nipple discharge is bloody, brownish or green, and occurs in one breast only, this may be an important sign of malignancy. In this case, or any case which disturbs you, a smear of the discharge can be sent for a Pap smear to detect any malignant cells. In addition, mammography can be done if there is no palpable mass and the woman is over age forty.

176. Fibrocystic disease of the breast

Fibrocystic disease of the breast usually occurs in women over twenty-five and probably results from a hormonal imbalance that can be triggered by a vast range of causes. It is believed that the imbalance allows estrogen to predominate in the body and stimulate the growth of the glands and fibrous tissue of the breast, creating a number of small lumps and distentions, usually in the outer areas of the breast. Some women will experience the growth of cysts that seem to come and go; some will experience growths in the fibrous tissues.

The major symptom is both the visible swelling *and pain* (a pretty good indication that the condition is *not* cancer. Padded bras with very good support are essential treatment. If the cysts grow large, aspiration (see #172 above) in the physician's office may be a good treatment. Usually, fibrocystic disease comes in spurts and goes away. It is not dangerous in itself, but a woman who suffers from it is considered a higher than average risk for breast cancer and should have herself checked routinely. In severe cases, danocrine (see p. 344) has been shown to have good results. (Ref. 46) An interesting recent report shows that cutting down on foods containing xanthines (coffee, tea, colas, chocolate) can reverse or reduce cystic disease. (Ref. 47) Try this method, coupled with examinations by your doctor.

177. Fibroadenomas: benign tumors of the breast

These are the most common tumors in young women. Characteristically they are firm, round, and movable, and feel like a marble under the skin of the breast. These can usually be removed simply under local anesthesia. The only significance of these benign tumors is that they *may* indicate a somewhat higher risk for cancer at a later time. (Ref. 48)

178. Breast abscess

Some masses in the breast and discharges from the nipple occur because of infections in the glands and ducts of the breast. These are common after childbirth or during breast-feeding. They can be treated with antibiotics but occasionally have to be drained surgically.

CERVICAL CANCER AND OTHER TUMORS OF THE REPRODUCTIVE TRACT

Breast cancer is the most common cancer in American women. After that comes gastrointestinal (approx. 88,000 cases annually), endometrial (37,000), lung (30,000), and cervical (16,000 cases of the invasive type), according to the National Cancer Institute. (Ref. 49)

Cancer of the cervix is unique in that an easy test—the Pap smear—(see ※182 below) makes early detection sure and simple, allowing complete cure in almost 100 per cent of cases.

Other tumors and cysts, both cancerous and non-cancerous, are common in the reproductive tract: almost all are curable through drugs and/or surgery. In general, the two major ways that a woman can guard herself against these diseases is to have regular examinations with Pap smear, and to be most attentive to any deviation from her normal menstrual cycle.

179. Cervical cancer

Approximately 16,000 new cases of cervical cancer are detected each year; about 7,400 women die of the disease yearly, almost always because they neglected the routine examinations that could have led to early detection and treatment. About 1 per cent of all American women get cancer of the cervix. Carcinoma-in-situ is excluded from these statistics. (See ※184 below)

180. Cervical cancer is related to sexual activity

Cervical cancer almost never occurs in sexually *inactive* women.

It seems to occur more frequently in women who

a. Started sexual activity at an early age;

b. Had an early first pregnancy;

c. Have multiple sexual partners.

Only 10 per cent of the women who contract the disease have never been pregnant. Jewish women show lower rates of cervical cancer than women from other cultural backgrounds. At one time, this was attributed to the fact that Jewish men were always circumcised. Today, however, even when almost *all* American men are circumcised, the ethnic differentiation in the disease mysteriously remains the same.

181. Herpes II virus may cause cervical cancer

The herpes II virus (see ✕31 above) is now widely held to be a factor in developing cervical cancer. The exact cause and effect is not clear, except that women with positive blood tests for herpes II show a higher incidence of cervical cancer. (Ref. 7) A woman who has had herpes is by no means a sure victim of cervical cancer; any more than a woman who has had cystic mastitis will surely get breast cancer. However, if you have had herpes, have a Pap smear every six months. The relationship between herpes and cervical cancer has led many physicians to now classify cancer of the cervix as a venereal disease, that is, one that is transmitted through sexual activity.

182. Pap smear: the way to detect cervical cancer early

George Papanicolaou was born and educated in Greece and was working in the Pathology Department of New York Hospital when he published his revolutionary book on the cytology—the cell structure— of the female genital tract in 1943. In this book he described the changes in the cells of the cervix and the vagina in response to 'hormones at different stages of the menstrual cycle. He also described early changes in the cells of the cervix among women who had cervical cancer. His work became the basis for a simple laboratory test. Named for Papanicolaou, the Pap smear detects cancer of the cervix in its earliest stages.

During her regular examination, scrapings are taken from the external part of the woman's cervix, as high up in the canal as possible (this causes a small cramp at most). Then the scrapings are analyzed in a lab; if cancer is present, the cell changes on the slide will show it. The Pap test detects cancer in its earliest and most frequently curable stage. *The Pap test should be a routine part of the gynecologic exam in all women, and should be performed at least once a year.* If abnormalities have been noted in the past, the test should be performed more frequently. The test is not 100 per cent accurate, with a small number of false negatives and positives. (Pap smears can also be done on cells from the breasts, lungs, and other organs to look for malignancy.)

183. The "do-it-yourself" Pap smear

For women who cannot or will not have regular gynecologic examinations, "do-it-yourself" vaginal lavage kits are available for Pap smears. (Call your local Health Department for information.) You squirt a small amount of water up into the cervix, then suck it back out with the same device and mail it to the lab for a reading. This test is not as accurate as the standard Pap smear (40 per cent vs. 90–95 per cent) *and it is only recommended for women who find themselves unable to obtain gynecologic care for long periods of time.* This test does not detect uterine or ovarian cancer; like the cervical Pap test it is specifically for cervical cancer.

184. The several stages of cervical cancer

The disease passes through several stages before it becomes invasive and begins to metastasize. In the earliest stages, there are no symptoms at all. The Pap test is used to detect the disease prior to invasive cancer and can be supplemented by colposcopy. (See ✕187 below)

a. The earliest stage is *dysplasia* (dis-PLAYS-ya). The most superficial cells have begun to change and are mildly abnormal. Some women with dysplasia will develop more severe changes, others will return to normal. No one can predict who will fall into which group *so all cases of dysplasia are treated or watched closely with repeat Pap smears.*

b. The second stage is called *carcinoma-in-situ* (*sigh-too*): a cancer is present, but limited to the outside layers of the cervix. (This is the latent stage, see ✕141 above.) This stage is not reversible, but is completely curable. Treatment is cone biopsy in the young (see ✕186 below) or hysterectomy in a woman whose family is complete.

c. The third stage of cervical cancer is called *invasive.* The disease has metastasized beyond the outer layers of the cervix and invaded the pelvis. Treatment is either radiation and/or surgery, depending on the extent of the tumor.

185. Steps after an abnormal Pap smear

The first thing to do after a Pap smear turns up abnormal is to do it over, just to make sure the laboratory has not made an error. Lab results are classified as follows:

A Class 1 result—test is normal; no cancer.

A Class 2 result—test indicates either infection of the cervix or mild dysplasia. Most of these cases will revert back to *Class 1,* so a repeat Pap smear is done.

If the Class 2 reading persists, then colposcopy is frequently done to localize and remove the abnormal areas.

A Class 3 Pap smear signifies moderate to severe dysplasia.

Class 4 and 5 Pap smears indicate carcinoma-in-situ, or invasive cancer.

Women with Class 3 tests or worse *must* have colposcopy and in some cases cone biopsy.

186. Cone biopsy of the cervix

In order to determine the full extent of the abnormality, a cone-shaped wedge of tissue is removed from the cervix and sent to the lab to be examined by the pathologist. This will be final proof that invasive cancer is not present. The biopsy is done in the hospital under anesthesia.

Cone biopsy of the cervix is a relatively safe procedure, but has a degree of complications, such as bleeding, stenosis of the cervix (see p. 362), infertility and incompetent cervix (see p. 166). RECOMMENDATION: *Where possible, colposcopy is preferable.*

187. Colposcopy: a new method of diagnosis and biopsy for cervical cancer

In colposcopy, a new procedure in which many physicians are becoming skilled, the cervix is cleansed and observed directly through a microscope in the office. Any abnormal areas are biopsied and sent for pathological report. In 75 per cent of the cases, colposcopy bypasses the need for hospital admission and cone biopsy. However, if the entire suspicious area of the cervix is not visualized, a cone biopsy must be done.

188. Steps to be taken if dysplasia is noted on biopsy

If dysplasia is noted on the Pap smear and colposcopy is adequate for evaluation and treatment, then follow-up Pap smears should be taken every three months for the first year and every six months thereafter. Some physicians are treating dysplasia with cryosurgery (see p. 309) that freeze-cauterizes the lining of the cervix and allows removal of affected tissues. Women who undergo this procedure should have themselves checked thereafter to make sure that dysplasia does not recur.

WARNING: *Cryosurgery to treat dysplasia must always be performed by a specialist in cancer therapy who will use the colposcope to identify the correct areas. It is a risky procedure if used improperly to treat more advanced stages than dysplasia.* Even in the treatment of dysplasia by cryosurgery, long-term studies are not yet available to show whether this is a safe treatment.

In cases of severe dysplasia, where carcinoma-in-situ seems a very likely next stage, hysterectomy may be suggested. This removes the risk of cervical cancer entirely, but it is a major abdominal operation that involves risks of its own. Think it over carefully, and seek an additional opinion.

189. What to do if carcinoma-in-situ is discovered

If the disease has progressed to the stage of carcinoma-in-situ, have a cone biopsy to rule out invasive cancer. If all the tumor seems to have been removed, and if the woman desires more children, she can go ahead and have them *if she is very closely watched by her doctors.*

If she has completed her family, hysterectomy is usually suggested. However, if a woman wants to avoid hysterectomy, and the doctor thinks that all the tumor was removed with cone biopsy, then it is quite safe to have frequent Pap smears (every three months). If the carcinoma-in-situ returns, the woman should proceed with hysterectomy.

Some physicians are using therapy with laser beams in the treatment of carcinoma-in-situ. Again this is an experimental method with no long-term studies available.

190. Opinion: Simple hysterectomy is recommended treatment for cervical cancer in-situ if hysterectomy is needed at all

Simple hysterectomy (see ⚹109 above), vaginal or abdominal, is the proper treatment for cervical in-situ cancer. *The ovaries need not be removed.* Afterward, a woman will still experience normal hormone cycles, with all that these mean to general well-being. Pap smears are a vital part of postoperative care, for a small number of women will also develop carcinoma-in-situ of the upper vagina, also detectable by the Pap smear.

191. Steps to be taken if invasive cancer is discovered

A woman with invasive cancer should, if at all possible, seek treatment at a center, usually a university hospital, which specializes in Gynecologic Oncology. Here she will find physicians who have passed examinations in a superspecialty—cancer of the female genital tract. They are simply better trained in the newest and most effective treatments than the woman's regular gynecologist. Treatment usually involves radiation and/or surgery. Chemotherapy is not as well developed as radiotherapy and surgery. A list of such centers in your locality may be obtained from the State Medical Society or from the American College of Obstetrics and Gynecology, 1 East Wacker Drive, Chicago, IL 60601. Women should remember that even at this more advanced stage, cervical cancer can be controlled sometimes for years and in many cases, cured completely.

192. Cancer of the uterus/endometrium

Cancer of the endometrium, the lining of the uterus, is the most common cancer of the female reproductive tract (37,000 new cases and 3,300 deaths yearly). It occurs mostly in postmenopausal women and is more common in women who have not ever been pregnant. *This cancer seems to be associated with*

a. *excess estrogen production, for instance in women who are not ovulating regularly, and with*

b. *general metabolic and endocrine imbalance, as in diabetes, hypertension, and obesity.* Women who do not ovulate for long periods of time should receive progesterone for several days every three to six months, to prevent the constant effect of estrogen on the endometrium.

Recently, an increase of this type of cancer has been reported in women who have been receiving estrogen during menopause (Ref. 27, 28). Women using estrogen for menopausul symptoms should also take progesterone periodically to counter the effects of estrogen on the endometrium. (See p. 291)

193. Bleeding is a major symptom of endometrial cancer

In the earliest stages of this tumor, a woman will frequently experience heavy menstrual bleeding, bleeding between periods, or bleeding after menopause. In this phase, it is impossible to determine whether cancer, polyps, or just hormonal imbalance causes the bleeding, so a D & C should be performed for diagnosis.

194. Stages of endometrial cancer and the treatment for each

a. The earliest stage is *hyperplasia,* the equivalent of the dysplasia stage in the cervical cancer. In young women, in women who have been taking estrogen, or in women who are not good risks for surgery, high doses of progesterone (or progestogens) may be used for three to six months in an effort to reverse the hyperplasia. Estrogens should be stopped. After this time, have a repeat D & C to make sure that the hyperplasia has disappeared, followed by endometrial biopsies or washings (see ✕195 below). If the hyperplasia is severe or does not respond to progesterone therapy, a total hysterectomy is the usual treatment.

b. The next stage is carcinoma-in-situ, when the tumor is in the uppermost layers of the endometrium. Treatment is hysterectomy and removal of the ovaries.

c. *If the tumor is invasive,* the woman should be treated at a regional oncology center, with radiation and/or surgery, depending on the extent of the spread.

Chemotherapy with hormones, particularly progestogens, is frequently used.

195. Endometrial biopsy and washing

Endometrial cancer is not always detected by the routine Pap test. However, several types of mini-suction or lavaging (washing) devices can obtain cells from the lining of the uterus for pathologic reading. Some physicians prefer using endometrial biopsy (mini-curettage) to obtain these samples. (See p. 104) These tests can be performed in the office, with minimal discomfort. *Certain women should have these routinely:*

    a. Those in high-risk groups (see ✕192 above) starting estrogen therapy

    b. Those already on estrogen therapy more than one year

    c. Those who have had hyperplasia

    d. Those with mildly irregular bleeding at menopause

196. Good news: Cure rates for cancer of the cervix and uterus are excellent

Even when the disease becomes invasive, chances of its being controlled and reversed through surgery and/or radiation and possible chemotherapy are excellent. No woman with either disease should feel hopeless. She should welcome the treatment suggested to her and prepare to live on for a long time.

197. Ovarian cancer should be checked for after menopause

Women who are postmenopausal should continue to have routine gynecologic examinations, for at the present time this is the only way to detect early cancer of the ovary. Most tumors of the ovary are benign, not malignant, but any abnormal enlargement should be evaluated.

198. Cancer of the vagina

    a. *Squamous cell cancer of the vagina* is a rare tumor found mainly in older women.

    b. *Clear-cell adenocarcinoma* is a cancer of the glandular tissue of the vagina that has been found in the daughters of women who took DES (diethylstilbestrol—die-ethyl-still-BES-troll) and related compounds during early pregnancy.

DES

---

199. Warning: Girls whose mothers took DES in early pregnancy should be checked for vaginal cell changes

DES is an artificial estrogen, which has been given to women early in pregnancy in an effort to prevent miscarriage. It was mainly used between 1948 and 1960, with peak use in the early 1950s.

    a. In 1971, Drs. Arthur Herbst, Howard Ulfelder, and David Poskanzer of the Gynecology Department at Massachusetts General Hospital reported a startling new rise in the incidence of *clear-cell adenocarcinoma* of the vagina among girls whose mothers had received the drug. (Ref. 24) About 350 cases of this tumor have been reported.

b. The other abnormality of the cervix and vagina occurring in DES-exposed girls is *adenosis,* a proliferation of the glandular tissue of the cervix, extending into the vagina. This change is much more common than the cancer and occurs in as many as 90 per cent of the exposed girls. (Cancer occurs in about 1/1000 to 1/10,000.) *The adenosis does not appear to progress to the clear-cell cancer in most cases.* However, all young women whose mothers were exposed to DES should be evaluated and followed closely.

c. Very disturbing recent reports have shown that as many as 75–85 per cent of young women with DES exposure may have abnormalities of the uterus as well. (Ref. 50) In addition, women exposed to DES in utero, appear to have a higher incidence of incompetent cervix (see p. 166) when they get pregnant. (Ref. 51)

d. There are also worries that DES-exposed women may be at higher risk for cervical dysplasia. (Ref. 52, 53) So Pap tests every six months are essential. These reports await confirmation.

200. Evaluation of women exposed to DES

Any woman who took DES or related drugs during pregnancy should get her daughter to a special gynecologic oncology center for at least one examination by colposcopy. (See ✗187 above) The test can usually be done in the office; if this is not possible, then under general anesthesia. Biopsies of the cervix or any abnormal areas in the vagina are done at this time. A girl should be examined first at about age fourteen or whenever she starts having any vaginal bleeding.

If adenosis or any other abnormalities are noted to confirm the DES exposure, Pap smears are recommended every six months. If any abnormalities are noted on the Pap smears, then the colposcopy will be repeated. If any malignancy, or premalignant condition is detected, make sure this is treated at a cancer center. Surgery is not the proper treatment of adenosis.

The proper way of evaluating DES daughters for abnormalities of the uterus has not been established. Within a year or so, if the reports of uterine abnormalities are corroborated, it may well be that certain women with DES exposure will be evaluated with hysterograms as well. (See p. 105)

Other recent reports suggest that the mothers who took DES may be at higher risk for the development of breast cancer. (Ref. 54) These women should be very careful to do routine self-breast exams and to have routine screening examinations. (See ✗167 above)

The management of DES-exposed women will probably change

greatly over the next few years. The women involved should keep in close touch with their nearest DES center (or cancer center) to keep up on the news.

201. Psychologic aspects of DES exposure

A woman who discovers that by taking DES during pregnancy, she endangered her daughter, is in for a dreadful duel with painful, self-defeating guilt. The girl herself is probably at an age when gynecologic examinations are not yet routine, where she is developing a normal awareness of her own genitals; it is a terrible time indeed to be faced with the fear of cancer and all the probing that goes with it. Some centers are using video cameras or mirrors to allow the young women to see the lesions directly—*this is very helpful, because the adenosis is not deforming;* the girl and her parents usually have had much worse fantasies.

Psychologic counselors are available at all centers. *Use them!* Discuss your fears and feelings with them. Contact DES-Watch and other patients' organizations dealing with this same problem; these are groups of women and their daughters who have become very knowledgeable about DES exposure. They will provide the comfort of informed counsel. This is a time when, at all costs, the love of mother and daughter, one for the other, must be preserved.

202. Boys may be affected by DES too

Some studies show that males exposed to DES in the uterus may have a significant increase in genital abnormalities such as cysts, small testicles, and low sperm counts. (Ref. 55, 56) They should have careful urologic examinations.

203. The medical irony of the DES problem

It will be many years before the entire spectrum of DES damage is detected. The medical irony is that this drug probably was not effective in preventing miscarriage, although it was given in good faith by many physicians. This should be enough to warn women and physicians alike to avoid *any* medications, if at all possible, during pregnancy (especially in the first three months).

204. Opinion: Fight to remove DES from animal feed!

People who eat beef are chronically exposed to DES, which is still being used in feed to fatten cattle before slaughter. While there is no proof that enough DES gets to someone eating the meat to do damage, in principle this is an outrage! All citizens fight to get this agent out of cattle feed.

For information booklet on DES, write for DHEW Publication ✗ (NIH) 76-1118 "Questions and Answers about DES exposure Before Birth," U. S. Department HEW, National Institutes of Health, Bethesda, MD. Also lists all similar drugs which might have affected the children.

ANEMIA

Anemia refers to a shortage of red blood cells. The strength of the body depends on the reliability and quality of its blood supply, and when the blood is deficient, the body is not getting the oxygen and other nutrients it needs to function well. Because healthy women bleed every month, anemia is always a threat; it can result from something as simple as one overly heavy menstrual flow. Sometimes anemia is the *principal* disease process, sometimes, the secondary result of another disease or injury.

205. Blood count: the principal test for anemia

There are two ways to perform a blood count.

a. A blood sample is taken and measured for hematocrit—the percentage of red blood cells in the total volume of blood taken. For healthy women who are not anemic, the red blood cell count is between 36 and 44 per cent.

b. *Hemoglobin* is a protein in the red blood cells that carries oxygen. Another kind of blood test shows the hemoglobin value in the sample of blood taken—a woman is not anemic if the hemoglobin value is over 12.0 grams per 100 cubic centimeters of blood.

One of these tests should be part of a routine medical exam of any kind, including a gynecological exam. Many other types of tests can be performed on blood samples, so *always know why the blood is being drawn.*

206. Bone marrow: the source of red blood cells

Red blood cells are manufactured in the bone marrow. For this process to occur, many elements must be present. The bone marrow must have adequate supplies of iron and certain vitamins such as folic acid (which can be found in green leafy vegetables and liver) and Vitamin B-12. In addition, the genes which govern the formation of the protein hemoglobin must be normal.

207. General symptoms of anemia

Symptoms characteristic of anemia, no matter what the cause, include: fatigue, light-headedness, headaches, pale nail beds and, occasionally, numbness and tingling in fingers and toes.

208. Types of anemia relevant to women
  a. Hereditary anemias
  b. Vitamin-deficiency anemias
  c. Iron-deficiency anemia

209. Hereditary anemias

The four most common types of hereditary anemia found in the United States are

  a. *Thalassemia,* in which the production of the hemoglobin molecule is not totally synchronized. Parts of the molecule are underproduced, leaving an excess of other parts. This excess (alpha-chains) clutter up the red blood cells, making them abnormal and causing them to get stuck in the spleen and bone marrow as they pass through the circulation. Here the cells are destroyed causing an enlarged spleen and other effects such as jaundice;

  b. *Spherocytosis,* in which the red cells are perfectly round, a shape which makes them get stuck in the spleen. As in thalassemia the spleen enlarges and the person becomes anemic because of the loss of red cells;

  c. *Glucose-6-phosphate-dehydrogenase deficiency* (*G-6-P-D deficiency*) in which an enzyme is missing from the red cells so that they are destroyed if certain drugs are taken; and

  d. *Sickle-cell anemia* the most common hereditary anemia in the United States.

210. Sickle-cell anemia, a hereditary anemia affecting American blacks

A recessive gene (see p. 215) is inherited from ancestors long gone and carried by some of their descendants. Along with the other anemias mentioned above (⚹209), sickle-cell anemia is a recessive-gene disease and approximately 5–10 per cent of black Americans carry the trait for it.

A person with sickle-cell trait has one normal and one abnormal gene for producing hemoglobin. Such a person may not be anemic—but can pass the trait on to children. If both father and mother have sickle-cell trait, the odds are one to four that their child will have sickle-cell anemia.

Sickle-cell *trait* is not, therefore, dangerous in itself.

In *sickle-cell anemia,* the hemoglobin molecule in the red cells is abnormal. When enough of the hemoglobin molecules have a low-oxygen content, the red cells tend to form into a sickle shape in the blood stream. The abnormal cells get stuck in the small blood vessels, the liver, and the spleen, and break down there, causing anemia. Unfortunately, treatment and control of this disease is very limited and people with sickle-cell anemia have a chronic debilitating disease which usually causes an early death.

211. How to prevent sickle-cell anemia

Because of the severe nature of the disease and the current lack of good treatment methods for sickle-cell anemia, black men and women may want to consider being tested for sickle-cell trait. A simple blood test will determine whether you carry the trait. These are readily available at all labs and public health centers. If both partners have sickle trait, there is a one in four chance that this couple would have a child with sickle-cell anemia.

Watch for news: Within the next year or so, it may be possible to routinely detect sickle-cell anemia prenatally by amniocentesis (see pp. 216–17) so that abortion will be an option if it is determined that the fetus is affected by the disease. Couples who both have sickle trait may also want to consider artificial insemination as a preventive method. (See pp. 112–113)

212. Vitamin-deficiency anemias

In women, these anemias are most commonly caused by a lack of folic acid or a lack of Vitamin B-12. They are called megaloblastic anemias (*megalo* meaning big; *blast* for cell) because on a blood smear, the cells show larger than normal.

213. Folic-acid-deficiency anemia

Folic acid comes from green leafy vegetables and liver.

A lot of people hate liver and some don't like salad either. If you won't eat lettuce, try to eat spinach, cabbage, broccoli, or escarole. If you eat neither greens nor liver, take supplements of folic acid. (See p. 268 for MDR)

Folic-acid deficiency is quite common during pregnancy (see p. 176) when the fetus is drawing on the total supply in a woman's body. In addition, there are reports of folic-acid deficiency among women on the pill. OPINION: Pregnant women and women on the pill should routinely take a folic-acid supplement—0.8 mg per day is adequate.

Certain drugs such as phenytoin (Dilantin) used for seizures cause folic-acid-deficiency anemia if a supplement is not taken. Alcoholic women suffer from this anemia as well.

214. Vitamin B-12 deficiency anemia

More common in older women, this disease occurs when a substance in the stomach (intrinsic factor), which normally allows B-12 to be absorbed, runs into short supply. This is "pernicious anemia." Other diseases such as regional ileitis may cause poor absorption of B-12 from the digestive tract. Treatment requires monthly B-12 *shots;* pills of B-12 are not absorbed by these women.

In very rare cases, vegetarians who eat no eggs or milk (in addition to no meat) also become deficient in B-12. These women need supplemental B-12, and for them pills are fine.

215. Remember: good nutrition can prevent and cure most vitamin-deficiency anemias

Somehow, good nutrition often stops after childhood. This silly mistake can take a severe toll on a woman's health. *A woman must feed herself as well as she feeds anyone in her family.*

216. Iron-deficiency anemia

This type of anemia is the most common among women.

Bone marrow contains more than enough iron to supply a normally menstruating woman who eats properly. Menstrual flow normally carries iron out of the body, but the iron is usually replenished during the weeks of the cycle when the woman is not bleeding.

However, a number of other factors can interrupt this course of events.

a. During pregnancy, iron-deficiency anemia is common as the fetus makes inroads into the woman's iron supply.

b. If for any reason menstrual flow is very heavy, too much iron can be lost and the manufacture of red blood cells slowed down so that anemia results.

c. Surgery or serious injury, with accompanying severe loss of blood, can cause this anemia.

Iron-deficiency anemia differs from vitamin-deficiency anemia in that the red blood cells become abnormally small instead of abnormally large.

217. Who runs a high risk of iron-deficiency anemia?

Women with poor diets, heavy menses, pregnant women, women using IUDs, women who have had major surgery or sustained a severe injury are all at a high risk for iron-deficiency anemia. These women should ask their doctors to check for anemia, and, if present, iron supplements should be used.

ARTHRITIS

Arthritis refers generally to a whole group of diseases which cause painful swelling, redness, and sometimes damage to joints. Aches and pains in the joints do not signify arthritis unless there is swelling, heat, redness, or changes which show up on the X ray of the joint. In the public mind, arthritis is more associated with age than sex. However, some forms affect women particularly.

218. Types of joint disease common in women
  a. Rheumatoid arthritis
  b. Degenerative joint disease or osteoarthritis.
  c. Lupus erythematosus and rheumatic fever
  d. Tendonitis—"tennis elbow," "housemaid's knee"
  e. Infectious—gonorrhea, rubella

219. Rheumatoid arthritis
Rheumatoid arthritis occurs three times more often in women than in men, more often in northern climates, and increasing in incidence with age. At one time, it was thought to be passed on genetically—this theory is now discounted. It is estimated that 3 per cent of adult women have some form of this disease.

220. Rheumatoid arthritis is an autoimmune disease
In this disease as well as in other autoimmune diseases such as lupus and rheumatic fever, the body manufactures antibodies that work against its own normal functioning. The antibodies of this autoimmune disease can attack the membranes covering the joints (called synovia —sin-OH-via), the membrane covering the heart—the pericardium (perr-ih-CARD-ium)—the lungs and their coverings (pleura), and the abdominal cavity (peritoneum—per-ih-toe-NEE-um).

Rheumatoid arthritis affects the joints specifically; in severe cases, it can affect the heart and/or kidneys. *It is an inflammation, not an infection: it cannot be cured* but it can be controlled.

221. Course of rheumatoid arthritis
The synovia, membranes that cover and lubricate the joints so that they move easily and painlessly, become inflamed, usually in the fingers, knees, hips, spine. When the inflammation becomes severe, the

cartilage, ligaments, and tendons (joint supports) around the joint also become inflamed and begin to degenerate. The course of the disease varies with the individual: it can affect one joint, it can affect many; it can be very painful for a time; then for no apparent reason, the discomfort will stop until the next attack, which likewise may occur for no apparent reason. Rheumatoid arthritis can get worse or can remain about the same for years. It all depends on the individual. Most people have the mild form of rheumatoid arthritis, where the joint supports are not involved.

222. How rheumatoid arthritis is diagnosed

Any swelling, redness, and pain in the joints should be checked out. Rheumatoid arthritis is typically indicated by swelling in the finger joints closest to the palm and by the presence in the blood of a protein called "rheumatoid factor."

223. Treatment of rheumatoid arthritis

The principle of treatment is to prevent the inflammation from spreading to the cartilage, tendons, and ligaments that support the joints, and to relieve the pain and swelling so the arthritis sufferer can live more or less comfortably with the disease.

There are several elements to treatment:

a. Aspirin and aspirin compounds and several new anti-inflammatory drugs;

b. Regular periods of rest during the day; coupled with regular activity;

c. Application of heat to the affected areas.

For severe cases, treatments may be:

d. Injections of gold salts;

e. Anti-malarial drugs;

f. Corticosteroids;

g. Phenylbutazone, indomethacin, and other drugs;

h. Surgery

224. Aspirin as a treatment for rheumatoid arthritis

Aspirin is far and away the most successful therapy for mild rheumatoid arthritis, for it fights inflammation while dulling pain. Depending on the individual's needs, a doctor may allow a dosage of up to sixteen pills a day. (Never decide yourself how many aspirin per day is your limit, consult with a doctor, for even this most common remedy can be overindulged, with bad side effects.)

The cheapest aspirin is as good as any aspirin on the market. National advertising notwithstanding, the *essential* ingredients in aspirin are always the same, by law. Other ingredients may be added but these deal with other disorders besides arthritis—for example, ingredients may be added to aspirin to prevent stomach discomfort.

Rheumatoid arthritis sufferers take a lot of aspirin and may have difficulty tolerating it in such large amounts. It may produce stomach upset or at the worst, actual stomach bleeding.

Try taking the aspirin with some antacid liquid or on a full stomach. If that doesn't work, try coated aspirin, which is easier on the stomach, or an aspirin with antacid right in it. Most arthritis sufferers find a way to live with large amounts of aspirin; if they don't, they must resort to stronger, more expensive combination anti-inflammatory drugs that have their own side effects. (See ⸸225 below)

Other signs of aspirin-overdose are ringing in the ears or temporary hearing loss. This condition reverses itself as soon as the dosage is cut back. The side effects of aspirin mean essentially that there is a limit on how much you can take. That in turn means there is a limit on how much pain you can alleviate.

Other pain-killers, such as Darvon or codeine, may be used along with the aspirin, *but these drugs do not relieve the inflammation,* only the pain.

225. New drugs that can be used instead of aspirin

There are several new drugs which are now used widely with great success in treating arthritis. The most widely used of these is ibuprofen (Motrin), which, like aspirin, is an anti-inflammatory as well as an-tipain agent. In fact, some people find it works better than aspirin. The side effects are similar to aspirin and apparently no more severe. Fenoprofen calcium (Nalfon) is very similar to Motrin. Another new drug with much potential is Naproxen (Naprosyn). All these drugs await long-term-usage data, but at present seem very useful especially for rheumatoid arthritis and osteoarthritis. They are the anti-pros-taglandin drugs, which may work for dysmenorrhea as well. (See ⸸84 above) Another drug, sulindac (Clinoril) is being widely pro-moted but has no great advantages at present.

226. Periods of rest each day are essential for arthritis sufferers

The more motion, the more inflammation. If the joints get a rest, the inflammation is controlled. Rest may not be a simple matter to arrange, especially if your arthritis affects the joints you need to work with: a typist with arthritic fingers, for example, has a problem that wouldn't be so bad if she were a sales executive. In such a case, more aspirin will probably not help; you may just have to change your job.

227. Local heat as relief for arthritis

A warm soak or an infra-red lamp may ease the pain, as may a hydroculator (high-DROC-u-lator), a device for applying *moist* heat, which can be purchased at a medical-supply store. After applying heat, try gently exercising the joint.

228. Muscle weakness: the role of physical therapy

Arthritis sufferers tend to sit still, to rest their aching joints. *Too much* rest may lead to a loss of tone in the muscles around the joints. When a woman returns to the activity she had given up because of arthritis, she may find she can't do it anymore—this time because she isn't strong enough. This is why a program of physical therapy should be set up for all arthritis sufferers. This will include range-of-motion exercises, isometrics, and heat treatments. Ask your physician for a referral to a physical therapist if you have moderate or severe arthritis.

229. Gold-salts injections: a treatment for severe rheumatoid arthritis

It is unclear why injections of gold salts reduce the pain and spread of severe arthritis, but they do, and if careful attention is paid to possible side effects, they may be very helpful. Before regular therapy begins, a small test dose should be given to test for possible allergy. If there is no allergy, then the shots are usually given once a week. It takes six to eight weeks, generally, to get a response. If the spread of the arthritis is stopped, then a monthly shot may suffice as maintenance. Oral gold salts may be available in this country soon; they are currently being tested in Europe.

Gold salts cause some *rare* side effects, including kidney damage and bone marrow damage. Therefore, have blood counts and urinalysis before each injection. Other side effects, also rare but not so dangerous, are skin rash and the appearance of small ulcers in the mouth. If any side effect appears, notify your doctor, who will probably stop the medication.

Penicillamine is a drug with similar effects and side effects as gold salts. It is currently being used widely in England and by many doctors in this country, although the FDA has not yet approved its use for arthritis. It seems to work for some women who do not respond to gold. (Ref. 57)

230. Antimalarial drugs as a treatment for severe rheumatoid arthritis

Certain drugs commonly used to treat malaria also seem to have good anti-inflammatory effect when used against rheumatoid arthritis. These include chloroquine (Aralen) and hydroxychloroquine (Plaquenil). Like gold salts, they need some time to begin working: four to six weeks. Some individuals experience side effects—nausea, vomiting, and skin rashes, loss of hair color. More serious is dimness of vision or photophobia, an abnormal sensitivity to light, or the sensation of seeing halos around lights. Women who are using these drugs to treat arthritis should have eye examinations every three to six months, so that any accumulation of the drug in the eye can be discovered, and the dosage cut down or out.

231. Corticosteroids: useful as treatment only for severe rheumatoid arthritis

The corticosteroids are a group of drugs which can be highly effective in relieving pain and stopping the spread of arthritic inflammation through the joint supports. *However, they should only be used in very severe cases: they have dangerous known side effects.* Low-maintenance doses can usually be taken safely, but in higher doses, steroids can cause unhealthful weight gain, stomach ulcers, and bone degeneration. *A patient using steroids must be under the constant observation of a physician.* Any sign of incipient side effects should be reason enough to try something else.

OPINION: In fact, unless you are being *crippled* by arthritis, this treatment is probably excessive. If your doctor prescribes corticosteroids as the first or only course of therapy, get another opinion before consenting.

232. Phenylbutazone, indomethacin, and tolmetin as treatment for severe arthritis

These strong anti-inflammatory drugs should be used only in very severe cases and only for a very short time, because prolonged use can lead to rash, stomach ulcer, and deterioration of the bone marrow leading to anemia. Tolmetin seems to have fewer side effects and so is probably the best of these. Again, before accepting these drugs as a first therapy, get another opinion and if you are on them for even a brief time, get frequent blood counts.

233. Opinion: Surgery is sometimes the safest treatment for severe arthritis

Although surgery is usually the treatment of last resort, in the case of severe arthritis, it is sometimes less dangerous and more sure of success than some of the stronger drugs. Because of enormous recent advances in orthopedic (bone and skeleton) surgery, damaged joints can be fixed mechanically; total replacement of hip and knee joints is now quite feasible. If you are so crippled by arthritis that it has put you on the inactive list for the foreseeable future, and you are being advised to try powerful drugs, consider surgery as a possibly safer alternative. But make sure you consult with orthopedic surgeons who have performed the particular operation you may need many times: orthopedic surgery is as highly specialized as open-heart surgery, perhaps even more so. You will find upon inquiry that you can probably count the number of recommended practitioners on your fingers. Research their reputations with such authorities as the Arthritis Foundation, with your local university medical school *and* your local medical association, and, very important, other arthritis sufferers.

Some specific surgical corrections of crippling arthritis include replacement of the hip joint, replacement of the knee joint and elbow, and repair of the kneecap, microsurgery on the tiny joints of the fingers and toes. The simplest form of surgery for arthritis is a synovectomy— removal of the inflamed membranes that cover the joint. This certainly gives temporary relief and, some physicians feel, may prevent the spread of the arthritis to the tendons, ligaments, and cartilage surrounding the joint. (This alleged prophylactic effect has not yet been proven.)

234. Experimental drugs as treatment for severe arthritis

Experiments are now being conducted with drugs which attack the autoimmune response that permitted the arthritis in the first place. They are called immunosuppressive drugs. Obviously, any therapy that affects the body's *autoimmune* reactions may also threaten its *immune* reactions, and the risk of infection is high. However, this line of research does hold out much hope.

235. Degenerative joint disease—osteoarthritis

About 40 million Americans have some form of osteoarthritis, degenerative joint disease. Unlike rheumatoid arthritis, it is not an autoimmune reaction but comes from the normal wear and tear of life.

Swelling and pain in the joints are similar to that of rheumatoid arthritis, but there is no rheumatoid factor in the blood, no inflammation that may spread to other organs. Osteoarthritis originates in the joint and stays there and is more common in the lower extremities and spine.

The single most important predisposing factor in osteoarthritis is overweight. There is no coincidence in the fact that the disease is so widespread when so many millions of Americans are overweight. (See Chapter 8, Everyday Good Health) Other orthopedic problems may cause the condition: for example, a crippled hip may force the body's weight onto the knee, creating an imbalance in the distribution of weight and overloading the knee joints. Trauma or injury to a specific joint may also lead to osteoarthritis. For example, a sports injury that

permanently hurts the knee may make the knee weaker, less capable of
carrying the weight which cannot be shifted onto another joint.

236. Treatment of osteoarthritis

Treatment should be to lose weight, if you are heavy, and to *keep*
yourself light. Rest frequently; use a firm mattress and a bed board to
give your body extra support. Sometimes, crutches or a cane can help
take the pressure off the joint. Aspirin is the first order of treatment for
pain; Sulindac may help as well. In severe cases, surgery may be
needed. Some physicians inject steroids into the joint to relieve the pain
and swelling, but this is of limited use and the side effects (see ✂248
below) may make it counterproductive.

237. Lupus erythematosus (generally called lupus)

Lupus (in Latin, it means wolf) occurs 90 per cent of the time in
women (two to three times more frequently in black women). It generally affects women in their twenties and thirties. The cause is still unknown.

It is another autoimmune disease, in which the body builds antibodies against the ribonucleic acids which are important in cell metabolism and the genetic material. (See p. 212) Antibodies against the
nucleic acids are found circulating in the blood of lupus patients and
serve as the basis for the tests which diagnose the disease (called LE
preps and antinuclear antibody tests).

As with the other autoimmune diseases, there is virtually no way at
present to see lupus coming or to prevent it. WARNING: Some drugs
cause a reaction indistinguishable from lupus; this is called "drug-in-
duced lupus." The drug which most commonly causes this side effect is
procainamide (Pronestyl), used for severe irregularities of the heartbeat. Other drugs such as *phenothiazines* (a group of tranquilizers) and
several antihypertensive medications such as hydralazine can cause this
reaction. If you develop any lupuslike symptoms after starting a new
drug, notify your physician.

238. Symptoms of lupus

These include:

a. Fever

b. Weakness and fatigue

c. Arthritis (in 90 per cent) which is usually not as severe as
rheumatoid arthritis

d. There may be a rash on face, neck, and arms

e. Sometimes there is anemia

Except for the rash, these are rather non-specific symptoms so that the disease must be verified by tests. (See ✕237 above) In most cases of lupus, the disease is very mild, limited to rash, arthritis and intermittent fever. In the more severe cases, circulating antibody-antigen complexes interact with certain cell parts, usually in the lining of blood vessels. In the most severe cases there is damage to the kidneys, heart, and brain. However, even in the most severe cases there is a good chance, with drug therapy, for the sufferer to live a normal and quite comfortable life.

239. Treatment of lupus

Treatment with aspirin or antimalarial drugs (see ✕230 above) to control the arthritis, keeps lupus a non-debilitating disease in many cases. Steroids and experimental drugs (see ✕234 above) which block the immune response are being used for severe cases in which the kidneys or brain are involved.

240. Rheumatic fever

This disease begins as an infection and *develops* into an autoimmune disease. It does not primarily affect women but is included because it may be confused with rheumatoid arthritis. Rheumatic fever usually begins with infected (strep) throat that goes untreated. The highest-risk age group is ages five to fifteen: about 25–35 per cent of all sore throats and fevers in this age group are due to strep. The best way to diagnose and treat strep throats is currently debatable. Any severe sore throat is usually routinely cultured by pediatricians, and—if it is strep —treated with antibiotics.

If a strep infection goes untreated, a small number of people will develop rheumatic fever. Why only a small number, no one knows. In most people, the infection is cleared by the body itself. In those who develop rheumatic fever, the strep infection leads to the autoimmune reaction because the antibodies which the body forms to fight the strep infection also react against other body organs—the heart and the joints. Antibodies which react with the heart muscle can be detected in the blood stream of most victims of rheumatic fever. Once the autoimmune reaction sets in, rheumatic fever has started.

241. Symptoms of rheumatic fever

These include:

a. Arthritis moving from joint to joint
b. Fever
c. Chorea (Sydenham's) which is characterized by sudden involun-

tary movements in parts of the body, occurring most frequently in children (See p. 52)

d. Skin rash and nodules under the skin

e. A history of a recent cold and sore throat

The disease is confirmed by the presence of a heart murmur or other evidence of heart disease, and by blood tests detecting a recent strep infection and the presence of an ongoing autoimmune reaction. Don't allow the diagnosis to be made without proof, because many viral illnesses can give aches and pains in the joints and fever.

242. Treatment of rheumatic fever

The infectious part of the disease can be treated with antibiotics. The autoimmune part of the disease is treated like rheumatoid arthritis, depending on severity. The attack may last six to twelve weeks. Restricted activity is required for all sufferers and total rest for those with severe heart involvement. Aspirin is used to control the symptoms of arthritis. In the most severe cases, steroids are needed to keep the inflammatory response under control. The final outcome of the disease is variable. Usually, the disease resolves without remaining heart disease. Sometimes, there is severe damage to the valves of the heart, which may show up at a later time and is a major cause of heart trouble for women during pregnancy. People who have had rheumatic fever are more prone to develop it again, so that everyone who has had the disease should take prophylactic penicillin or sulfa until at least age eighteen if there is no evidence of heart damage and for the rest of their lives if there is heart damage.

243. Tendonitis ("tennis elbow")

Tennis elbow is an old term come into use again because of the extraordinary recent popularity of tennis. It is actually *tendonitis,* a form of bursitis, involving inflammation of the tendon of the lateral portion of the elbow. It comes from repeated strain on the tendons of the elbow, which is often caused more by poor tennis form than by the rigors of competition. There is a debate over treatment—some say "Rest," others say "Continue to play." The symptoms seem to go away within six months no matter what the treatment.

244. Infections that can cause arthritis

Some infectious diseases which invade the body generally can also invade the joints, causing the pain, swelling, and heat symptomatic of arthritis.

a. Gonorrhea, when not discovered early, may cause very painful arthritis. The treatment for gonorrhea at this stage is usually hospitalization and antibiotics by intravenous drip.

b. Bacterial endocarditis is an infection of the lining of the heart which may also be accompanied by arthritis.

c. Hepatitis, a viral infection of the liver, is often preceded by arthritis symptoms.

d. Lyme arthritis is caused by a virus spread by a tick. It was recently discovered in Connecticut, but has been reported in other states. Some of the severe cases resembled rheumatic fever with rash, and heart involvement. (Ref. 58)

245. Rubella can cause arthritis symptoms

Rubella, so dangerous to the fetus in early pregnancy (see p. 221), can cause arthritis during its acute stages in adults. The joint pain usually disappears when the disease has run its course. Many adults who get rubella vaccine experience pain and occasionally swelling in their joints afterward.

246. Other diseases sometimes accompanied by arthritis

Psoriasis (sore-EYE-a-sis) is a common skin disease in both men and women. About 7 per cent of those who have it also have arthritis. The joints involved and the treatment is very similar to rheumatoid arthritis. Ulcerative colitis and regional ileitis are bowel disorders which may be accompanied by arthritis.

247. Joint tap: a diagnostic test for type of arthritis

In a joint tap, a physician removes some fluid from a joint to see which type of arthritis is present. The fluid can be cultured to discover an infection and otherwise analyzed. This is a very safe procedure when done under sterile conditions and is very essential for diagnosis. The skin over the joint must be cleansed carefully and then a small needle is placed into the joint and fluid withdrawn. This same procedure should be used for injecting steroids into the joints.

248. Use of steroid injections into the joints to treat arthritis

Some physicians recommend injections of steroids directly into the joints to relieve arthritis inflammation and pain. This treatment usually affords only temporary relief. It should be used *only* when the pain is crippling and all less powerful treatments have failed to relieve it. Steroid injections should never be used if infection is present and should only be administered under the most sterile conditions. The recipient must be checked frequently for undesirable reactions.

249. If you have any form of arthritis, consult the Arthritis Foundation

So much about arthritis is still unknown that virtually all cases should be treated by rheumatology specialists. Avail yourself of the enormous resources of the Arthritis Foundation. Your local chapter can usually be found in the phone book. If not, write the Arthritis Foundation, 1212 Avenue of the Americas, New York, NY 10036 for information and recommendations on physicians in your area who are especially well qualified to treat this disease. You can also consult your local medical society for specialists in rheumatology.

VARICOSE VEINS

250. What are varicose veins?

There are two types of blood vessels in the body—*arteries,* which carry the blood from the heart, and *veins,* which carry the blood back to it. Veins have much thinner walls than arteries generally, and are somewhat more easily damaged.

The farther away the veins are from the heart, the greater the force of gravity against the flow of blood—imagine, what an uphill fight it is for the leg veins with the help of the leg muscles, for example, to push the blood back to the heart. Sometimes the force of gravity, along with extraneous pressure, can cause the veins in the legs and the rectogenital area to swell. The valves that help the blood along are not strong enough to do their job. This means that the blood does not move along on its upward course but rather rolls back, like the backup in a flooded pipe, and the veins bulge outward. These bulges are called varicosities—varicose veins (the word comes from the Latin "varix," which means a dilated vein).

Varicose veins are actual weaknesses in the walls of the vein, and not related to blood pressure or the temporary distention of the veins as during athletic activity.

251. Varicosities occur in the outer veins close to the skin surface

The body has two vein systems—the *superficial veins,* which are close to the surface of the skin, and the *deep veins.* Varicosities develop in the superficial veins, usually in the legs.

252. Causes of varicose veins

a. Heredity is a major factor. If your mother or father had them, you may have inherited thin-walled veins and should take care not to aggravate pressure on your legs.

b. If a woman suffers from phlebitis (clots in the deep veins of the legs that are, in themselves, a much more serious disorder than varicose veins), this can add pressure on the superficial veins and cause varicosities. (See p. 49)

c. Prolonged standing over many years can put too great pressure on the veins of the legs and cause varicosities.

d. Prolonged pressure on the veins through many years of wearing tight girdles and garters that cut into the upper leg can contribute to varicosities.

e. Pregnancy or abdominal tumors can block the return of blood through the pelvic area to the heart, causing pelvic varicosities.

f. High levels of estrogen produced during pregnancy may dilate the veins and cause varicosities. Often the varicosity will disappear after childbirth; sometimes it is there to stay.

g. Some women react to the birth-control pill with varicosities. This means that the pill should be stopped, or at the very least, changed to a lower-hormone combination. (See p. 49)

253. Varicose veins of the vulva during pregnancy

The sheer pressure of gravity in carrying a child, coupled with the high hormone levels, may cause painful varicosities in the vulva during pregnancy. Buy special elastic supports from medical-supply stores to relieve this condition.

254. Hemorrhoids are varicose veins of the anus

Few women get through pregnancy without a bout with hemorrhoids —varicosities in the veins of the anus caused by pressure, constipation (especially after childbirth), and complicated in some women by heredity.

255. Symptoms of varicose veins in the legs

Varicosities in the legs become more frequent as a woman grows older and the accumulated wear and tear on her body begins to have its effect. Varicosity symptoms are

a. A feeling of heaviness in the legs (literally the pressure of blood unable to resist the downward pull of gravity);

b. Swelling (edema);

c. Sometimes by dryness of the skin over the area of the veins. The severity of the varicosities can range from little spidery marks to severely disfiguring, tortuous veins covering the entire leg.

256. Treatment of varicose veins

a. Although it is hard to avoid the predestination of heredity, women can do a lot to avoid varicose veins. If either of your parents suffers from varicosities, start wearing stockings or support hose, early in life; put your feet up when you are sitting; try not to choose a career which will keep you on your feet all day. Wear good solid shoes that exercise your calf muscles properly.

b. The injection of irritating materials directly into the vein (sclerosing agents) is another method of treatment. Injections are usually made into areas where the veins bulge significantly. A reaction is set up inside the vein and a clot forms which closes off that area of the vein and decreases the bulging. These injections generally give only temporary relief, for at times the vein can open again and the problem recur. Another problem is the severe irritation which occurs if some of the sclerosing agent gets outside of the vein into the leg tissues. Make sure you are treated by a physician who has performed this procedure often.

c. Stripping of the veins: this is performed under general anesthesia and involves making several incisions at various places along the veins of the leg. A wire is threaded throughout the entire length of the vein (or as far as possible) and a knob is placed over the end, in the region of the groin. The thick wire is then pulled and the entire vein comes out with the device. Elastic bandages are immediately placed to prevent bleeding. The woman will have to wear elastic stockings for several weeks after surgery, to allow for healing. The postoperative period involves little discomfort and there are few complications, the main one being bleeding from the torn ends of the veins. This procedure helps cosmetically, but the varicosities may recur as other vessels dilate from the same factors which caused the problem in the first place.

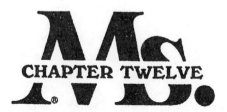

CHAPTER TWELVE

SEXUAL HEALTH

The notion of what is "normal" in sex changes from age to age, from culture to culture, from generation to generation. Mothers and daughters may differ radically on the subject; private citizens may be astounded at the views on sex held by the law. The line between public acceptance of a sexual practice and private consent is always unclear. What *is* clear, however, is that a satisfactory sex life is important in the overall physical and mental health of a woman. This aspect of health has long been overlooked by physicians and lay people alike.

It is far beyond the scope of this book to discuss the infinite variety of normal sexual practices. We have suggested several readings in the reference section. We will discuss the normal sexual reponse of women and a few of the major sexual problems. Also, when certain sexual activities may have associated medical problems we will discuss these.

In general, the normal range of sexual expression includes abstinence, masturbation, heterosexuality, and homosexuality. There is nothing inherently dangerous, either physically or psychologically, in any of these practices. What is *not* normal or healthy in sex is a situation in which a woman is forcing herself or being forced by others to assume a role for which she has no respect, which makes her feel uncomfortable or anxious, or which makes her dislike herself. Sex should be enjoyable and contribute to a woman's feeling of well-being. Sex is not normal if it becomes compulsive or ritualistic. And violence in sex, whether between consenting parties, or rapist and victim, is not normal at all.

NORMAL SEXUAL RESPONSE

1. Female sexual arousal and orgasm

Although sexual arousal may start with an emotional-psychological impulse—for example, a fantasy—it involves specific physical responses in all parts of the body, particularly the nervous system, the endocrine system and the genital organs. (We all owe a great debt to the researchers Masters and Johnson for finally recording the physiological parameters of female orgasm.)

a. *The first stage: excitement*

In the early stages of sexual excitement, the blood vessels of the genital and pelvic area begin to enlarge and lubrication of genital area begins. The vagina expands, enough to accept a penis virtually regardless of size. (This expansion occurs even if a penis is not inserted into the vagina.) The walls of the uterus become engorged with blood and the uterus enlarges, pushing slightly out of the pelvic cavity. (This movement of the uterus places the cervix in a position that generally heightens the chances of fertilization.)

b. *Second stage: the plateau phase*

As sexual arousal builds to what Masters and Johnson call "the plateau stage," vascular tissue of the pelvis grows congested along with the tissues and muscles surrounding the entrance to the vagina. Vaginal lubrication occurs. Heart rate and breathing speed up.

Unless these changes take place, a woman will not find intercourse especially pleasurable. Thus, it is essential to allow sufficient time for sexual arousal before attempting intercourse.

c. *Third stage of sexual reponse cycle: orgasm*

A series of rapid contractions occur in the muscles around the vagina and pelvic floor. Throughout the body muscles tense then relax, producing a sensation of intense pleasure.

d. *Last stage of sexual reponse cycle: resolution*

After orgasm, body tissues gradually return to normal. Heart rate and breathing slow to their usual rate.

2. The clitoris—the most sensitive of all female genital structures

The clitoris is a small hump of erectile tissue near the upper rim of the vagina and over the pubic bone, which is the most sensitive of all the female genital organs. Both the first stage of sexual arousal and the orgasm itself are triggered by sensations which are most intense in the clitoris. *Thus, there is no physiological difference between "vaginal orgasm" and "clitoral orgasm."*

Women who have felt sexually deficient because they cannot achieve orgasm simply through the friction of penile thrusting should know that they are normal. At least 30–50 per cent of women need additional clitoral stimulation, usually manual, in addition to intercourse to achieve orgasm. Penile thrusting causes *indirect* stimulation to the clitoris which may not be enough for some women. (See ✕15 below)

3. Lubrication of the vagina during sexual arousal

The amount of vaginal lubrication during sexual arousal varies from woman to woman, and an individual woman can experience more or less at various times of the menstrual cycle or at different times of her life. If there is no lubrication at all, intercourse can be very painful and not pleasurable. If this is an occasional problem, additional lubricants available without prescription may be used. If this is a chronic problem, and you suspect a psychosexual basis, consider therapy.

Some women on certain oral contraceptives complain of decreased lubrication. If this is your problem, try changing your birth-control method. During or after menopause, severe vaginal dryness may stem from estrogen deficiency. Try non-prescription lubricants. If these fail, consider a low-dose estrogen cream. (See p. 283)

4. All orgasms are not the same

Although all orgasms are physiologically the same, the intensity of contractions may vary considerably, depending on the stimulus, the time of the cycle or the woman's mood.

5. Multiple orgasm

Some women at certain stages of their lives are capable of having multiple orgasms. (Physiologically, all women are capable, but many women simply do not experience this reaction.) A woman who can have multiple orgasms is in no way more mature or more healthy than a woman who only has one orgasm.

6. Sexual arousal without orgasm

If a woman is sexually aroused but does not reach her climax, she does not experience "resolution" and her blood vessels may be engorged, her body tense for hours afterward.

Many women find that intercourse is pleasurable even if they do not have an orgasm. However, prolonged and repeated sex without the relief of orgasm may produce pelvic congestion with persistent backache and abdominal and genital pain. (See pp. 327–28)

7. Fantasies during sex are normal

Fantasies often heighten sexual arousal. Many people fantasize about other people besides their partners during sex; many people fantasize about violence. Remember, as peculiar as a fantasy may seem to you, it endangers no one as long as it is only in your mind. A woman who finds she is *acting out* her more dangerous fantasies—e.g., engaging in actual violence during sex—should seek counseling. And any woman who finds that her partner is acting out violent fantasies should send him for therapy or end the relationship.

8. Oral-genital and anal sex

These are both normal and widely practiced sexual activities. There are some cautions, however. If one partner has a herpes infection (cold sores) of the mouth, oral-genital sex should be avoided because the virus can be spread to the genital area. (See p. 307) Vaginal intercourse immediately following anal sex can result in vaginal infections if the penis has not been washed very carefully before insertion into the vagina. Lubricants should be used during anal sex to avoid tearing of the anus resulting in fissures.

9. Swinging sex or group sex

These practices of sex for physical pleasure only are on the rise and for short periods of time may well suit a woman's needs and be considered normal. There are definite risks to sex with a large number of partners, mainly the many types of venereal disease. (See p. 312) If this is your sexual pattern, make sure to get regular gynecologic examinations and VD testing.

10. Vibrators

These are battery or electrically operated devices used by many women during masturbation and in lovemaking between partners. These produce intense, rapid orgasms which individual women may or may not enjoy. There are some reports of vaginal bruising or lacerations mainly caused by inserting the device into the vagina before turning on the power—turn it on before insertion. The vibrators which strap onto the hand or are handheld and used for general body massage and clitoral stimulation are very safe.

SEXUAL DYSFUNCTION

11. What is sexual dysfunction?

Sexual dysfunction (diss-function), the inability to have satisfying sexual relations, can be caused by a number of emotional or physical problems, many of which can be improved or cured by recently developed therapy techniques.

The word "frigidity" has been used to describe sexual dysfunction in women. Like calling menstruation "the curse," calling an unsatisfied woman "frigid" is pejorative; it blames a woman for something which may not be anyone's "fault," certainly not hers. *It is time to stop using this word.*

12. What causes sexual dysfunction?

a. Ignorance—about one's own or one's partner's sexual physiology and anatomy

b. Miseducation—for example, childhood taboos about sex that linger, consciously or subconsciously, into adulthood

c. Specific, unresolved emotional conflicts—such as inordinate attachment to one parent

d. Current tensions between partners

e. Fear of losing control

f. Lack of confidence or, anxiety about one's own sexual performance

g. Fatigue

h. Physical illness

FEMALE SEXUAL PROBLEMS

---

13. Lack of sexual desire

Most women find that at one time or another in their lives, they do not feel the need for sexual activity. They lose interest in having sex with anyone; in masturbating; even erotic fantasies stop. How long this lack of interest has to last for it to be labeled abnormal is hard to say. If it persists for months in a previously good relationship, some new conflict between the partners may be the cause. Illness must always be suspected. Fatigue is a common cause; the harried homemaker raising small children may just be too tired for sex; likewise the overworked businesswoman. Disinterest in sex may also occur after severe trauma such as rape (see ✕26 below) or emergency hysterectomy.

If a woman has never had any interest in sex, this probably indicates a basic emotional conflict about sexuality—and if she is unhappy about her state, she should see a therapist.

Only when the lack of interest is prolonged over many months should it be considered unhealthy.

14. Inhibited sexual excitement

Some women, though mentally interested in sex, find that they sometimes cannot become physically aroused; others, though highly aroused during sexual activity, cannot achieve orgasm. Very few women are orgasmic 100 per cent of the time, and this is normal. Lack of orgasm should only be considered a "problem" if it persists. A woman can try masturbation or seek additional clitoral stimulation from her partner. If this does not work, consider sex therapy.

15. Many women need additional clitorial stimulation to achieve orgasm

Thirty to fifty per cent of all women have this entirely normal sexual need. Some women have orgasms only when the partner is stimulating the clitoris (with mouth or hands). If the couple finds this pattern upsetting or boring, they can alter it by longer foreplay and manual stimulation of the clitoris during intercourse by either the woman herself or her partner.

16. Vaginismus (involuntary muscle spasm at the entrance to the vagina)

Vaginismus (vadge-in-IS-mus) occurs when the muscles of the vagina contract so forcefully that a woman is unable to have intercourse. Some women with this problem also find that they cannot insert a tampon or a diaphragm. A gynecologic examination can make the diagnosis, for the muscles will be able to be observed and palpated in spasm. Treatment is usually begun by teaching the woman to dilate her own vaginal muscles with her fingers or dilators. The object is to make the woman relax and gain control over her pelvic muscles. OPINION: Surgery is not recommended for this problem! Many women who actually have vaginismus are operated upon to "open a rigid hymen." Of course, the surgery does not work for vaginismus. Make sure the diagnosis and treatment are begun by reliable physicians. Always get a second opinion if surgery is recommended.

17. Dyspareunia: pain during intercourse

Dyspareunia (diss-pa-ROON-e-ah) can be caused by several physical problems such as endometriosis (see p. 342), pelvic infection (see p. 312), and occasionally by a retroverted (tipped backward) uterus. A woman experiencing pain repeatedly during intercourse, should have a gynecologic examination. If the doctor finds no abnormality, the pain can frequently be traced to one of the above causes of sexual dysfunction. (See ⚥12 above) Occasionally, ovaries are bumped during intercourse, which can cause a severe, sharp pain. A change of position during sex will help this problem.

SEXUAL PROBLEMS OF MEN

18. Common sexual problems of men

a. *Premature ejaculation* occurs when a man does not have voluntary control over the timing of ejaculation, usually causing ejaculation before he desires. This becomes a problem if he ejaculates within the first few minutes of sex play and before the woman has had time to become sexually aroused. If this happens regularly, it can lead to mutual recrimination between partners and real misery. This problem can be caused by anxiety or by a man's early sexual experience, which may have created in him a desperate need to hurry. Therapy for this disorder has been highly successful and should be sought. (See ⚕20 below)

b. *Impotence* (IM-po-tense), the inability to have an erection, afflicts virtually every man at some time or another, and if it happens occasionally, it is nothing to worry about. If men are tired, worried, drunk, "not in the mood," they may become impotent as a result. Unfortunately, however, men tend to be terribly frightened by impotence. Victimized by a notion of machismo that dictates they must always be able to perform, they can feel so defeated by an occasional bout of impotence that they worry themselves into a permanent siege. The answer is to discuss the cause of the impotence (to rule out fatigue and anxiety) and take steps to alleviate it; one of these may be marital or sex therapy.

c. *Retarded ejaculation.* Some men cannot ejaculate inside the vagina. They are able to maintain an erection but must masturbate to achieve ejaculation. Very rarely, the problem may have anatomical causes—for example, if the vagina becomes so enlarged that the man experiences reduced friction. But most of the time, it is psychological in origin, and for couples seeking to have a child, it can be most distressing. First, the man should see a doctor for an examination. Then, *the couple* should seek sexual counseling.

TREATMENT OF SEXUAL PROBLEMS

19. How to deal with sexual dysfunction

a. Read. This is the best cure for ignorance, the source of much sexual dysfunction in couples, and today, there are innumerable books on the market which give explicit advice. Men particularly tend to be ignorant of the geography of a woman's genitals; in fact, an awful lot of men and women manage to reach sexual maturity without knowing that the clitoris exists, much less where it is.

b. Talk. People have to tell each other their needs. If a relationship is warm, this should be possible without undue embarrassment. However, sometimes loving partners do not wish to hassle each other with sexual demands, and just let a growing problem lie silent between them. Say what you need: that is probably the best way of getting it.

c. If a woman doesn't understand her own sexual needs, masturbation may be a good way to find out about them—so that later she can communicate her feelings to her partner. She should also use a mirror to examine her genital area and locate various structures.

d. Rule out physical illness. Consult your doctor. Your problem may have a simply physiological cause which can be discovered by examination and cured quickly.

e. If your partner has a sexual problem, don't automatically blame yourself. A frightened man may blame his partner for his impotence, for example, but he is not necessarily right. Don't assume that he is having trouble because you are a bad lover or because you have thin thighs.

f. Try to change the outward circumstances of sexual relations. Maybe you're both too tired to make love at night; try having sex after a good night's sleep. Try sleeping someplace else. Try changing the atmosphere. There is much truth to the reports that people who stopped having sex altogether in their apartments, with the children softly snoring down the hall and the bathroom faucet dripping, rediscovered their passion for each other in the Caribbean, or for that matter, in the motel down the road.

g. Sex therapy—a relatively new counseling specialty—should be considered.

20. Warning: When seeking a good sex therapist, be careful!

Since Masters and Johnson made the first real scientific breakthroughs in sex research in many years, and since books by a few other sexologists have popularized sexual self-awareness, all kinds of unqualified and semiqualified people have entered the field. There are quick-cure clinics, weekend blitz programs, sexual encounter groups and enrichment programs, which may help some people but may not help you at all. Even when a therapist is working alone, it is hard to judge whether he or she is good—because the field is so new, and still so widely experimental.

Guide yourself to a really qualified counselor by following these steps:

a. The following professional associations certify therapists:

1. The American Association of Sex Educators, Counselors, and Therapists (AASECT) 5010 Wisconsin Avenue N.W., Suite 304, Washington, D. C. 20016 certifies sex therapists.

2. The Eastern Association for Sex Therapy (EAST) 2040 Abington Road, Cleveland, Ohio, 44106 certifies sex therapists.

3. The American Association of Marriage and Family Therapists (AAMFT) 924 West Ninth Street, Upland, California, 91786 certifies marital and family therapists.

Contact one of these organizations for reputable therapists in your area.

b. Make sure the therapist you use has had training at least to the masters degree level and, preferably, has a medical degree or a Ph.D. in a particular auxiliary field such as psychology or social work. Some members of the clergy are certified marital counselors.

21. What will a good therapist do, and not do?

a. take a long, detailed history of your relationship, if you seek treatment as a couple (which is preferable), or your individual sex life;

b. make sure you and your partner have both had a thorough physical examination recently;

c. discuss anatomy and physiology;

d. seek to discover emotional problems which may be contributing to the dysfunction;

e. possibly suggest exercises which can be done at home, in private.

A good therapist will not suggest

a. that he or she observe you while you are making love;

b. that he or she have sex with you or your partner.

Some sex therapists—only those who are M.D.s—suggest a foursome physical examination, in which two physicians, one male, one female, conduct an examination on each partner with the other partner present in order to demonstrate physical anatomy. This examination should be no more sexually arousing than an ordinary pelvic exam. *It should never be done by anybody except a physician.*

22. Exercises to treat sexual problems

Most treatment programs for sexual dysfunction are modifications of the Masters and Johnson "sensate focus exercises." The partners will be instructed to take the focus off intercourse and place it on other forms of sexual pleasuring for each other. Privacy and relaxation are absolutely prerequisite. These exercises are used most often to treat persistently non-orgasmic women and men who suffer from impotence, or premature ejaculation. (See Bibliography for completely descriptive material.)

23. Avoid surgical treatment for sexual dysfunction unless it is recommended by a very reputable sex therapist, and verified by other medical opinions

In most cases, sexual dysfunction is *not* caused by anatomical problems in the genital area—so that surgery to somehow alter the genitals is a very dangerous suggestion.

Watch out for any doctor who suggests the fad therapy, now catching on in the popular magazines, which suggests that the skin over the clitoris be surgically loosened so that the clitoris will be more stimulated during intercourse. This is a nonsense operation; it doesn't work for most women any better than additional manual or oral stimulation of the clitoris during lovemaking. Do not have it.

Watch out for any doctor who suggests surgery to "open the hymen." A rigid hymen is very rare; when it is diagnosed, the woman can usually dilate it herself; and very often, the diagnosis is mistaken—the woman really has vaginismus (see ⚹16 above). Never accept this surgery, unless yours is one of the very rare cases which can be corroborated by several physicians.

24. Warning: Never consider transsexual surgery until you have had a careful trial of psychotherapy

Transsexuals are different from homosexual women in that they are not happy with their identity as women (which homosexuals are) but actually think of themselves as men.

Any woman who believes she is a transsexual should seek counseling only from a therapist working at a center which specializes in these problems. For information contact the Janus Information Facility of Texas Medical Branch, Galveston, Texas, 77550.

The general practice is to require intensive counseling for several years, and then to suggest that the woman live as a man for at least a year before surgery is contemplated. *No reputable surgeon would perform the transsexual operation without assurance that the patient had spent a very long time in therapy, and without the recommendation of a qualified psychiatrist.*

25. How physical illness and its treatment can cause sexual dysfunction

a. Almost any severe or prolonged illness can cause sexual problems. Kidney disease or diabetes, for example, which affect the endocrine system, are almost sure to decrease sexual interest.

b. Pain, even from an illness which is not otherwise serious except for its discomforts, may decrease sexual appetite; and the pain-killers needed to alleviate the discomfort may decrease it even more.

c. A person who is recovering from a serious illness may be afraid that sex will cause a recurrence, and therefore avoid sex altogether, sometimes quite needlessly. Heart-attack victims are a classic example. Although capable of sexual arousal, they fear the exertion of sex will lead to another heart attack. *Check with your doctor for assurance of exactly when sexual exertion is not dangerous after major illness or surgery.*

e. Medication used to treat a disease may cause orgasm problems or impotence. Medications sometimes having this effect include antidepressants, tranquilizers, sedatives, and drugs used to treat hypertension. If you note a sudden change in sexual function after starting a certain drug, check with your doctor. *A physician should always tell you beforehand if a drug can be expected to cause sexual problems.*

f. Illness may touch off emotional/relational problems between partners which can lead to sexual dysfunction. Women who are having severe emotional reactions to mastectomy or hysterectomy, for example, may feel so bad about their bodies that they cannot resume sex. (See p. 353) Very often, the woman's fears of rejection are unfounded; she feels worse about her appearance than does her partner. Talking, plain communication, may alleviate the problem. Time as well as love and understanding often solve it. Seek outside help first from the patient self-help organizations; go to psychological therapy as a final resort.

RAPE

The crime of rape (along with other sexual assaults) is on the increase in the United States and in other countries as well. It is clearly a violent crime of male aggression against women. It is a means of humiliating and injuring women, made yet worse by the fact that those involved with the rape victim after the assault (doctors, lawyers, and police) are caught up in sexist attitudes too and often contribute to the humiliating and misogynous aspects of the crime. Things are changing, but not quickly enough.

26. Rape fantasies: male and female

The prevalent belief about rape in this and other countries is that women cannot be raped unless they want to be. This is a nonsensical male fantasy. Many men have fantasized about raping women, about overcoming the resistance of an unwilling woman who finally gives in to the overwhelming power of the male. It is a power fantasy. The vast majority of men never act on it—but just because they have had the fantasy, they may lack sympathy with the rape victim.

It is no easier for a woman to resist an armed rapist than for a bank teller to resist an armed robber. Because the robber gets away with the money, the teller is not accused of collusion; why then should the woman be accused of collusion if the attacker gets away with the rape? There is, thus, no logic to the power fantasy; but it can only be knocked out of the societal subconscious if the parents of boys give careful instruction which will eventually help the power fantasy to be replaced by a more egalitarian view of sex.

Women have fantasies about rape too, usually because they have somehow accepted the notion that men must be overpowering to be excitingly virile. This is another manifestation of conditioned self-hatred among women. It has no bearing on the actuality of rape, for it is a romantic fantasy and rape is not a romantic crime, it is a violent crime.

27. Who is a rapist?

There are many different kinds of mental and emotional calamities that cause a man to rape women: however, in general, rapists have a few things in common. They are immature. They are violent. They hate women and cannot control their desire to humiliate and intimidate their victims. They are sexually disoriented and believe they cannot attain sexual satisfaction in any context except the context of violence. They get little sexual pleasure from subjection and control of another human being. In fact, many rapists show sexual dysfunction, such as impotence or retarded ejaculation, during the attack. (Ref. 1) Rapists are generally people who feel put down and humiliated elsewhere in their lives and must vent their anger by an attack on those unable to defend themselves.

28. How to avoid being raped

Try not to be alone in high-risk areas; avoid streets where gangs hang out. A rapist who might be too frightened to try an attack on his own may get all the courage he needs from two or three equally unbalanced cronies. If someone is following you, get out into the middle of the street where the cars are and run, scream. When people rush out of their apartments, the man may say that he gave you no cause for such hysterical behavior. People may laugh at you. Let them laugh; their presence prevented you from being attacked. *Never at any time of day get into your parked car without looking into the back seat. Do not leave your car unlocked.* It is terrifying how many women unwittingly drive rapists home with them from the supermarket. Do not open the door to any serviceman who does not have an ID that you can read. It is a common *modus operandi,* especially in suburban neighborhoods, for men to knock at the door, posing as gas inspectors, etc., and rape a woman in her own home.

If your assailant is unarmed, scream and fight, you may be able to get a finger in his eye or a knee in his groin that will enable you to get away from him, *and most important, you may be able to raise some help with your yelling.*

If he is armed, do not underestimate the danger. Not resisting may save your life. Unless you are sure of your karate, it is not a good idea to struggle with a weapon.

Remember always that in dealing with a rapist, you are dealing with someone who is enraged and violent.

No normal man needs to rape women!

29. What to do if you have been raped

a. *Report the crime.*

Social pressures, legitimate and illegitimate, must never keep a woman from reporting a rape. Any man who is sick enough to attack one woman is almost surely sick enough to attack another. By not reporting rape, women are contributing to possible assaults on others and perhaps inviting a second assault on themselves.

b. Call a friend, if you can, to be with you for the next few hours.

c. Contact the police.

d. See a doctor as soon as possible, certainly within the first twelve to twenty-four hours, if not sooner.

e. Do not wash or change clothes until after the medical examination and the police statement.

f. Keep a friend or relative with you at all times. Contact the rape crisis center or a local women's group for advice.

g. Try to notice every single thing you can about your assailant— features, height, weight, peculiarities in speech.

h. Do not go home alone after making your report; do not stay at home by yourself. If you are afraid the rapist may know where to find you, go to a friend's house and notify the police of your whereabouts.

30. Medical examination after rape

a. In large cities, the examination will frequently be done by physicians working closely with the police department. These doctors examine many rape victims and will be well acquainted with the tests to be done and the method to preserve the chain of evidence for court later on. In areas where a private gynecologist or family physician must be consulted, a woman should insist that the doctor do specific tests to make sure that he or she is establishing enough evidence for the later court case.

b. First, you should have a general examination (inspection) of your entire body. Make sure that the doctor writes down descriptions of any bruises, lacerations, redness, or pain anywhere on your body. If any evidence of trauma appears after you have left the hospital or doctor's office, make sure that you return and have the doctor note these and enter them into the medical record.

c. Secondly, a pelvic examination should be performed, again to look for any evidence of trauma. This may be very upsetting: the last thing most women want after being raped is a vaginal examination. However, most are also happy to be reassured that there has been no damage done, or if there has, to have it repaired. Approximately 25–50 per cent of women have some physical trauma from the rape incident, so the general examination and the pelvic examination are *very* important.

d. In addition, during the pelvic examination, samples of the vaginal secretions should be taken for sperm and acid phosphatase (FOSS-fatase) a component of seminal fluid which would be present even if a man had no sperm (e.g. if he had had a vasectomy). *It is a very important corroborating piece of evidence in many cases and must be tested for.*

e. Tests for gonorrhea should be done if the assault was more than twenty-four hours before the examination. Some examiners do these tests routinely, more as a public health measure than for their actual relevance to the case.

f. The anus and mouth must be examined if the attack involved these areas.

g. Most rape victims would like to receive preventive treatment for VD and pregnancy. If the woman desires it, she can receive two shots of procaine penicillin and probenecid (a drug to make the blood level of penicillin higher). Of course, it is her option to wait and have the tests for gonorrhea and syphilis repeated at three and six weeks (and again, in twelve weeks, for syphilis). If you are allergic to penicillin, report this to the examiner and request tetracycline or spectinomycin. (See p. 314)

h. Pregnancy prevention may be obtained in the form of the "morning-after pill" (see p. 71), unless you were taking birth-control pills or were otherwise protected against pregnancy at the time of the attack. Menstrual extraction is another option if the period is delayed, and does not involve the side effects of the "morning-after pill." (See.p. 193)

i. Always get the name, address, and phone number of the examining doctor before you leave, so you can phone back if any problems arise.

j. Much of the above requires cool decision-making at a time of great crisis, and may be difficult. If a friend is with you at this time, the decisions may be much easier.

31. Physical aftereffects of rape

a. Vaginal discharge and itching may occur. This can be due to monilia infection (see p. 302) if a woman received penicillin or tetracycline. (If you have a tendency toward moniliasis ask for a prescription to prevent this.) Some women will contract trichomoniasis (see p. 305) from the rapist, or any of the other vaginal infections that are spread by sexual contact. If a discharge develops, seek medical help. It is very unlikely to be syphilis or gonorrhea if you received the prophylactic antibiotics.

b. Bruises, swelling, pain not apparent immediately after the rape may show up later on. Go back to the same doctor you saw after the rape and make sure these are noted on his or her report. If you didn't like that doctor, go to another doctor—but make sure the information about latent injury is reported to the police.

c. Lacerations of the rectum may accompany rape cases which involve anal sodomy. Sometimes they do not bleed until you move your bowels. Report these to the physician you are consulting. If there is anal pain but no bleeding, report this as well. For treatment sometimes vaseline or Nupercainal ointment will be helpful.

d. A follow-up medical examination should be scheduled for four to six weeks after the assault. At this time tests for venereal disease and pregnancy should be taken, if indicated. It will also be a reassurance that all things are medically well.

32. Psychological aftereffects of rape

Initially, many women are stunned and appear calm, as though they cannot believe this assault has happened to them. Most women suffer tension, anxiety, even hysteria eventually. It is normal to be afraid to be alone, even for a few minutes; normal to be sleepless; normal to want to run away and disappear off the face of the earth. In time, these psychological reactions pass—and if friends, family, and police are sympathetic, they will pass much more quickly.

The trouble is that people are so conflicted about rape victims that they often fail a woman when she needs them the most. Police and doctors are not reliably sympathetic; you may not want to tell your family because they would be too upset. If it's a choice between your mother and your brother, try to think which of them will care most about you and least about the rape.

The women's groups and rape crisis centers are enormously helpful to the rape victim—because they are understanding strangers. After calling the police, the doctor, and a close friend, call them—they can counsel you, comfort you, give legal advice, and help guide you past serious psychological trauma. It is probable that most adult women can come out of a rape without serious psychological therapy, provided they have early input from advocate groups and good friends.

The most helpful emotion to have after a rape is rage. Too many women are afraid to get as angry as they would like.

The least helpful emotion after a rape is guilt. Too many women feel that they were somehow to blame for the incident.

The rage is justified; the guilt is groundless. Qualified counselors at the rape crisis centers and in the women's groups can help you cope with both emotions.

33. Sex crimes against children

The younger the woman, the more severe the psychologic trauma in general after a rape. Children who are raped or otherwise sexually molested suffer the most—especially because the attacker is frequently a relative. *It is very important not to try to handle a case of child molestation without professional guidance.* If your child, boy or girl, has been assaulted in this way, seek referral to a qualified counselor through the rape crisis center or family physician. In such a case, the mother may be the last person able to get the child to speak frankly and master the nightmare.

34. Legal aspects of rape

In most states, rape is defined as contact between the penis and the vagina that is against the will of the victim. The aspect of force is the most difficult to prove, if there is no bodily injury. That is why the careful medical examination is so important. By legal definition, fear of body injury is also force, so the victim must be able to prove in court, that she did not willingly engage in sexual activities.

If semen or sperm are present, this is good corroborating evidence. However, if the attacker did not ejaculate (as happens in as many as one third of cases [Ref. 1]) the medical exam will not be helpful unless there is evidence of trauma. If you do not think the man ejaculated, inform the doctor and the police.

The police statement, taken at the time of reporting the crime, should contain only questions surrounding the assault and the details, some of which may be very embarrassing. Ask to be interviewed in a private room, and by a female investigator, if one is available. If you think that the investigator is becoming offensive in his attitude, tell him so. It is very important, if possible, to have a second person with you during these proceedings.

The trial, if the case gets to trial, will be very tedious for the woman. However, it is reassuring that many states are changing their laws of evidence to prohibit questions concerning a woman's sex life which are not pertinent to the case. Women's groups may have volunteers available to accompany victims to court, and by all means take a friend.

Juries are known for their prejudice against uninjured rape victims, and defense attorneys will cite historical precedent for women falsely accusing men of rape. (The trial of the Scottsboro boys in Alabama is the most frequently cited example.)

In spite of all the problems, report the crime. Get angry that someone invaded your personal freedom and do your best to convict him. Enlist the help of other women and men in the process.

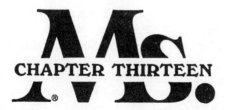

CHAPTER THIRTEEN

ROUTINE
HEALTH CARE for
WELL WOMEN

A rather typical thirty-seven-year old woman whom we know has had a gynecological examination every year of her life since the age of twenty-one. She has had Pap smears, breast-exams, pelvic-exams routinely. She has lived in three different American cities and traveled abroad, and everywhere that she has been, she has taken the trouble to know about a local gynecologist who was reputed to be competent. She has had three children and a laparoscopic sterilization. And for each of these events, she shopped for the doctor and the hospital she used until she was quite sure she had the best.

The only time she was really *sick* in all those years was when she got the chicken pox from her children—and then she had absolutely no idea what to do.

Her fever was well over 100 degrees and persisting. She ached and burned. Because she had been unable to prepare for her illness, and because she was sick simultaneously with her children, her household and her job were plunged into chaos. She was very ill, and she had no doctor.

Her gynecologist recommended that she call an internist or family practitioner and gave her several names. All happened to be unavailable that day. She called the emergency room of the local hospital, just for advice. They told her to stay in bed, where she already was. Ultimately, the only doctor she knew personally who could help at all was her children's pediatrician.

After the pox receded and she could reflect on what had happened, this woman concluded several things: first, that she could have prepared for the disease (so much more serious in adults than in children) if she had only kept her own pediatric records and known what childhood diseases she had *not* had. It turned out that these records were beyond retrieval, her own pediatrician having long since retired to sunny places unknown, and her mother having been unable to remember which child had what. (Her mother-in-law couldn't remember either. But since her husband was the only family member not to get the chicken pox, it was assumed that he had had it.) Wiser, the woman looked at her own slow-fading spots and wondered if he had ever had the mumps. Or the measles.

She resolved to preserve the medical records of her own children in duplicate and in safe places, where they would be accessible long after she was dead.

And then she found herself an internist.

This woman's story is a comedy of errors we can all avoid. Gynecology is not enough. There is much much more to a woman's body than her urogenital tract, and she should take as much care to maintain her general health as she does to check and maintain the organs that make her particularly female. *We recommend that, wherever possible, women seek primary care from an internist or a family practitioner, not a gynecologist.*

These physicians will often take care of general medical problems, perform routine general examinations and routine pelvic exams and Pap smears as well. If an abnormality is noted in the genital tract, then a referral to a gynecologist is in order.

Throughout this book we have suggested that a woman ought to have a personal process to cope with each event in her health history—with menarche; with pregnancy; with change of life; with illness. This process should be as routine, as comforting, and useful as a fire drill.

Many of us already have a process for being sick. But we must all make sure that we have a thought-through process for being and staying *well* that maintains general as well as gynecological health.

The following are recommendations for the *process,* as standardized here as possible, by which well women may guard their good health and make a lifelong practice of preventive medicine.

1. Assume primary responsibility for your own health care

This is not to say that you should doctor yourself.

But you must assume personal responsibility for researching the alternatives and obtaining the best care available.

Never passively accept any treatment, no matter how simple or routine, without knowing exactly what it is and why it is being suggested.

You can count on no one to protect you against bad medical choices —not your physicians, your friends or your government—for all of these are essentially advisers. Concentrate all your resources on choosing what is best for you and ultimately, trust yourself.

2. A woman must practice preventive medicine throughout her life

The best preventive medicine is to always protect your body against outside assaults. Eat properly. Do not allow yourself to become obese. Exercise regularly. Get adequate sleep. Do not smoke. Do not drink excessively. Never take drugs for pleasure and treat marijuana gingerly, like liquor. Fight like a demon to keep the environment clean. Avoid any medicines except those absolutely needed for treatment. Pass your concern about health on to children and friends, and make sure that the major medical issues of these changing times are not decided without your attentive participation.

3. Read! Keep yourself informed on issues that affect your health

Don't leave medicine to the specialists. It's too important.

Know as much about your body as possible. For starters, know what is normal for you so you can immediately detect any deviations from the norm. Keep up on all the major issues of health care which might affect you or yours (remember that what affects someone else today may affect you tomorrow, so don't be exclusive). Never imagine, for example, that industrial poisons only affect the health of those who work in industry. Find a regular source of medical news that you enjoy and respect, and read it—regularly.

4. Maintain a record of your own health history

Know the health history of your family. For example, are there any diseases which run in the family (e.g., diabetes, hypertension), for which you and your descendants should be screened in routine examinations? Keep a record of any serious illnesses and surgery. Know exactly what was done during surgery. (For example, did the hysterectomy include removal of the ovaries?) Find and keep your pediatric records. A doctor who has your current medical records must give them to you if you put your request in writing. Do so! Do not take "no" for an answer. This is vital information that everyone must have for herself.

If you have any problem which might cause an emergency, such as allergies to specific medications or bad reactions to insect stings, carry this information with you. Carry your blood type on a card in your wallet. (Write to Medic Alert, P.O. Box 1009, Turlock, California 95380 or 3 East 54th St., New York, New York 10022 for information on warning bracelets or neck chains.)

5. The following routine examinations and screening tests are important to maintain your health: (see Table 8, p. 410)

a. *General physical examinations* should be obtained at periodic intervals—although there is considerable debate as to whether *complete* examinations are necessary routinely for people with no complaints. These should be done by your internist or family practitioner; in some areas of the country, a gynecologist may perform the entire examination.

b. *Blood pressure* should be taken yearly below age forty and every six months after that. Hypertension—high blood pressure—is a common disease which can *only* be detected by blood pressure testing. A nurse, gynecologist, or family physician can do this.

c. *Urine* should be tested for protein and sugar at least once a year. This simple screening test is used to detect diabetes and kidney disease, as well as other conditions, and can be done with the gynecologic exam.

d. *Women should examine their breasts once a month.* (See p. 356) Most breast tumors can be detected at a very early stage if women are careful to perform this examination.

e. A physician should examine your breasts every six months after age forty, and yearly before then as part of the regular gynecologic exam. You must be completely undressed and examined both while you are sitting and lying down. Your breasts cannot be adequately examined inside your bra. *Mammography* should be considered by women over fifty. (See p. 356)

f. *A pelvic examination* is in order at least once a year (twice a year after age forty). The examiner should place a speculum into the vagina to visualize the cervix and to take a *Pap smear* and *tests for venereal disease*. (The Pap smear will detect cancer of the cervix at a very early stage as well as other conditions.) Then the examiner should place one or two fingers into the vagina and press on the abdomen to evaluate the size of the uterus and ovaries.

Routine pelvic examinations should be started when a woman is sixteen to eighteen years old or whenever she becomes sexually active. The Pap smear does not need to be taken more than once a year unless there are high-risk factors. (See p. 362)

g. *A rectal examination* should be performed yearly in conjunction with the pelvic examination. The examiner inserts a finger into the anus, to rule out any rectal problems and in some cases to facilitate palpation of the ovaries.

h. *Stool* should be analyzed at least once a year after age forty, to test for the presence of blood and to screen for intestinal cancer. This should be done in conjunction with the routine pelvic and rectal examinations.

i. Some physicians recommend routine *proctosigmoidoscopy* for all people over age sixty. In this test, usually done by an internist or surgeon, a small tube is inserted into the anus, and the lower part of the bowel is visualized for any abnormalities.

j. *A blood test for anemia* should be performed once a year for all women from childhood on. This can be done by drawing blood from the arm or by sticking the finger with a needle and determining either hemoglobin content or hematocrit. (See p. 370) These are routine tests that should accompany all general examinations, whether they are performed by an internist, a gynecologist or a pediatrician.

k. *Cholesterol* and other blood fat levels should be determined yearly after age fifty. (See pp. 257–58) This involves a simple blood test from the arm, but should be performed after a woman has *not* eaten for at least twelve hours.

l. Routine *eye examinations* should be obtained every two to three years before age forty and every year thereafter. Those who wear corrective lenses should have their eyes checked once a year from the time the lenses are prescribed. After age forty, your eye doctor should check interocular pressure as a screening test for glaucoma, a prevalent eye disease.

m. *Dental examinations* should be obtained every six months until age thirty. After that, once-a-year checkups are adequate.

n. *Testing for tuberculosis* should be considered on a routine basis for everyone who has contact with large numbers of people.

o. *Check your weight* on a good scale at home routinely. Cosmetic considerations aside, any precipitous gain or loss, or any steady weight loss without conscious dieting, should be further checked.

p. *Women who smoke should consider annual chest X rays.* Women who work with or near toxic substances should consult union and management health officials for screening tests that apply particularly to them.

THE ABOVE SCHEDULE OF EXAMINATIONS APPLIES TO WOMEN *WHO HAVE NO COMPLAINTS* AND WHO ARE NOT AT PARTICULARLY HIGH RISK FOR A DISEASE. THE TESTS WOULD CHANGE IF ANY DISORDER WERE SUSPECTED. FOR ROUTINE TESTS DURING PREGNANCY, SEE CHAPTER 5.

6. If a problem is detected and treatment or surgery is suggested, get a second opinion

If a diagnosis of a serious condition is made, and no emergency exists, you should take time to read up on the problem and question your doctor extensively. Determine whether there are alternative methods of treatment which might suit you better. If you do not feel completely satisfied, seek a second opinion. *This is especially important in non-emergency surgery.* (See p. 333)

7. If you are taking any medications, know exactly what they are and why you are taking them

If medications are prescribed for you, take the trouble to know all about them. How quickly should they afford you relief? How soon can you stop them? Are there short or long-term side effects? Do they interact with any other medications you may be taking or foods you may be eating? Consult your doctor as well as your pharmacist, and apply this process to over-the-counter as well as prescription drugs.

8. If you are using a number of medications, make sure that one pharmacy handles all your business

The pharmacist is a valuable adviser in helping you evaluate the possible interaction of medications which may have been prescribed by different doctors. In addition, he will be able to tell you a great deal about the potential side effects of drugs.

9. Use health care professionals as advisers, but take the major responsibility on yourself

Of course, we must all rely on the advice and expertise of health care professionals. But shop carefully for this advice.

Many of us think nothing of spending days shopping for clothes, months shopping for housing, for the best plumber, the best school, the best car. SHOP WITH EVEN MORE INTENSITY FOR THE BEST HOSPITAL AND THE VERY BEST PHYSICIANS.

Ignorance is only a comfort to those who can afford to let other people control their lives. No woman can afford ever again to be tempted by such spurious luxury. We have too much to gain—in liberty, in selfhood, in health—from the task and the joy of knowing our own way.

TABLE 8
SUGGESTED PROGRAM OF HEALTH MAINTENANCE FOR
WELL WOMEN

	Age 16–40 Every ___ mos.	Age 40–60 Every ___ mos.	Age 60+ Every ___ mos.
General physical examination	36	24	24
Blood pressure check	12	6	6
Urine test for protein and sugar	12	12	12
Self breast exam	1	1	1
Breast exam	12	6	6
Mammography (over age 50)	—	12–24	12–24
Pelvic exam	12	6	6
Pap smear	12	12	12
VD testing, when appropriate	6–12	6–12	6–12
Rectal exam and test for blood in stool	12–24	12	12
Proctosigmoidoscopy	—	—	12
Blood test for anemia	12	12	12
Cholesterol and other Blood Fats (over age 50)		12	12
Eye examination	24	12	12
Dental examination	6	12	12
Tuberculosis testing (If appropriate)	12–24	12–24	12–24

REFERENCES

CHAPTER TWO

1. Frisch, R. E. and Renelee, R. "Height and weight at menarche and a hypothesis of critical body weight and adolescent events." *Science* 169: 397, 1970.
2. Hafez, E. S. E. "Reproductive Life Cycle." In Hafez, E. S. E., and Evans, T. N. *Human Reproduction.* Hagerstown, Maryland: Harper & Row, 1973.
3. Peck, G. L., Olsen, T. G. *et al.* "Prolonged remissions of cystic and conglobate acne with 13-cis-retinoic acid." *New England Journal of Medicine* 300: 299, 1979.

General References

Romney, S. L., et al. *Gynecology and Obstetrics, the Health Care of Women.* New York: McGraw-Hill, 1975.

Nowak, E. R., Jones, G. S., and Jones, H. W. *Nowak's Textbook of Gynecology,* 8th edition. Baltimore: Williams and Wilkins, 1970.

Kappelman, M. *What Every Parent Should Know about Sex and the American Teenager.* New York: Reader's Digest Press, 1977.

Zackler, J. Brandstadt, W. *The Teenage Pregnant Girl.* Springfield, Illinois, Charles Thomas, 1975.

CHAPTER THREE

1. Potts, M., van der Vlug, T. T., et al. "Advantages of orals outweigh disadvantages." *Population Reports* Series A, ⚥2, 1975.
2. Miale, J. B., and Kent, J. W. "The effects of oral contraceptives on the results of laboratory tests." *American Journal of Obstetrics and Gynecology* 120: 264, 1974.
3. Royal College of General Practitioners' Oral Contraceptive Study, "Mortality among oral-contraceptive users." *Lancet,* p. 727, October 8, 1977.
4. Lyon, F. A., and Frisch, M. J. "Endometrial abnormalities occurring in young women on long-term sequential oral contraception." *Obstetrics and Gynecology* 47: 639, 1976.
5. Cohen, C. J., and Deppe, G. "Endometrial carcinoma and oral contraceptive agents." *Obstetrics and Gynecology* 49: 390, 1977.
6. Kane, F. J. "Evaluation of emotional reactions to oral contraceptive use." *American Journal of Obstetrics and Gynecology* 126: 968, 1976.
7. Rinehart, W., Piotrow, P. T., "OCs—Update on usage, safety and side effects." *Population Reports* Series A, ⚥6, 1979.

8. Jain, A. K. "Cigarette smoking, use of oral contraceptives, and myocardial infarction." *American Journal of Obstetrics and Gynecology* 126: 301, 1976.

9. Vana, J., Murphy, G. P., Aronoff, B. L., Baker, H. W. "Primary liver tumors and contraceptives: results of a survey." *Journal of the American Medical Association* 238: 2154, 1977.

10. Greenblatt, D. J., and Koch-Weser, J. "Oral contraceptives and hypertension." *Obstetrics and Gynecology* 44: 412, 1974.

11. Laraugh, J. H. "Oral contraceptive-induced hypertension—nine years later." *American Journal of Obstetrics and Gynecology* 126: 141, 1976.

12. Brenner, P. F., and Mishell, D. R. "Contraception for the woman with significant heart disease." *Clinical Obstetrics and Gynecology* 18: 155, 1975.

13. Robboy, S. J., and Welch, W. R. "Microglandular hyperplasia in vaginal adenosis associated with oral contraceptives and prenatal diethylstilbestrol exposure." *Obstetrics and Gynecology* 49: 430, 1977.

14. Rifkin, I., Nachtigall, L. E., and Beckman, E. M. "Amenorrhea following use of oral contraceptives." *American Journal of Obstetrics and Gynecology* 113: 420, 1972.

15. Van Campenhout, J., Blanchet, P., Beauregard, H., Papas, S. "Amenorrhea following the use of oral contraceptives." *Fertility and Sterility* 28: 728, 1977.

16. Sandmire, H. F., Austin, S. B., and Bechtel, R. C. "Carcinoma of the cervix in oral contraceptive steriod and IUD users and nonusers." *American Journal of Obstetrics and Gynecology* 125: 339, 1976.

17. Kennedy, B. J. "Appearance and spread of human breast cancer." In Griem, M. L., et al. *Breast Cancer: A Challenging Problem, Recent Results in Cancer Research* 42: 31, 1973.

18. Kastrup, E. K., Boyd, J. R., Eds. *Facts and Comparisons.* St. Louis: Facts and Comparisons Inc., 1977, p. 107f.

19. Rosenfield, A. G. "Injectable long-acting progestogen contraception: a neglected modality." *American Journal of Obstetrics and Gynecology* 120: 537, 1974.

20. Reihnart, W., and Winter, J. "Injectable progestogens—officials debate but use continues." *Population Reports* Series K, ⌗1, 1975.

21. Dickinson, R. L. *Control of Conception.* Baltimore, Williams and Wilkins Co., 1938.

22. Sagiroglu, N. "Local effects of polyethylene IUDs in Women." Abstract in program of "Third International Conference on Intrauterine Contraception." The Population Council. New York: 1974, p. 38.

23. Tatum, H. J. "Metallic copper as an intrauterine contraceptive agent." *American Journal of Obstetrics and Gynecology* 117: 602, 1973.

24. Mishell, D. R. "Assessing the intrauterine device." *Family Planning Perspectives* 7: 103, 1975.

25. Ory, H. W. "A review of the association between intrauterine devices and acute pelvic inflammatory disease." *Journal of Reproductive Medicine* 20: 200, 1978.

26. FDA. "Pelvic inflammatory disease in IUD users." *FDA Drug Bulletin* 8: 19, 1978.

27. Laufe, L. E., Gibor, Y., McClanahan, B. J., Wheeler, R. F. "Volume and copper concentration of menstrual discharge of women employing

Copper-7 and other types of contraceptives." In Lewit, S., ed. *Advances in Planned Parenthood* 9: 38, 1974.

28. Huber, S. C., Piotrow, P. T., Arlans, B., and Kommer, G. "IUDs Reassessed—a Decade of Experience." *Population Reports* Series B, ⋕2, 1975.

29. Implementation of the Medical Device Amendments of 1976. *Federal Register* 41: 22620, June 4, 1976.

30. Stopes, M. C. *Contraception, Birth Control, Its Theory, History and Practice,* 3rd ed. London: Putnam, 1931.

31. Wortman, J. "The diaphragm and other intravaginal barriers—a review." *Population Reports* Series H, ⋕4, 1976.

32. Ryder, N. B. "Contraceptive failure in the United States." *Family Planning Perspectives* 5: 133, 1973.

33. Belsky, R. "Vaginal contraceptives, a time for reappraisal?" *Population Reports* Series H, ⋕3, 1975.

34. Gale, T. F., and Ferm, V. H. "Embryopathic effects of mercuric salts." *Life Sciences* 10: 1341, 1971.

35. Cutler, J. C., Nickens, O. J. and Balisky, H. "Pro-con vaginal contraceptives as venereal disease prophylactic agents." *Advances in Planned Parenthood* 11: 43, 1974.

36. Aref, I., Hafez, E. S. E. "Postcoital contraception: physiological and clinical parameters." *Obstetrical and Gynecological Survey* 32: 417 1977.

37. Rinehart, W. "Postcoital contraception—an appraisal." *Population Reports* Series J, ⋕9, 1976.

38. Lippes, J., Malik, T., and Tatum, H. J. "The postcoital copper-T." *Advances in Planned Parenthood* 11:24, 1976.

39. Himes, N. E. *Medical History of Contraception.* New York: Gamut Press, 1963.

40. Glass, R. K., Vessey, M., and Wiggins, P. "Use-effectiveness of condom in selected family planning clinic population in the United Kingdom." *Contraception* 10:591, 1975.

41. Bremner, W. J., and De Kretser, D. M. "The prospects for new, reversible male contraceptives." *New England Journal of Medicine* 295: 1117, 1976.

42. Frick, J. "Control of spermatogenesis in men by combined administration of progestion and androgen." *Contraception* 8: 191, 1973.

43. Rock, J., and Robinson, D. "Effect of induced intrascrotal hyperthermia on testicular function in man." *American Journal of Obstetrics and Gynecology* 93: 793, 1965.

44. Fahim, M. S., et al. "Ultrasound as a new method of male contraception." *Fertility and Sterility* 28: 823, 1977.

45. Ross, C., and Piotrow, P. T. "Birth control without contraceptives." *Population Reports* Series I, ⋕1, 1974.

46. Billings, J. J. *Natural Family Planning: The Ovulation Method.* Collegeville, Maryland: Liturgical Press, 1973.

47. "A vaccine against pregnancy." *People,* 3: 29, 1976.

48. Evans, T. N. "Sterilization in Women." In Hafez, E. S. E., and Evans, T. N. *Human Reproduction.* Hagerstown, Maryland: Harper & Row, 1973.

49. Wortman, J. "Tubal sterilization—review of methods." *Population Reports* Series C, ⚥7, 1976.
50. Berkman, S. "Late complications of tubal sterilization by laparoscopy." *Contemporary Obstetrics and Gynecology* 9: 118, 1977.
51. Wortman, J., and Piotrow, P. T. "Colpotomy—the vaginal approach." *Population Reports.* Series C, ⚥3, 1973.
52. Darabi, K. F., Richard, R. M. "Collaborative study on hysteroscopic sterilization procedures." *Obstetrics and Gynecology* 49: 48, 1977.
53. Wortman, J., and Piotrow, P. T. "Vasectomy—old and new techniques." *Population Reports* Series D, ⚥1, 1973.
54. Wortman, J. "Vasectomy—what are the problems?" *Population Reports* Series D, ⚥2, 1975.

CHAPTER FOUR

Behrman, S. J., and Menge, A. C. "Immunologic Aspects of Infertility. In *Human Reproduction,* ed. by Hafez, E. S. E., and Evans, T. N., Hagerstown, Maryland: Harper & Row, 1973.

Eliasson, R. "Parameters of Male Fertility." In *Human Reproduction,* ed. by Hafez, E. S. E., and Evans, T. N., Hagerstown, Maryland: Harper & Row, 1973.

CHAPTER FIVE

1. Gabbe, S. G., Ettinger, B. B., Freeman, R. K., Martin, C. B. "Umbilical cord compression associated with amniotomy: laboraory observations." *American Journal of Obstetrics and Gynecology* 126: 353, 1976.
2. LeBoyer, F. *Birth Without Violence.* New York: Alfred A. Knopf, Inc., 1975.
3. MacMahon, B., Cole, P., Brown, P. "Etiology of human breast cancer: a review." *Journal of the National Cancer Institute* 5: 21, 1973.
4. Collea, J. V., Rabin, S. C., Weghorst, G. R., Quilligan, E. J. "The randomized management of term frank breech presentation: Vaginal delivery vs. cesarean section." *American Journal of Obstetrics and Gynecology* 131: 186, 1978.
5. Niswander, K. R., and Gordon, M. *The Women and Their Pregnancies* Philadelphia: W. B. Saunders Company, 1972, p. 101.
6. Bowman, J. M. "Suppression of Rh isoimmunization: a review." *Obstetrics and Gynecology* 52: 385, 1978.
7. FDA, "Fetal alcohol syndrome." *FDA Drug Bulletin* 7: 18, 1977.
8. Clarren, S. K., and Smith, D. W. "The fetal alcohol syndrome." *The New England Journal of Medicine* 298: 1063, 1978.
9. Meyer, M. B., and Tonascia, J. A. "Maternal smoking, pregnancy complications, and perinatal mortality." *American Journal of Obstetrics and Gynecology* 128: 494, 1977.
10. Pirani, B. B. K. "Smoking during pregnancy." *Obstetrical and Gynecological Survey* 33: 1, 1978.

General References and Suggested Readings

Bing, E. *Six Practical Lessons for Easier Childbirth.* New York: Bantam Books, 1969.

Greenhill, J. P., and Friedman, E. A. *The Biological Principles and Modern Practice of Obstetrics.* Philadelphia: W. B. Saunders, 1974.

Karmel, M. *Thank YOU, Dr. Lamaze.* Garden City, New York: Dolphin Books, 1959.

Kitzinger, S. *The Experience of Childbirth.* Harmondsworth, Middlesex, England: Pelican Books, 1967.

Klaus, M. H., and Kennell, J. H. *Maternal-Infant Bonding.* St. Louis, Missouri: C. V. Mosby Company, 1976.

Olds, S. W., and Eiger, M. S. *The Complete Book of Breast Feeding.* New York: Workman Publishing Co., 1972.

Pryor, K. *Nursing Your Baby.* New York: Pocket Books, 1972.

Romney, S. L., Gray, M. J., et al. *Gynecology and Obstetrics: The Health Care of Women.* New York: McGraw-Hill, 1975.

CHAPTER SIX

1. Rudel, H. W., Kincl, F. A., Henzl, M. R. *Birth Control, Contraception and Abortion,* Chapter 6. New York: Macmillan, 1973.
2. U. S. Department of HEW, Center for Disease Control. "Abortion Surveillance, 1976." August 1978.
3. Tietze, C. "The effect of legalization of abortion on population growth and public health." *Family Planning Perspectives* 7: 123, 1975.
4. U. S. Department of HEW, Center for Disease Control. "Comparative risks of three methods of midtrimester abortion." *Mortality and Morbidity Weekly Report.* November 26, 1976, p. 370.
5. Grimes, D. A., Schulz, K. F., Cates, W., and Tyler, C. W. "Midtrimester abortion by dilatation and evacuation." *New England Journal of Medicine* 296: 1141, 1977.
6. Grimes, D. A., Cates, W., Jr. "Complications from legally-induced abortion: a review." *Obstetrical and Gynecological Survey* 34: 177, 1979.
7. "Maternal-infant mortality at all-time low, according to latest U. S. Data." *Contemporary Obstetrics and Gynecology* 8: 113, 1976.
8. Richardson, J. A., Dixon, G. "Effects of legal termination on subsequent pregnancy." *British Medical Journal* 1: 1303, 1976.

General References and suggested readings

Callahan, D. *Abortion: Law Choice and Morality.* New York: Macmillan, 1970.

Denes, Magda. *In Necessity and Sorrow.* New York: Basic Books, 1976.

Family Planning Perspectives, a bimonthly publication of the Planned Parenthood Federation of America. Alan Guttmacher Institute, 515 Madison Avenue, New York 10022.

Group for the Advancement of Psychiatry. *The Right to Abortion: A Psychiatric View.* New York: Charles Scribner's Sons, 1969.

Schwarz, R. H. *Septic Abortion.* Philadelphia: Lippincott, 1968.

CHAPTER SEVEN

1. Cavalieri, L. "New strains of life-or-death." The New York *Times Magazine,* August 22, 1976, p. 8.
2. Saxen, L. "Embryonic induction." *Clinical Obstetrics and Gynecology* 18: 149, 1975.
3. Smith, A. *The Human Pedigree.* New York; Lippincott, 1975, p. 126.
4. NICHD National Registry for Amniocentesis Study Group. "Midtrimester amniocentesis for prenatal diagnosis: safety and accuracy." *Journal of the American Medical Association* 236: 1471, 1976.
5. Simpson, N. E., et al. "Prenatal diagnosis of genetic disease in Canada: report of a collaborative study." *Canadian Medical Association Journal* 115: 739, 1976.
6. Mennuti, M. "Prenatal genetic diagnosis: current status." *New England Journal of Medicine* 297: 1004, 1977.
7. Golbus, M. S., et al. "Prenatal genetic diagnosis in 3000 amniocenteses." *New England Journal of Medicine,* 300: 157, 1979.
8. Rorvik, D. M., and Shettles, L. B. *Your Baby's Sex: Now You Can Choose.* New York: Bantam Books, 1970.

For information:

National Foundation March of Dimes
Box 20
White Plains, New York, 10602

National Genetics Foundation
250 West 57th Street
New York, NY, 10019

CHAPTER EIGHT

1. Chase, D. *The Medically Based No-nonsense Beauty Book.* New York: Alfred A. Knopf, 1975, ch. 11–15.
2. Garfinkel, J., Selvin, S., Brown, S. M. "Possible increased risk of lung cancer among beauticians." *Journal of the National Cancer Institute* 58: 141, 1977.
3. Menck, H. R., et al. "Lung cancer risk among beauticians and other female workers." *Journal of the National Cancer Institute* 59: 1423, 1977.
4. Farah, A. P. "Be armed against perspiration." *Family Health/Today's Health,* 8: 58, 1976.
5. Wilson, L. A., Julian, A. J., Ahern, D. G. "The survival and growth of microorganisms in mascara during use." *American Journal of Ophthalmology* 79: 596, 1975.
6. Department of HEW, Food and Drug Administration. "Proposal to establish monographs for OTC nighttime sleep-aid, daytime sedative, and stimulant products." *Federal Register* Vol. 40 ⚡236, p. 57292, December 8, 1975.
7. Department of HEW, Food and Drug Administration, "Proposal to establish monographs for OTC laxative, antidiarrheal, emetic, and antiemetic products." *Federal Register* Vol. 40 ⚡56, p. 12902, March 21, 1975.

8. Finn, R., Wainscoat, J. S. "Laxan Nephropathy." *Lancet*. May 25, 1975, p. 1202.
9. Chase, D. *op. cit.*, p. 89.
10. "Saccharin and chemical carcinogenesis." *The Medical Letter on Drugs and Therapeutics* 19: 75, 1977.
11. Leff, D. N. "Megavitamin therapy: does it work?" *McCall's*. September 1974, p. 47.
12. "Myths of Vitamins." *FDA Consumer*. March 1974. DHEW Publication No. (FDA) 74-2053.
13. Committee on Nutrition of the Mother and Preschool Child. "Oral contraceptives and nutrition." *National Academy of Sciences*. Washington, 1975.
14. U. S. Department of HEW, Food and Drug Administration. "Liquid protein and sudden cardiac deaths—an update." *FDA Drug Bulletin* 8: 18, 1978.
15. Michiel, R. R., et al. "Sudden death in a patient on a liquid protein diet." *New England Journal of Medicine* 298: 1005, 1978.
16. "Bypass operation for obesity." *The Medical Letter on Drugs and Therapeutics* 20: 33, 1978.
17. "Stapling creates mini-stomach for obese patients." *Medical World News* October 16, 1978, p. 17.
18. Cohen, S., Booth, G. H. "Gastric acid secretion and lower-esophageal-sphincter pressure in response to coffee and caffeine." *New England Journal of Medicine* 293: 897, 1975.
19. "Coffee and cardiovascular disease." *The Medical Letter on Drugs and Therapeutics* 19: 65, 1977.
20. "Another look at coffee." *The Harvard Medical School Health Letter* 3, ⚹6: 5, 1978.
21. "High density lipoproteins (HDL)." *The Medical Letter on Drugs and Therapeutics* 21: 1, 1979.
22. "Update on coronary artery disease." *The Harvard Medical School Health Letter* 3, ⚹4: 1, 1978.
23. Mendeloff, A. K. "Dietary fiber and human health." *New England Journal of Medicine* 297: 811, 1977.
24. Mayer, J. "How to eat right and live longer." *U.S. News & World Report*. August 9, 1976, p. 37.
25. Jukes, T. H. "Food additives." *New England Journal of Medicine* 297: 427, 1977.
26. "A holiday check list." *The Harvard Medical School Health Letter* Vol. 3, ⚹2, 1977, p. 1.
27. Slone, D. et al. "Relation of cigarette smoking to myocardial infarction in young women." *New England Journal of Medicine* 298: 1273, 1978.
28. Stolley, P. D. "Lung cancer: an unwanted equality for women." *New England Journal of Medicine* 297: 886, 1977.
29. "Heavy smokers reach menopause earlier than nonsmokers." *The Female Patient*, November 1977, p. 53.
30. Califano, J. A., Jr. National Cancer Program Special Communication on Smoking. March 28, 1978.
31. Luce, B. R. and Schweitzer, S. O. "Smoking and alcohol abuse: a comparison of their economic consequences." *New England Journal of Medicine* 298: 569, 1978.

32. "Marijuana." *The Medical Letter on Drugs and Therapeutics* 18: 69, 1976.
33. Levine, R. "Dangers of Stress." Bergen *Record*. January 9, 1977, p. A-1.
34. Wilson, E. D., Fisher, K. H., Fuqua, M. E. *Principles of Nutrition,* 3rd ed. New York: John Wiley and Sons, 1975.

Suggested references

  The Medicine Show. Mount Vernon, New York: Consumers Union, 1974.

  Chase, D. *The Medically Based No-nonsense Beauty Book*. New York: Alfred A. Knopf, 1975.

  Mayer, J. *A Diet for Living*. New York: Pocket Books, 1977.

  "Dietary Goals for U.S." 2nd edition-pamphlet available for 95¢ from the Superintendent of Documents, U. S. Government Printing Office. Washington, D.C. 20402

Brochures on How to Stop Smoking
  "Cleaning the Air: a Guide to Quitting Smoking." Free
  Office of Cancer Communications
  National Cancer Institute
  Building 31, Room 10A18,
  9000 Rockville Pike,
  Bethesda, Maryland 20014.

  "If you must smoke" Free
  Office on Smoking and Health
  Park Building, Suite 1–58,
  12420 Parklawn Drive,
  Rockville, Maryland, 20857.

  "Slim and Smokeless: a Guide to Weight Control After Quitting Cigarettes." Free
  Order ⚹ DHEW(CDC) 77-8346
  Office on Smoking and Health
  Address above.

CHAPTER NINE

1. Money, J. and Ehrhardt, A. K. *Man and Woman, Boy and Girl*. Baltimore, Maryland: Johns Hopkins Press, 1972.

CHAPTER TEN

1. Friederich, M. A. "Psychophysiology of menstruation and the menopause." In Romney, S. L., et al., eds. *Gynecology and Obstetrics: The Health Care of Women,* New York, McGraw-Hill, 1975, p. 603.
2. Rybo, G., and Westerberg, H. "Symptoms in the postmenopause: a population study. A preliminary report." *Acta Obstetrica Gynecologica Scandinavia* 50: 25, 1971.

3. Ballinger, C. B. "Psychiatric morbidity and the menopause: screening of general population sample." *British Medical Journal* 3: 344, 1975.
4. Connell, E. B. "The pill revisited." *Family Planning Perspectives* 7: 62, 1975.
5. Morrison, J. C., Givens, J. R., Wiser, W. L., Fish, S. A. "Mumps Oophoritis: a cause of premature menopause." *Fertility and Sterility* 6: 655, 1975.
6. Coulam, C. B., and Ryan, R. J. "Premature menopause. I. Etiology." *American Journal of Obstetrics and Gynecology.* 133: 639, 1979.
7. Meema, S., Bunker, M. L., and Meema, H. E. "Preventive effect of estrogen on postmenopausal bone loss." *Archives of Internal Medicine.* 135: 1436, 1975.
8. Stadl, B. V., and Weiss, N. "Characteristics of menopausal women: a survey of King and Pierce countries in Washington. 1973–1974." *American Journal of Epidemiology* 102: 209, 1975.
9. Ziel, H. K., and Finkle, W. D. "Increased risk of endometrial carcinoma among users of conjugated estrogens." *New England Journal of Medicine* 293: 1167, 1975.
10. Smith, D. C., Prentice, R., Thompson, D. J., Herrman, W. L. "Association of exogenous estrogen and endometrial cancer." *New England Journal of Medicine* 293: 1164, 1975.
11. Mack, T. M., Pike, M. C., et al. "Estrogens and endometrial cancer in a retirement community." *New England Journal of Medicine* 294: 1262, 1976.
12. Gray, L. A., Christopherson, W. M., Hoover, R. N. "Estrogens and endometrial carcinoma." *Obstetrics and Gynecology* 49: 385, 1977.
13. Gordon, J., Reagan, J. W., Finkle, W. D., and Ziel, H. K. "Estrogen and endometrial cancer: an independent pathology review supporting original risk estimate." *New England Journal of Medicine* 297: 570, 1977.
14. Antunes, C. M. F., et al. "Endometrial cancer and estrogen use: report of a large case-control study." *New England Journal of Medicine* 300: 9, 1979.
15. Jick, H., et al. "Replacement estrogens and endometrial cancer." *New England Journal of Medicine* 300: 218, 1979.
16. Horwitz, R. I., and Feinstein, A. R. "Alternative analytic methods for case-control studies of estrogen and endometrial cancer." *New England Journal of Medicine* 299: 1089, 1978.
17. Gordon, T., Kannel, W. B., Hjortland, M. C., and McNamara, P. M. "Menopause and coronary heart disease. The Framingham study." *Annals of Internal Medicine* 89: 157, 1978.
18. Nachtigall, L. E., Nachtigall, R. H., Nachtigall, R. D., Beckman, E. M. "Estrogen replacement therapy I: a 10-year prospective study in the relationship to osteoporosis." *Obstetrics and Gynecology* 53: 277, 1979.
19. Avioli, L. V. "Senile and postmenopausal osteoporosis." *Advances in Internal Medicine* 21: 391, 1976.
20. National Institutes of Health. "Over-the-counter antacid preparations can have adverse effects on bone." *Journal of the American Medical Association* 238: 1018, 1977.

Suggested reading:

Sheehy, Gail. *Passages: Predictable Crises in Adult Life.* New York: E. P. Dutton, 1974.

CHAPTER ELEVEN

1. Fleury, F. J., et al. "Single dose of two grams of metronidazole for *Trichomonas vaginalis* infection." *American Journal of Obstetrics and Gynecology* 128: 320, 1977.
2. Weltman, R. "New metronidazole study: some reassuring findings for now." *Journal of the American Medical Association* 239: 1371, 1978.
3. Pheifer, T. A., et al. "Nonspecific vaginitis: the role of *Haemophilus vaginalis* and treatment with metronidazole." *New England Journal of Medicine* 298: 1429, 1978.
4. Schacter, J. "Chlamydial infections." *New England Journal of Medicine* 298: 428, 490, 540, 1978.
5. Osborne, N. G. "The significance of mycoplasma in pelvic infection." *Journal of Reproductive Medicine* 19: 39, 1977.
6. "Herpes simplex viruses and cervical cancer." *Journal of the American Medical Association* 238: 1614, 1977.
7. Rawls, W. E., Gardner, H. L., and Kaufman, R. L. "Antibodies to genital herpes virus in patients with carcinoma of the cervix." *American Journal of Obstetrics and Gynecology* 107: 710, 1970.
8. Handsfield, H. H., et al. "Asymptomatic gonorrhea in men: Diagnosis, natural course, prevalence and significance." *New England Journal of Medicine* 290: 117, 1974.
9. Singh, B., Cutler, J. C., and Utidijian, H.M.D. "Studies on the development of a vaginal preparation providing both prophylaxis against venereal disease and other genital infections and contraception." *British Journal of Venereal Diseases* 48: 57, 1972.
10. Henzl, M. L., Buttram, V., Segre, E. J. Bressler S. "The treatment of dysmenorrhea with naproxen sodium." *American Journal of Obstetrics and Gynecology* 127: 818, 1977.
11. Corson, S. L., Bolognese, R. J. "Ibuprofen therapy for dysmenorrhea." *Journal of Reproductive Medicine* 20: 246, 1978.
12. Dalton, K. *Premenstrual Syndrome.* Springfield, Illinois, Thomas, 1964.
13. Masters, W. H., Johnson, V. E. *Human Sexual Response.* Boston: Little, Brown, 1966, pp. 119–22.
14. Dyck, F. J., et al. "Effect of surveillance on the number of hysterectomies in the province of Saskatchewan." *New England Journal of Medicine* 296: 1326, 1977.
15. "Danazol—a new drug for endometriosis." *The Medical Letter on Drugs and Therapeutics* 19: 62, 1977.
16. MacMahon, B., Cole, P., Brown, P. "Etiology of human breast cancer: a review." *Journal of the National Cancer Institute* 50: 21, 1973.
17. Hoover, R., Gray, L. A., Cole, P. MacMahon, B. "Menopausal estrogens and breast cancer." *New England Journal of Medicine* 295: 401, 1976.
18. Vorherr, H., Messer, R. H. "Breast cancer: potentially predisposing and protecting factors." *American Journal of Obstetrics and Gynecology* 130: 335, 1978.
19. Department of H.E.W. "Multiple fluoroscopies and breast cancer." *FDA Drug Bulletin* 6: 38, 1976.
20. Shimkin, M. B. "Epidemology of breast cancer." In Griem, M. L., et

al. "Breast cancer: a challenging problem." *Recent Results in Cancer Research* 42: 6, 1973.

21. Sarkar, N. H., Moore, D. H. "Viral transmission in breast cancer." in Griem et al. op. cit., p. 15.

22. Mavligit, G. M., Gutterman, J. U., Hersh, E. M. "Immunologic aspects of human cancer." In Castro, J. R., Meyler, T. S., and Baker, D. C., eds. *Current Concepts in Breast Cancer and Tumor Immunology*. New York: Medical Examination Publishing Company, 1974, p. 237.

23. Oettgen, H. F. "Immunotherapy of cancer." *New England Journal of Medicine* 297: 484, 1977.

24. Herbst, A. L., Ulfelder, H., Poskanzer, D. C. "Adenocarcinoma of the vagina. Association of maternal stilbestrol therapy with tumor appearance in young women." *New England Journal of Medicine* 284: 878, 1971.

25. Herbst, A. L., et al. "Age-incidence and risk of diethylstilbestrol-related clear cell carcinoma of the vagina and cervix." *American Journal of Obstetrics and Gynecology* 128: 43, 1977.

26. Lyon, F. A., Frisch, M. J. "Endometrial abnormalities occurring in young women on long-term sequential oral contraception." *Obstetrics and Gynecology* 47: 639, 1976.

27. Ziel, H. K., Finkle, W. D. "Increased risk of endometrial carcinoma among users of conjugated estrogens." *New England Journal of Medicine* 293: 1167, 1975.

28. Smith, D. C., Prentice, R., Thompson, D. J., and Herrman, W. L. "Association of exogenous estrogen and endometrial cancer." *New England Journal of Medicine* 293: 1164, 1975.

29. Lipsett, M. B. "Hormonal induction of breast cancer." In Griem et al., op. cit., p. 28.

30. Kennedy, B. J. "Appearance and spread of human breast cancer." In Griem et al., op. cit. p. 31.

31. Fasal, E., and Paffenbarger, R. S. "Oral contraceptives as related to cancer and benign lesions of the breast." *Journal of the National Cancer Institute* 55: 767, 1975.

32. Siiteri, P. "Endocrine aspects of breast cancer." In Castro et al., op. cit., p. 61.

33. Henderson, B. E., et al. "Elevated serum levels of estrogen and prolactin in daughters of patients with breast cancer." *New England Journal of Medicine* 293: 790, 1975.

34. Meites, J. "Relation of prolactin and estrogen to mammary tumorigenesis in the rat." *Journal of the National Cancer Institute* 48: 1217, 1972.

35. Boston Collaborative Drug Surveillance Program. "Reserpine and breast cancer." *Lancet* 2: 669, 1974.

36. McGregor, D. H., et al. "Breast cancer incidence among atomic bomb survivors, Hiroshima and Nagasaki, 1950–1969." *Journal of the National Cancer Institute* 59: 799, 1977.

37. Simon, N. "Breast cancer induced by radiation: relation to mammography and treatment of acne." *Journal of the American Medical Association* 237: 789, 1977.

38. McGuire, W. L., Carbone, P. P., Vollmer, E. P., eds. *Estrogen Receptors in Human Breast Cancer*. New York: Raven Press, 1975.

39. Young, R. C., et al. "Perspectives in the treatment of breast cancer: 1976." *Annals of Internal Medicine* 86: 784, 1977.
40. Lou, M. A., Mandel, A. K., Alexander, J. L. "The pros and cons of outpatient breast biopsy." *Archives of Surgery* 111: 668, 1976.
41. Witkin, M. H. "Sex therapy and mastectomy." *Journal of Sexual and Marital Therapy* 1: 290, 1975.
42. Watts, G. T. "Restorative prosthetic mammaplasty in mastectomy for carcinoma and benign lesions." *Clinics in Plastic Surgery* 3: 177, 1976.
43. Asken, M. J. "Psychoemotional aspects of mastectomy: a review of recent literature." *American Journal of Psychiatry* 132: 56, 1975.
44. Department of HEW. "Thermography restriction." *FDA Drug Bulletin* 6: 32, 1976.
45. Moskowitz, M., et al. "Lack of efficacy of thermography as a screening tool for minimal and Stage I breast cancer." *New England Journal of Medicine* 295: 249, 1976.
46. Aksu, M. F., Tzingonnis, V. A., Greenblatt, R. B. "Treatment of benign breast disease with Danazol: a follow-up report." *Journal of Reproductive Medicine* 21: 181, 1978.
47. "Benign breast disease tied to coffee, tea, cocoa, cola." *Medical World News* 20: 11, 1979.
48. Scarpelli, D. G., Murad, T. M. "Recent contributions to our knowledge about the pathology of breast cancer." In Griem et al., op. cit. p. 42.
49. "Cancer statistics 1979." *CA—A Cancer Journal for Clinicians* 29: 6, 1979
50. Kaufman, R. H., Binder, G. L., Gray, P. M. M., and Adam, E. "Upper genital tract changes associated with exposure in utero to diethylstilbestrol." *American Journal of Obstetrics and Gynecology* 128: 1977: 51.
51. Goldstein, D. P. "Incompetent cervix in offspring exposed to diethylstilbestrol in utero." *Obstetrics and Gynecology* 52: 73s, 1978.
52. Fowler, W. C., Edelman, D. A. "In utero exposure to DES." *Obstetrics and Gynecology* 51: 459, 1978.
53. Robboy, S. J. "Squamous cell dysplasia and carcinoma in situ of the cervix and vagina after prenatal exposure to diethylstilbestrol." *Obstetrics and Gynecology* 51: 528, 1978.
54. Bibbo, M., et al. "A twenty-five-year follow-up study of women exposed to diethylstilbestrol during pregnancy." *New England Journal of Medicine* 298: 763, 1978.
55. Gill, W. B., Schumacher, G. F. B., Bibbo, M. "Structural and functional abnormalities in the sex organs of male offspring of mothers treated with diethylstilbestrol (DES)." *Journal of Reproductive Medicine* 16: 147, 1976.
56. Bibbo, M., et al. "Follow-up study of male and female offspring of DES-exposed mothers." *Obstetrics and Gynecology* 49: 1, 1977.
57. "Penicillamine for rheumatoid arthritis." *The Medical Letter on Drugs and Therapeutics* 20: 73, 1978.
58. Steere, A. C., Hardin, J. A., Malawista, S. E. "Lyme arthritis: a new clinical entity." *Hospital Practice* April 1978, p. 143.

General References and Suggested Readings

Committee of the American Rheumatism Association of the Arthritis Foundation. *Primer on the Rheumatic Diseases,* 7th edition, New York: The Arthritis Foundation, 1973.

Conn, H. F., ed. *Current Therapy 1979*. Philadelphia: W. B. Saunders, 1979.

Gardner, H. L., and Kaufman, R. H. *Benign Diseases of the Vulva and Vagina*. St. Louis: Mosby, 1969.

Thorne, G. W., et al., eds. *Harrison's Principles of Internal Medicine*. New York: McGraw-Hill, 1977.

Cancer and the Worker. New York: The New York Academy of Sciences, 1977. (Available at The New York Academy of Sciences, 2 East 63rd St., New York, New York, 10021.)

CHAPTER TWELVE

1. Groth, A. N., and Burgess, A. W. "Sexual dysfuncton during rape." *New England Journal of Medicine* 297: 764, 1977.

Information to sex

Boston Women's Health Collective. *Our Bodies, Our Selves*. New York: Simon & Schuster, 1976. (Paperback)

Gadpaille, W. J. *The Cycles of Sex*. New York: Scribner's, 1975. (Paperback)

Friday, N. *My Secret Garden*. New York: Pocket Books, 1974. (Paperback)

Masters, W. H., and Johnson, V. E. *Human Sexual Response*. Boston: Little, Brown, 1966. (Paperback)

Brecher, R., and Brecher, E., eds. *An Analysis of Human Sexual Response*. New York: Signet, 1966. (Paperback)

Sexual Dysfunction

Barbach, L. G. *For Yourself*. Garden City, New York: Doubleday, 1975, Anchor, 1976 (Paperback)

Kline-Graber, G., and Graber, B. *Women's Orgasm*. New York, Popular Library, 1976. (Paperback)

Kaplan, H. S. *The Illustrated Manual of Sex Therapy*. New York: Quadrangle/New York Times Book Co., 1975.

Masters, W. H. and Johnson, V. E. *Human Sexual Inadequacy*. Boston: Little, Brown, 1970. (Paperback)

Belliveau, F. and Richter, L. *Understanding Human Sexual Inadequacy*. New York: Bantam Books, 1970. (Paperback)

Marriage

Gottner, J., Notarus, C., Gonso, T., Markman, H. *A Couple's Guide to Communication*. Champaign, Illinois, Research Press, 1976. (Order from Research Press, 2612 N. Mattis Ave., Champaign, Illinois 61826).

Divorce

Women in Transition. New York: Scribner's, 1976. (Paperback)

Weiss, R. *Marital Separation*. New York: Basic Books, 1977. (Paperback)

General Mental Health

Park, C. C., and Shapiro, L. *You Are Not Alone.* Boston: Atlantic, Little, Brown, 1976. Available in paperback through Consumers Union, 256 Washington St., Mount Vernon, New York, 10550.

Miller, J. B., ed. *Psychoanalysis and Women.* Baltimore: Penguin Books, 1973. (Paperback)

Rape

Amir, M. *Patterns in Forcible Rape* Chicago: University of Chicago Press, 1971.

Brownmiller, Susan. *Against Our Will: Men, Women and Rape* New York: Simon & Schuster, 1975.

CHAPTER THIRTEEN

Suggested readings

Consumers Union, 256 Washington St., Mount Vernon, New York, publishes many books and pamphlets of interest to the health care consumer.

The Food and Drug Administration publishes a monthly magazine called the *FDA Consumer.* A subscription is $8.55 per year and is obtainable from the Government Printing Office, Superintendent of Documents, Washington, D.C. 20402

The National Cancer Institute, Bethesda, Maryland 20014, publishes frequent news bulletins.

Harvard Medical School publishes a monthly newsletter for the public. The subscription is $12.00 per year and is obtainable from *The Harvard Medical School Letter,* 79 Garden Street, Cambridge, Massachusetts 02138.

Family Health is a reliable magazine. A subscription is $9.95 per year and may be obtained by writing Family Health Subscription Department, 149 Fifth Avenue, New York, New York 10010.

INDEX

Abdominal cancer. *See* Stomach cancer
Abdominal hysterectomy, 333–34, 335, 336
Abdominal muscles, postpartum exercises for, 157
Abdominal pains and cramps (*see also* Cramps): abnormal in pregnancy, 135–36; pregnancy and, 135–36
Abortions, 188–206; choosing a safe clinic, 204; complete, 165; complications, 200–6; counseling, 205–6; death rate, 202; earliest as safest, 200; emotional effects, 203; habitual, infertility and, 94, 97, 98; immature delivery, 165–67; incomplete, 165; insurance, 190; legality, availability, and increased safety, 190, 191; long-term effects, 203; medical reasons for, 190–91; as method of last resort, 189–90; methods, 191–92ff.; missed, 165; normal postabortion course, 198–200; out-of-town, 204–5; routine pre-abortion procedures, 192; secret, avoiding, 205; spontaneous (miscarriage), 135, 164–65; statistics, 191, 202
Abruptio placenta, 178
Abscess: Bartholin's, 341; breast, 359; Skene's glands, 342
Abstinence, sexual, 386; as birth-control method, 89
Acetaminophen, 138, 238, 240
Acidophilus replacement, lactose intolerance and, 259
Acne, 31–34; antibiotics for, 32–33; avoiding radiation for, 348; blackheads, 31; cryotherapy for, 33; dermatologists and, 32–33; estrogen and steroids for, 33–34; facial make-up and allergies and, 233; mild, treatment for, 32; the pill and, 45, 47; surgery for, 33; vitamin A acid for, 33; whiteheads, 31–32
ACTH (adrenocorticotropic hormone), 18
Additives. *See* Food additives and preservatives
Adenomas, 51
Adenosis, 366, 367
Adolescence (teen-agers), 25–34 (*see also* Children); acne, 31–34; anemia, 176; and athletics, 27; and discipline, 27; gynecological exams, 27–28; homosexual attachments, 26; masturbation and self-exploration, 27; menstrual irregularity, 330; neurotic dieting, 30–31; nutrition, 30; parents and, 25ff.; pregnancy (*see* Pregnancy, adolescent); puberty (*see* Puberty); sexual activity, 26–27ff.; venereal disease, 30
Adoption, child, 114
Adrenal glands (adrenals), 31 (*see also* Androgen); and acne, 31; and breast cancer, 349; in fetus, 185; menopause and, 281
Adrenalin and anxiety in labor, 151–52
"After-birth," 145
Air pollution. *See* Environmental pollution
Air-swallowing, gas pains and, 241
Al-Anon, 263
Alcohol (alcoholism), 262–63; avoiding drunkenness, 262; medical risks, 262–63; moderate use of, 262 (*see also* Alcoholic beverages); organizations that help, 263; pregnancy risks, 182; symptoms of problem, 262; tranquilizers and, 264
Alcoholic beverages (wine), 262; for menstrual pain, 326; to stop premature labor, 171
Alcoholics Anonymous, 263
Allergies (allergic reactions): and anesthesia in abortions, 202; contact dermatitis, 235; drugs and cosmetics and, 233, 235, 241; over-the-counter drugs and, 241; recording, 406; and vaginitis-vulvitis symptoms, 309
Alpha-fetoprotein, amniocentesis for, 219–20
Aluminum hydroxide, 292–93
Aluminum salts, 235
Amenorrhea, 24, 287 (*see also* Menopause); the pill and, 53; in puberty, 24
American Association of Marriage and Family Therapists (AAMFT), 394
American Association of Sex Education, Counseling, and Therapists (AASECT), 394
American Board of Obstetrics and Gynecologists, 102, 204
American College of Midwifery, 123
American College of Obstetrics and Gynecology, 363
American Fertility Society, 102
American Medical Association, 6
Amino acids, 120
Ammonium chloride, 243
Amniocentesis, 140, 179, 186, 216–20; alpha-fetoprotein and brain and spinal cord defects, 219–20; cystic fibrosis and, 220; genetic testing and, 216–20; limits of, 218; risks of, 217–18; sex-linked genetic disorders and, 218, 219; sickle-cell anemia and, 220, 370; Tay-Sachs disease and, 218–19; what it is, 217; who should consider having, 218
Amniogram (amniography), 186, 217, 220
Amnioscopy, 185–86
Amniotic fluid (amniotic sac), pregnancy and labor and, 118, 120, 141–42; amniocentesis and genetic testing and, 186, 217ff.; amniogram test, 186, 217, 220–21; amnioscopy test, 185–86;